T0275472

Disorder Contained

Disorder Contained is the first historical account of the complex relationship between prison discipline and mental breakdown in England and Ireland. Between 1840 and 1900 the expansion of the modern prison system coincided with increased rates of mental disorder among prisoners, exacerbated by the introduction of regimes of isolation, deprivation and hard labour. Drawing on a range of archival and printed sources, the authors explore the links between different prison regimes and mental distress, examining the challenges faced by prison medical officers dealing with mental disorder within a system that stressed discipline and punishment and prisoners' own experiences of mental illness. The book investigates medical officers' approaches to the identification, definition, management and categorisation of mental disorder in prisons, and varied, often gendered, responses to mental breakdown among inmates. The authors also reflect on the persistence of systems of punishment that often aggravate rather than alleviate mental illness in the criminal justice system up to the current day. This title is also available as Open Access.

CATHERINE COX is Associate Professor of History at University College Dublin and director of UCD Centre for the History of Medicine in Ireland. She is the author of *Negotiating Insanity in the Southeast of Ireland, 1820–1900* (2012) and with Susannah Riordan edited *Adolescence in Modern Irish History* (2015).

HILARY MARLAND is Professor of History at the University of Warwick and founder director of Warwick's Centre for the History of Medicine. She is the author of *Dangerous Motherhood: Insanity and Childbirth in Victorian Britain* (2004) and *Health and Girlhood in Britain 1874–1920* (2013).

Disorder Contained

*Mental Breakdown and the Modern Prison
in England and Ireland, 1840–1900*

Catherine Cox
University College Dublin

Hilary Marland
University of Warwick

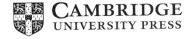
CAMBRIDGE
UNIVERSITY PRESS

CAMBRIDGE
UNIVERSITY PRESS

University Printing House, Cambridge CB2 8BS, United Kingdom

One Liberty Plaza, 20th Floor, New York, NY 10006, USA

477 Williamstown Road, Port Melbourne, VIC 3207, Australia

314–321, 3rd Floor, Plot 3, Splendor Forum, Jasola District Centre,
New Delhi – 110025, India

103 Penang Road, #05-06/07, Visioncrest Commercial, Singapore 238467

Cambridge University Press is part of the University of Cambridge.

It furthers the University's mission by disseminating knowledge in the pursuit of
education, learning, and research at the highest international levels of excellence.

www.cambridge.org
Information on this title: www.cambridge.org/9781108834551
DOI: 10.1017/9781108993586

First published 2022

A catalogue record for this publication is available from the British Library.

Library of Congress Cataloging-in-Publication Data
Names: Cox, Catherine, 1970- author. | Marland, Hilary, 1958- author.
Title: Disorder contained : mental breakdown and the modern prison in England and
    Ireland, 1840-1900 / Catherine Cox, University College Dublin, Hilary Marland,
    University of Warwick.
Description: Cambridge, United Kingdom ; New York, NY : Cambridge University Press,
    2022. | Includes bibliographical references and index.
Identifiers: LCCN 2021044723 (print) | LCCN 2021044724 (ebook) | ISBN
    9781108834551 (hardback) | ISBN 9781108995191 (paperback) | ISBN
    9781108993586 (epub)
Subjects: LCSH: Prisoners–Mental health–England–History–19th century. | Prisoners–
    Mental health–Ireland–History–19th century. | Mentally ill prisoners–England–History–
    19th century. | Mentally ill prisoners–Ireland–History–19th century. | BISAC:
    MEDICAL / History
Classification: LCC RC451.4.P68 C695 2022 (print) | LCC RC451.4.P68 (ebook) | DDC
    365/.608740941–dc23
LC record available at https://lccn.loc.gov/2021044723
LC ebook record available at https://lccn.loc.gov/2021044724

ISBN 978-1-108-83455-1 Hardback

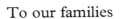
To our families

Contents

Figures

Acknowledgements

Writing this book has been a fascinating and troubling process, one that has led us into many archives and libraries and involved numerous interactions with scholars from many disciplines. Our research and writing took place alongside many public engagement activities, which brought us into contact with people in prison or who have been in prison, making us ever more aware of the enduring nature of many of the issues that we discuss in this book. It has led us to reflect on the continuing high rates of mental illness in prisons, and, despite the efforts of prison services and organisations working to reform prisons and improve care and conditions, the ongoing challenges of providing effective responses and treatment. We have also been made aware of the obstacles involved – both current and historical – in removing prisoners experiencing mental ill health from the prison system and of preventing them entering the system in the first place. One of our intentions in writing this book was to offer the backstory of the emergence of prison psychiatry and an exploration of the experiences of prisoners suffering from mental disorders in the past. It also provides an examination of the impact of prison disciplines in the modern prison, initially introduced under a banner of reform and effective rehabilitation, on the minds of those experiencing these regimes and on the medical staff tasked with implementing them.

First and foremost, we would like to acknowledge the generous support of the Wellcome Trust in funding our Investigator Award, 'Prisoners, Medical Care and Entitlement to Health in English and Irish Prisons, 1840–2000' (1003341/Z/13/Z and 1003351/Z/13/Z), which provided support for the research that underpins this book and allowed us the time to write it. It also gave us the opportunity to work with an exceptional team of scholars. Fiachra Byrne, Oisín Wall and Holly Dunbar at University College Dublin (UCD), Margaret Charleroy, Rachel Bennett, Max Hodgson and Becky Crites at the University of Warwick, William Murphy at Dublin City University, and Virginia Berridge and Janet Weston at the London School of Hygiene and Tropical Medicine, offered feedback, evidence and leads discovered while conducting their own research and enabled us to build a strong sense of community and collaboration around the project. Nicholas Duvall worked at both Warwick and UCD, and ably assisted us in our archival research during the first two years of the project. Henrietta Ewart, Louise Hide and David Durnin provided research support in the early stages of our project, while Lynn Kilgallon conducted additional research as we neared the end of the book project. Our wonderful public engagement officers, Flo Swann at Warwick and Sinead McCann at UCD, gave truly outstanding support, advice and expertise in developing our public engagement projects in tandem with the book. They enriched our experiences of public engagement, as did our many partners in the arts, policy, prison reform and prisons. Much of our public engagement was based on our research on mental illness in prison, which in turn fed back into the framing of our ideas for the book.

We have also both been fortunate in having excellent support beyond the project team from our two host research centres and universities. Colleagues at UCD's Centre for the History of Medicine and School of History provided ongoing practical support and expert knowledge as well as great enthusiasm and interest in our work: thanks to Sarah Feehan, Roy Fletcher, Robert Gerwarth, James Grannell, Mary Hatfield, Sara Honarmand Ebrahimi, Jen Keating, Emma Lyons, Alice Mauger, Ciarán McCabe, Ivar McGrath, William Mulligan, Elizabeth Mullins, Tadhg Ó hAnnracháin, Susannah Riordan, Michael Staunton, Fionnuala Walsh, Jennifer Wellington and Sandy Wilkinson. Beyond the UCD Centre and the School of History, Ian O'Donnell and Deirdre Healy in Law, Lynsey Black, now in Law at Maynooth University, and Justin Synnott, Máire Coyle and colleagues in UCD Research and Innovation engaged with and supported our work with great interest. Colleagues at Warwick's Centre for the History of Medicine have been a source of knowledge, expertise, and ongoing support and conviviality: Roberta Bivins, Andrew Burchell, Michael Bycroft, Tania Cleaves, Jennifer Crane, Kelly-Ann Couzens, Faby Creed, Angela Davis, Hannah Elizabeth, Jane Hand, Sheilagh Holmes, Sophie Mann, Gareth Millward, Michelle Nortey, James Poskett, Claire Sewell, Claire Shaw, Chris Sirrs, Elise Smith, Claudia Stein and Mathew Thomson, and our fantastic PhD community, and beyond our Centre for the History of Medicine, Anna Hájková, Sarah Hodges, Maria Luddy and Charles Walton in History, Jackie Hodgson in Law, Ana Chamberlen in Sociology, and David Duncan, James Green, Katie Klaassen, Liese Perrin and Emma Roberts in Research and Impact Services.

Over the years we have been researching and writing the book we have had many opportunities to present at seminars, workshops and conferences, and to share and discuss our work with colleagues from many institutions. We would like to thank the audiences at these events for their questions, comments and feedback, particularly Clare Anderson, Catharine Coleborne, Ian Cummins, Margot Finn, Barry Godfrey, Louise Hide, James Kelly, Laura Kelly, Kathleen Kendall, Hamish Maxwell-Stewart, Alice Mills, James Moran, Laura Sellers, Sonu Shamdasani, Len Smith, Matt Smith, Barbara Taylor, Nancy Tomes and David Wright.

We would like to thank many archivists and librarians for supporting our research on visits to the Modern Records Centre at Warwick University, particularly Helen Ford and Elizabeth Wood, The National Archives, the National Archives of Ireland, particularly Brian Donnelly and Gregory O'Connor, who sadly passed away in December 2020, the Wellcome Library, the British Library, the National Library of Ireland, the London Metropolitan Archives, Dublin City Archives, Royal College of Physicians of Ireland, Liverpool Record Office, Berkshire County Record Office, Lancashire Archives and Wakefield County Record Office.

Our research and public engagement activities have brought us into contact with many outstanding organisations and individuals working in prison reform and the arts, too many to list here, but including Anita Dockley at the Howard League, Kimmett Edgar at the Prison Reform Trust, Fíona Ní Chinnéide and all the team at the Irish Penal Reform Trust, Annie Bartlett at St George's, University of London, Sharon Shalev at the Oxford Centre for Criminology, Derek Nisbett, Peter Cann and the actors and production team of Talking Birds Theatre Company, Feidlim Cannon and Gary Keegan of Brokentalkers Theatre Company and their production team and cast, including Rachel Bergin and Willie White, Saul Hewish at Rideout and his colleagues, theatre maker Helena Enright, Andy Watson, Liz Brown and the rest of the team at Geese Theatre Company, Kate McCrath, Molly Sharpe and their colleagues at Fuel, the team at the Bridge Project, Dublin, who supported the artistic work of Sinead McCann, Anne Costello and her colleagues at the Education Unit, Mountjoy Prison, Dublin, the governors at Mountjoy Prison, the team at PACE, and Brian Crowley and Niall Bergin at Kilmainham Gaol Museum, Dublin. Many thanks too to the staff at HMP Hewell, HMP Peterborough and HMP Stafford, in particular Governor Gareth Sands, Governor Ralph Lubkowski and Fran Southall, and to the men and women in prison who contributed so much to our projects. In addition to support from the Wellcome Trust, our public engagement work was awarded further funding from UCD Research Seed Funding and Warwick University's Impact Fund.

We would like to thank Lucy Rhymer, Rachel Blaifeder, Stephanie Taylor and Dhanuja Ragunathan and the rest of the team at Cambridge University Press for guiding us through the production process, Matthew Seal for his meticulous copyediting and Kate McIntosh for compiling such a comprehensive index, and the anonymous referees for their insightful comments and feedback on our manuscript. We would like to acknowledge the British Library, Howard League for Penal Reform, Irish Architectural Archive, The National Archives, New York Public Library and Wellcome Collection for permission to reproduce illustrative material.

Last, and most importantly, we would like to thank our families, Sebastian, Sam, Daniel and Catherine, and William, Damian and Michelle for their enormous support, advice and encouragement.

1 Introduction

Mental Disorder and the Modern Prison in England and Ireland, 1840–1900

> Now regarding the prisoner as a moral patient, the paramount object is to render him as amenable as possible to the reformatory process.... The isolation that depresses the animal nature of the prisoner, and lowers the whole tone of the nervous system, produces a corresponding effect upon the mind.... In consequence of the lowering of the vital energies, the brain becomes more feeble, and, therefore, more susceptible. The chaplain can then make the brawny navvy in the cell cry like a child; he can work on his feelings in almost any way he pleases; he can, so to speak, photograph his own thoughts, wishes, and opinions, on his patient's mind, and fill his mouth with his own phrases and language.[1]

Referring to his close observations of the convict system in England and Ireland and of prisoners undergoing the solitary system of separate confinement, Reverend W.L. Clay highlighted the anticipated, and desired for, impact of cellular isolation: to break down and then re-form the minds of prisoners or, as he put it, 'patients'. The discipline of separate confinement dominated English and Irish prison regimes from the mid-nineteenth century to the early part of the twentieth. The reformers who supported its uptake, not least Clay's father, Reverend John Clay, chaplain at Preston Gaol, underlined its potential to produce deep-seated redemption among prisoners. John Clay collected detailed evidence demonstrating the success of the regime in the form of notes based on his conversations with prisoners, revealing how the process of redemption was shaped – or, perhaps more precisely, manipulated – by the ministrations of the chaplain in the cell.[2] This disturbing quotation also starkly illuminates the risks of this strategy for the mental wellbeing of the many deeply vulnerable and isolated people confined in prison.

---

[1] Reverend W.L. Clay, *Our Convict Systems* (Cambridge: Macmillan and Co., 1862), pp. 43–4.

[2] John Clay's son, Walter, published the biography *The Prison Chaplain: A Memoir of the Reverend John Clay* (Cambridge: Macmillan, 1861) after his father's death in 1858.

The prisoners who were the subjects of separate confinement provided very different but equally disturbing interpretations of cellular isolation, referring to it as a form of torture designed to undermine the will and weaken the faculties that for many resulted in complete mental breakdown. Convict E.F., who served time in Mountjoy Convict Prison, Dublin in the 1870s, claimed to have borne witness to the terrible effects of separate confinement. Among his fellow convicts, held in separation, were 'cases of violent insanity, for days and nights men had to be strapped down and strait jacketed and others refused to take food for weeks and had to be pumped'.[3] 'No one', declared Florence Maybrick, describing her fifteen-year prison sentence in Liverpool, Woking and Aylesbury prisons, 'can realize the horror of solitary confinement who has not experienced it … the voiceless solitude, the hopeless monotony, the long vista of tomorrow, tomorrow, tomorrow, stretching before her, all filled with desolation and despair.' 'The torture of continually enforced silence', she concluded, 'is known to produce insanity or nervous breakdown more than any other feature connected with prison discipline.'[4]

This book explores how, from the creation of the modern prison system in the mid-nineteenth century, prisons have stood accused of both producing and exacerbating mental despair and illness, their regimes functioning as detonators for pre-existing mental health problems, and their emphasis on enforcing discipline and punishment destroying the minds of prisoners and obstructing efforts to ameliorate conditions and to care for and treat those showing signs of mental breakdown.[5] From the era of Charles Dickens, who castigated prison reformers for introducing the cruel and mentally taxing system of separate confinement in the 1840s, through to that of Oscar Wilde, who experienced the discipline of the separate system firsthand towards the end of the century, the prison has been subject to continuous criticism for making its inmates mad and for doing very little to address this issue.[6] In the nineteenth century the prison became and remained a place where

---

[3] Royal Commission into Penal Servitude Acts, Minutes of Evidence [Kimberley Commission] (1878–79) [C.2368] [C.2368–I] [C.2368–II], p. 829.

[4] Florence Elizabeth Maybrick, *Mrs. Maybrick's Own Story: My Fifteen Lost Years* (New York and London: Funk & Wagnalls, 1905), pp. 68, 74–5, 81.

[5] Mary Gibson has argued that dating the emergence of the 'modern prison' to the early and mid-nineteenth century is accurate only for the Western/Anglo world: Mary Gibson, 'Global Perspectives on the Birth of the Prison', *American Historical Review*, 116:4 (2011), 1040–63.

[6] Charles Dickens, *American Notes for General Circulation, Vol. 1* (London: Chapman and Hall, 1842; with an Introduction and Notes by Patricia Ingham, London: Penguin Classics, 2002), pp. 111–24; Oscar Wilde, *Oscar Wilde: The Soul of Man and Prison*

the mentally disordered were incarcerated and retained in significant numbers in spite of their deteriorating mental health, a situation that endures today.[7]

This is the first historical study to offer a sustained and detailed exploration of the closely intertwined relationship between the modern prison and mental breakdown. It focuses on the 1840s, when the separate system was first introduced to Britain and Ireland, to the end of the nineteenth century when it was finally acknowledged, notably with the publication of the Gladstone Report in 1895, that prisons might have a detrimental effect on prisoners' mental health, initiating the slow and halting dismantling of this system. Drawing on a wide range of archival and official sources, and the accounts of prison administrators, reformers, prison doctors and prisoners, our book investigates the ways in which the English and Irish prison authorities attempted to mask, subdue and manage the high rates of mental illness that manifested themselves in their prisons. It seeks to understand the motivations of prison officers eager to disclaim the impact of prisons in causing mental breakdown, while at the same time attempting to deal with ever-increasing rates of insanity that confounded the order and discipline of the prison. As prison doctors spent more time dealing with mentally ill prisoners, our book argues that they positioned themselves increasingly as specialists in managing insanity in the particular setting of the prison, dealing with the distinct category of prisoner patients, creating new taxonomies and ways of describing mental illness, devoting themselves to the task of distinguishing real from feigned insanity, and authorising transfers of mentally disordered offenders within the prison estate or to criminal lunatic or public asylums.

In taking an approach that has investigated underutilised English and Irish prison archives in conjunction with official publications and reports and medical literature, our analysis, rather than reprising their

---

Writings, edited with an Introduction by Isobel Murray (Oxford: Oxford University Press, 1990).

[7] See, for example, Tony Seddon, *Punishment and Madness: Governing Prisoners with Mental Health Problems* (Abingdon: Routledge-Cavendish, 2007), which, while providing a brief historical overview, focuses largely on the relationship between the prison and mental illness between 1980 and 2005. There have been numerous inquiries into mental health in prisons in England and Ireland, including *The Bradley Report: Lord Bradley's Review of People with Mental Health Problems or Learning Disabilities in the Criminal Justice System* (London: Department of Health, 2009); Sharon Shalev and Kimmett Edgar, *Deep Custody: Segregation Units and Close Supervision Centres in England and Wales* (London: Prison Reform Trust, 2015); Michael Reilly, *Healthcare in Irish Prisons* (Nenagh: Inspector of Prisons, 2016); Agnieszka Martynowicz and Linda Moore, *Behind the Door: Solitary Confinement in the Irish Penal System* (Dublin: Irish Penal Reform Trust, 2018).

arguments, puts to an empirical test the conclusions of influential studies of the prison, particularly those of Michel Foucault, Michael Ignatieff and David Garland.[8] These authors have emphasised the imposition of penal power in nineteenth-century prisons and the ways in which new categories were produced in prisons through the discourses of the locally powerful. As psychiatry and medicine expanded their influence beyond nineteenth-century lunatic asylums, prisons became sites of intervention and 'mental disorders provided ways of constructing social deviance', blurring 'the lines between … medicine and … the jurisdiction of other authoritative bodies'.[9] Our evidence has highlighted the complex exercises of authority and decision-making within prisons, for example between chaplains and prison medical officers, key brokers in gauging and responding to mental illness, or between prison officials and local magistrates, who had an enduring influence in shaping the destinations of mentally disordered offenders. Exploring transfers between prisons and asylums, we ask how far these were prompted by law, pragmatism and the desire for effective prison management, as well as the assertion of professional authority and knowledge.

A study encompassing England and Ireland has offered rich opportunities for comparison. The Irish prison system was an expression of colonial power, and prison administrators were actors in the colonial apparatus answerable to the British administration in Dublin Castle. While sharing ideologies and similar systems of governance and administration, there was much variation in terms of implementation and interpretation in the two countries, notably in the way the separate system was adapted for Irish prisons. In the early 1860s the graduated marks system introduced by the Chairman of the newly established Directors of Convict Prisons, Sir Walter Crofton, made Ireland a model of penal management, and was pointed to for its impact in reducing crime, for its cheapness and for being '*curatively* deterrent and reformatory' in

[8] Michel Foucault, *Discipline and Punish: The Birth of the Prison*, translated from the French by Alan Sheridan (London: Allen Lane, 1977); Michael Ignatieff, *A Just Measure of Pain: The Penitentiary in the Industrial Revolution 1750–1850* (New York: Pantheon Books, 1978); David Garland, *Punishment and Modern Society: A Study in Social Theory* (Oxford: Clarendon, 1990).
[9] Jean Daniel Jacob, Amélie Perron and Dave Holmes (eds), *Power and the Psychiatric Apparatus: Repression, Transformation and Assistance* (London and New York: Routledge, 2014), p. 5. We have consciously used the terms 'psychiatry' and 'psychiatrist' as useful in describing the emergence of a distinct form of specialism focusing on the management and treatment of mental disorder in the second half of the nineteenth century, though prison medical officers might also refer in their publications to their engagement with medical psychology or morbid psychology.

contrast to England.[10] A comparison of the two countries provides opportunities for understanding how particular orders and regulations concerning prison administration, alongside penal philosophies and psychiatric theories, were reinterpreted and adjusted as they crossed the Irish Sea, and also significantly expands the scope to investigate a variety of prison contexts. Prison reformers, prison chaplains and doctors, magistrates, penologists and prison administrators, including Crofton, moved back and forth between England and Ireland, visiting and critiquing prisons. They went on to exchange ideas and theories in their publications and official reports and through such organisations as the Association for the Improvement of Prisons and Prison Discipline in Ireland, the Evangelical Society for the Improvement of Prison Discipline and the Reformation of Juvenile Offenders, the Social Science Association and the Howard Association, prompting debates on the impact of prison regimes on mental health, and the finer points of management in mitigating the negative effects of prison discipline on the mind. Those in a position to compare the two prison systems, like land reformer and Fenian Michael Davitt, argued that treatment in Irish prisons was more humane and less likely to produce insanity than English prisons. Our book also focuses on a period of significant legislative change across the two prison estates, which repeatedly saw adaptations in nomenclature and usage at different moments. For example, with the implementation of the English Prison Act of 1865, the term 'gaol' was replaced with 'prison' to denote local institutions, yet the older nomenclature continued to be widely used. Consequently we adhered to the labels found in our source material, which at times might be inconsistent with the official terminology.

While our book is not based on a case study approach, we draw extensively on the records of individual prisons, local and convict, that provide rich examples of their landmark status in introducing the system of separate confinement; the impact of particular prison officers, chaplains or doctors and the ways they interpreted prison policies; and the local conditions within which they operated. This approach has provided us with the opportunity to draw on a wealth of individual prison archives and evidence about how prison officials and doctors dealt with mental illness in a variety of prison settings, urban and rural, large and small, convict and local, male and female. Special provisions were devised for

---

[10] This inspired Wakefield Prison, for example, to adopt elements of the Irish system in 1861: Edward Balme Wheatley, *Observations on the Treatment of Convicts in Ireland with Some Remarks on the Same in England by Four Visiting Justices of the West Riding Prison at Wakefield* (London: Simpkin, Marshall and Co., 1862), pp. 124–5.

female prisoners that reduced the term they spent in separate confinement, given claims that they were poorly equipped to cope with long periods in isolation. Women were depicted as being particularly volatile and irrational in their conduct. As explored in Chapters 3 and 4, Liverpool Borough Prison was notable for receiving many Irish prisoners, and it also housed what was said to be the largest female prison population in Europe by the late nineteenth century.[11]

Taking as our sources not only the wealth of official reports, which provide rich and voluminous information on the viewpoints of prison administrators, inquiries into the discipline and running of prisons, the evidence and facts and figures on the rate of mental illness and the treatment and destinations of the mentally ill, the archives of individual prisons also offer important evidence. These are scattered, often scanty, and varied in form and content (notably between England and Ireland), and they include minute books and prison journals, reports, character and punishment books, prisoners' files, correspondence between prison officers and prison administrators and letter books.[12] Collectively, despite the fragmented status of the archival sources and variation in terms of what has survived, they provide us with new insights into the levels of mental illness in prison; official accounts tended to downplay rates of mental disorder, while prison archives provide detail on the impact of mentally disturbed prisoners on a day-to-day basis. They uncover great variation in the implementation of official policy and directives and in terms of the impact of individual prison medical officers on the management and treatment of prisoners. They also reveal individual stories of prisoners' mental breakdown and how it was dealt with, movements of prisoners within and between institutions, prisoners' efforts to feign mental illness and the attempts of prison doctors to detect this, alarm at prisoners' suicide attempts, and, in a small number of cases, the discharge of prisoners on medical grounds. Where possible, we have also drawn on asylum casebooks and reports to track the institutional careers of individuals removed to public and criminal asylums. Alongside archival material, the book draws on a diversity of print sources, the accounts and memoirs of prison chaplains, governors and prison doctors, as well

---

[11] For Liverpool Borough Prison, see Catherine Cox and Hilary Marland, '"Unfit for Reform or Punishment": Mental Disorder and Discipline in Liverpool Borough Prison in the Late Nineteenth Century', *Social History*, 44:2 (2019), 173–201.

[12] For Ireland, individual prisoners' stories can also be accessed using Convict Reference Files and other individual penal files. See Elaine Farrell, *Women, Crime and Punishment in Ireland: Life in the Nineteenth-Century Convict Prison* (Cambridge: Cambridge University Press, 2020), pp. 26–8; Catherine Cox, *Negotiating Insanity in the Southeast of Ireland, 1820–1900* (Manchester: Manchester University Press, 2012), pp. 97–132.

as a rich medical journal literature. By the late nineteenth century, prison doctors had begun to publish extensively on their work in prison medicine and psychiatry in leading medical journals, most notably for our purposes in the *Journal of Mental Science*, the premier journal for mental science and psychiatry in the late nineteenth century, setting out their distinctive approaches to practice and their thoughts on the criminal mind and on mental disorder in prison, their unique ways of describing and classifying mental illness in the context of the prison, and advancing their claims as a specialist group.

While the vast majority of prison archives prioritise prison officials and administrators, our study additionally draws on the various critics of the prison system, many of them ex-prisoners, who described its devastating impact on mental health. Dickens, Maybrick, Davitt and Wilde have already been referred to, and alongside these were the works of prison reformers such as Mary Gordon and W.D. Morrison, and a wealth of other prison memoirs, including those of political prisoners, produced mainly after the 1860s.[13] These appeared in book form, but also in pamphlets, periodicals and the press, and provide rich insights into prison practices, what it was like to be in prison, and the plight and management of the mentally ill. In the final decades of the nineteenth century, these accounts, penned largely by educated, middle-class prisoners, also helped shape changes in prison policy.[14] The Victorian public, concerned about the expanding prison population and increased rates of crime and recidivism, had a vested interest in the way that prisons were run, and many were concerned with the treatment of prisoners themselves. Towards the end of our period, reform organisations began to make their impact felt, and their records, reflecting on both English and Irish prisons, form a further rich resource for this study.

---

[13] William Douglas Morrison, 'Are Our Prisons a Failure?', *The Fortnightly Review*, 55:328 (Apr 1894), 459–69; Mary Gordon, *Penal Discipline* (London: Routledge, 1922). Among many influential prison memoirs are One Who Has Endured It, *Five Years of Penal Servitude* (London: Richard Bentley & Son, 1878); One Who Has Tried Them, *Her Majesty's Prisons: Their Effects and Defects*, vols 1 and 2 (London: Sampson Low, Marsten, Searle & Rivington, 1881); W.B.N., *Penal Servitude* (London: William Heinemann, 1903); Jeremiah O'Donovan Rossa, *Six Years in Six English Prisons* (New York: P.J. Kennedy, 1874). See also Sean T. O'Brien, 'The Prison Writing of Michael Davitt', *New Hibernia Review*, 14:3 (2010), 16–32.

[14] For overviews of prison memoirs, see Philip Priestley, *Victorian Prison Lives: English Prison Biography, 1830–1914* (London: Pimlico, 1985); Sarah Anderson and John Pratt, 'Prisoner Memoirs and Their Role in Prison History', in Helen Johnston (ed.), *Punishment and Control in Historical Perspective* (Houndmills: Palgrave Macmillan, 2008), pp. 179–98.

Institutions of Confinement

Despite the long-standing association of prisons with the deteriorating mental health of their inmates, there has been little historical work on this subject. Criminologists and historians of crime and prisons have produced an impressive scholarship examining nineteenth-century prisons and prisoners, though this is chiefly in the context of England. Irish prisons, despite a number of important contributions, have had less coverage, especially with regard to late nineteenth-century Irish penal policy.[15] Histories of the convict system and transportation in both contexts, the colonial character of the Irish convict system, women in prison and political prisoners have engaged little with matters of health and medicine in prison, and even less with mental illness.[16] However,

---

[15] See, for example, William James Forsythe, *The Reform of Prisoners 1830–1900* (London and Sydney: Croom Helm, 1987); Ignatieff, *A Just Measure of Pain*; Seán McConville, *A History of English Prison Administration, Vol. 1, 1750–1877* (London, Boston and Henley: Routledge & Kegan Paul, 1981); Seán McConville, *English Local Prisons 1860–1900: Next Only to Death* (London and New York: Routledge, 1995); Martin J. Wiener, *Reconstructing the Criminal: Culture, Law, and Policy in England, 1830–1914* (Cambridge: Cambridge University Press, 1990); Alyson Brown, *English Society and the Prison: Time, Culture and Politics in the Development of the Modern Prison, 1850–1920* (Woodbridge: Boydell, 2003); Helen Johnston, *Crime in England 1815–1880: Experiencing the Criminal Justice System* (London and New York: Routledge, 2015); Victor Bailey, *Policing and Punishment in Nineteenth-Century Britain* (Abingdon: Routledge, 2016); Victor Bailey (ed.), *Nineteenth-Century Crime and Punishment*, 4 vols (Abingdon: Routledge, 2021). For Ireland, see Patrick Carroll-Burke, *Colonial Discipline: The Making of the Irish Convict System* (Dublin: Four Courts Press, 2000); Tim Carey, *Mountjoy: The Story of a Prison* (Dublin: Collins Press, 2000); Cal McCarthy and Barra O'Donnabhain, *Too Beautiful for Thieves and Pickpockets: A History of the Victorian Convict Prison on Spike Island* (Cork: Cork County Library, 2016); Richard Butler, *Building the Irish Courthouse and Prison: A Political History, 1750–1850* (Cork: Cork University Press, 2020); Eoin O'Sullivan and Ian O'Donnell, *Coercive Confinement in Ireland: Patients, Prisoners and Penitents* (Manchester: Manchester University Press, 2012); Beverly A. Smith, 'The Irish General Prisons Board, 1877–1885: Efficient Deterrence or Bureaucratic Ineptitude?', *Irish Jurist*, 15:1 (1980), 122–36; Shane Kilcommins, Ian O'Donnell, Eoin O'Sullivan and Barry Vaughan, *Crime, Punishment and the Search for Order in Ireland* (Dublin: Institute of Public Administration, 2004).

[16] Carroll-Burke, *Colonial Discipline*; Lucia Zedner, *Women, Crime and Custody in Victorian England* (Oxford: Clarendon, 1991); Lucy Williams, *Wayward Women: Female Offending in Victorian England* (Barnsley: Pen & Sword, 2016); Farrell, *Women, Crime and Punishment in Ireland*; Elaine Farrell, '"Having an Immoral Conversation" and Other Prison Offenses: The Punishment of Convict Women', in Christina S. Brophy and Cara Delay (eds), *Women, Reform and Resistance in Ireland, 1850–1950* (Houndmills: Palgrave Macmillan, 2015), pp. 101–18; Beverly A. Smith, 'The Female Prisoner in Ireland, 1855–1878', *Federal Probation*, 54:4 (1990), 69–81; Clare Anderson and Hamish Maxwell-Stewart, 'Convict Labour and the Western Empires, 1415–1954', in Robert Aldrich and Kirsten McKenzie (eds), *Routledge History of Western Empires* (London and New York: Routledge, 2014), pp. 102–17; Hamish Maxwell-Stewart, 'Transportation from Britain and Ireland, 1615–1875', in Clare Anderson (ed.), *A Global History of*

there are some important exceptions to this. The studies of Joe Sim, Anne Hardy and Peter McRorie Higgins have drawn attention to the status and role of prison medical officers, and Higgins' work also examined the management and treatment of the mentally ill in English prisons before 1850.[17] Scientific criminology and the relationship between crime, degeneracy and mental unfitness have been interrogated by Neil Davie and Stephen Watson in the context of late nineteenth-century English prisons, with particular emphasis on assessing the ways in which English criminology varied in approach from continental theorists.[18] Overall, there has been far less historical research on health and prisons in Ireland; the few existing studies have been largely preoccupied with exploring how political prisoners and suffragists used their bodily health during campaigns to achieve specific goals, and, while we have worked closely with and greatly enhanced the existing scholarship on English prison health, our contributions to the Irish historiography are particularly novel.[19]

Convicts and Penal Colonies (London: Bloomsbury, 2018), pp. 183–210; Joan Kavanagh and Dianne Snowden, *Van Diemen's Women: A History of Transportation to Tasmania* (Dublin: The History Press, 2015); William Murphy, *Political Imprisonment and the Irish, 1912–1921* (Oxford: Oxford University Press, 2014); Seán McConville, *Irish Political Prisoners, 1920–1962: Pilgrimage of Desolation* (New York: Routledge, 2014).

[17] Joe Sim, *Medical Power in Prisons: The Prison Medical Service in England 1774–1989* (Milton Keynes and Philadelphia, PA: Open University Press, 1990); Anne Hardy, 'Development of the Prison Medical Service, 1774–1895', in Richard Creese, W.F. Bynum and J. Bearn (eds), *The Health of Prisoners* (Amsterdam and Atlanta, GA: Rodopi, 1995), pp. 59–82; Peter McRorie Higgins, *Punish or Treat?: Medical Care in English Prisons 1770–1850* (Victoria, BC and Oxford: Trafford, 2007). See also J.E. Thomas, *The English Prison Officer since 1850* (London and Boston: Routledge & Kegan Paul, 1972). For articles on health and medicine in the nineteenth-century Australian prison system, see the special issue of *Health and History*, 22:1 (2020), edited by Louella McCarthy, Kathryn Weston, Stephen Hampton and Tobias Mackinnon.

[18] Stephen Watson, 'Malingerers, the "Weakminded" Criminal and the "Moral Imbecile": How the English Prison Officer Became an Expert in Mental Deficiency, 1880–1930', in Michael Clark and Catherine Crawford (eds), *Legal Medicine in History* (Cambridge: Cambridge University Press, 1994), pp. 223–41; Neil Davie, *Tracing the Criminal: The Rise of Scientific Criminology in Britain, 1860–1918* (Oxford: Bardwell Press, 2006). For debates on the relationship between criminality and eugenics in the US, see Nicole Hahn Rafter, *Creating Born Criminals* (Champaign, IL: University of Illinois Press, 1997). Ian O'Donnell has explored prisoners' strategies for overcoming mental distress while endeavouring to deal with the rigours of solitude: Ian O'Donnell, *Prisoners, Solitude, and Time* (New York and Oxford: Oxford University Press, 2014). For a compelling study of the 'death-in-life' experience of solitary confinement in the US, see Lisa Guenther, *Solitary Confinement: Social Death and Its Afterlives* (Minneapolis, MN and London: University of Minnesota Press, 2013).

[19] Beverly A. Smith, 'Irish Prison Doctors – Men in the Middle, 1865–90', *Medical History*, 26:4 (1982), 371–94; William Murphy, 'Dying, Death and Hunger Strike: Cork and Brixton, 1920', in James Kelly and Mary Ann Lyons (eds), *Death and Dying in Ireland,*

This stands in stark contrast to the emphasis in the medical humanities over the last few decades on exploring the other institutions that contained and treated the mentally ill, notably public, district and criminal lunatic asylums, but also workhouses, private madhouses, and institutions and schools specialising in the care of those deemed mentally deficient.[20] These studies have focused intently on the processes and pressures that prompted large-scale confinement of the insane in the nineteenth century. They question how far this was driven by major demographic and socioeconomic shifts, the growth of towns, poverty and poor living conditions, and the migration of large groups of people from the countryside into urban centres, factors also deemed to be productive of high rates of crime and incarceration. These major disruptions took place alongside changes in family structure and in working lives, including regimented factory conditions that subjected the poor to rigid and lengthy working days. These conditions, it has been argued, meant that mentally ill family members were less likely to be cared for within the household and became more liable to institutional

---

Britain, and Europe: Historical Perspectives (Dublin: Irish Academic Press, 2013), pp. 297–316; Ian Miller, *A History of Force Feeding: Hunger Strikes, Prisons and Medical Ethics, 1909–1974* (Houndmills: Palgrave Macmillan, 2016); Ian Miller, *Reforming Food in Post-Famine Ireland: Medicine, Science and Improvement, 1845–1922* (Manchester: Manchester University Press, 2014), pp. 74–81; Ciara Breathnach, 'Medical Officers, Bodies, Gender and Weight Fluctuation in Irish Convict Prisons, 1877–95', *Medical History*, 58:1 (2014), 67–86.

[20] For example, out of a vast literature, see Andrew Scull, *The Most Solitary of Afflictions: Madness and Society in Britain 1700–1900* (New Haven, CT and London: Yale University Press, 2005); Roy Porter, 'Madness and Its Institutions', in Andrew Wear (ed.), *Medicine in Society* (Cambridge: Cambridge University Press, 1992), pp. 277–301; Peter Bartlett, *The Poor Law of Lunacy: The Administration of Pauper Lunatics in Mid-Nineteenth-Century England* (London and New York: Leicester University Press, 1999); Joseph Melling and Bill Forsythe (eds), *Insanity, Institutions and Society, 1800–1914* (London and New York: Routledge, 1999); Mark Finnane, *Insanity and the Insane in Post-Famine Ireland* (London: Croom Helm, 1981); Cox, *Negotiating Insanity*; David Wright, *Mental Disability in Victorian England: The Earlswood Asylum, 1847–1901* (Oxford: Oxford University Press, 2001); Mark Jackson, *The Borderland of Imbecility: Medicine, Society and the Fabrication of the Feeble Mind in Late Victorian and Edwardian England* (Manchester: Manchester University Press, 2000); Janet Saunders, 'Institutionalised Offenders: A Study of the Victorian Institution and Its Inmates, with Special Reference to Late Nineteenth Century Warwickshire' (unpublished University of Warwick PhD thesis, 1983) is unusual in exploring both the prison and asylum, and the passage of inmates between the two institutions. For Ireland, see Oonagh Walsh, '"A Person of the Second Order": The Plight of the Intellectually Disabled in Nineteenth-Century Ireland', in Laurence Geary and Oonagh Walsh (eds), *Philanthropy in Nineteenth-Century Ireland* (Dublin: Four Courts Press, 2015), pp. 161–80; Peter Reid, 'Children, Mental Deficiency and Institutions in Dublin, 1900 to 1911' (unpublished University College Dublin MLitt thesis, 2018).

confinement; many, including those committing minor offences, would end up moving between the prison, asylum and workhouse.[21]

Other scholarship has highlighted the role of reform and the optimism that permeated the provision of asylum care after the 1830s, with the introduction of new therapeutic approaches into specialised asylums, notably moral treatment, with its emphasis on routine, occupation of the patients and self-management, and the creation of a new group of specialists in the care of the insane.[22] Meanwhile, specific groups within the prison population, such as children and juveniles, whose minds required distinct consideration, were catered for in separate institutions with specialist care.[23] The large county and district asylums of the nineteenth century had been preceded by voluntary asylums and private asylums or madhouses. The latter, set up by entrepreneurial individuals or families, operated on a much smaller scale (particularly in the Irish context) though they demonstrated and further stimulated a growing market for asylum services. Set up initially to cater largely for well-to-do patients, in the nineteenth century private asylums in England provided an important back-up service to overstretched county asylums and to a lesser extent prisons.[24] In Ireland, due to different funding

[21] For the role of families in caring for mentally ill relatives, see Andrew Scull, *Museums of Madness: The Social Organization of Insanity in 19th Century England* (London: Allen Lane, 1979); Scull, *The Most Solitary of Afflictions*. John Walton has argued, however, that households continued to support and care for mentally ill family members for as long as possible: John K. Walton, 'Lunacy in the Industrial Revolution: A Study of Asylum Admissions in Lancashire 1848–50', *Journal of Social History*, 13:1 (1979), 1–22; John K. Walton, 'Casting Out and Bringing Back in Victorian England: Pauper Lunatics, 1840–70', in W.F. Bynum, Roy Porter and Michael Shepherd (eds), *The Anatomy of Madness: Essays in the History of Psychiatry*, vol. II (London and New York: Tavistock, 1985), 132–46; Mark Finnane, 'Asylums, Family and the State', *History Workshop Journal*, 20:1 (1985), 134–48.

[22] David Wright, 'Getting out of the Asylum: Understanding the Confinement of the Insane in the Nineteenth Century', *Social History of Medicine*, 10:1 (1997), 137–55. For moral treatment, see, for example, Anne Digby, *Madness, Morality, and Medicine: A Study of the York Retreat, 1796–1914* (Cambridge: Cambridge University Press, 1985). For a more critical take on moral treatment, see Andrew Scull, 'Moral Treatment Reconsidered: Some Sociological Comments on an Episode in the History of British Psychiatry', in Andrew Scull (ed.), *Madhouses, Mad-Doctors, and Madmen: The Social History of Psychiatry in the Victorian Era* (London: Athlone, 1981), pp. 105–20.

[23] Fiachra Byrne, '"In Humanity's Machine": Prison Health and History', *ECAN Bulletin: Howard League for Penal Reform*, 33 (July 2017), 14–20; Paul Sargent, *Wild Arabs and Savages: A History of Juvenile Justice in Ireland* (Manchester: Manchester University Press, 2014); Victor Bailey, *Delinquency and Citizenship: Reclaiming the Young Offender 1914–18* (New York: Oxford University Press, 1987); Barry Godfrey, Pamela Cox, Heather Shore and Zoe Alker, *Young Criminal Lives: Life Courses and Life Chances from 1850* (Oxford: Oxford University Press, 2017).

[24] Roy Porter, *Mind-Forg'd Manacles: A History of Madness in England from the Restoration to the Regency* (London: Athlone, 1987; Penguin edn, 1990), ch. 3; Leonard Smith, *Private*

structures, private asylums remained relatively distinct and continued to cater for wealthier patients. Voluntary asylums in both contexts, usually charitable, non-profit and in Ireland often holding religious affiliations, provided additional relief to less affluent patients.[25]

Prisons of course were never intended to be places of medical treatment and cure, and from the 1830s onwards legislation endeavoured to divert mentally ill offenders away from prisons to asylums, including Dundrum Criminal Lunatic Asylum after 1850 and Broadmoor, which took over the treatment of the criminally insane from Bethlem Hospital in 1863.[26] This had limited impact in practice, with, as Chapter 4 demonstrates, large numbers of mentally ill people still confined in English and Irish prisons by the late nineteenth century. Additionally, many mentally ill patients were housed in workhouse accommodation following poor law legislation, in England the New Poor Law in 1834 and in Ireland in 1838.[27] The Irish Poor Law, modelled on the English system, had greater emphasis on indoor relief.[28] That the English Poor Law continued to provide out relief, outside of the detested workhouse, became a factor in encouraging large-scale migration from Ireland in the post-Famine era, in turn pushing up the admission of mentally ill Irish migrants into workhouses, asylums and prisons.[29] Despite the huge scale of asylum provision, and the equally rapid expansion of workhouse accommodation, with many English and Irish workhouses having dedicated wards for lunatics and idiots after the 1840s, the pace of provision never kept up with demand. For much of the second half of the nineteenth century asylums were overcrowded and workhouses under pressure from mentally ill or weak-minded paupers.[30] Despite the pressure on these institutions, they, alongside Dundrum and Broadmoor criminal

---

Madhouses in England, 1640–1815: Commercialised Care for the Insane (Cham: Palgrave Macmillan, 2020).

[25] Alice Mauger, *The Cost of Insanity in Nineteenth-Century Ireland: Public, Voluntary and Private Asylum Care* (Cham: Palgrave Macmillan, 2018); Leonard D. Smith, *'Cure, Comfort and Safe Custody': Public Lunatic Asylums in Early Nineteenth-Century England* (London and New York: Leicester University Press, 1999).

[26] Pauline M. Prior, *Madness and Murder: Gender, Crime and Mental Disorder in Nineteenth-Century Ireland* (Dublin: Irish Academic Press, 2008); Brendan Kelly, *Custody, Care & Criminality: Forensic Psychiatry and Law in 19th Century Ireland* (Dublin: History Press, 2014); Mark Stevens, *Broadmoor Revealed: Victorian Crime and the Lunatic Asylum* (Barnsley: Pen & Sword, 2013).

[27] Barlett, *The Poor Law of Lunacy.*   [28] Cox, *Negotiating Insanity*, ch. 6.

[29] Catherine Cox, Hilary Marland and Sarah York, 'Emaciated, Exhausted and Excited: The Bodies and Minds of the Irish in Nineteenth-Century Lancashire Asylums', *Journal of Social History*, 46:2 (2012), 500–24.

[30] Ibid., p. 502; Scull, *The Most Solitary of Afflictions*; Catherine Cox and Hilary Marland, '"A Burden on the County": Madness, Institutions of Confinement and the Irish Patient in Victorian Lancashire', *Social History of Medicine*, 28:2 (2015), 263–87.

lunatic asylums, as explored in Chapter 4, became repositories for many mentally ill offenders over the course of the nineteenth century.

The Discipline of Separation and the Prison Cell

With new models of discipline introduced from the 1840s onwards, and explored in Chapter 2, the prison was intended to reform, rehabilitate and produce moral improvement in the isolation of the cell, directed largely by the prison chaplains, with prisoners entering a place 'of instruction and of probation rather than a GAOL OR OPPRESSIVE PUNISHMENT'.[31] This marked a significant shift in approach, which Michael Ignatieff has described as a new philosophy of punishment directed at the mind rather than the body, intended to replace the disorder, filth and arbitrariness rife in prisons, the whip and the gallows with a prison discipline based on rationality and order, supervised by the state.[32] While the late nineteenth century has been strongly associated with the process of centralisation, as Bill Forsythe has pointed out there was a 'decisive tilt towards the centre in the prison system of the 1830s', with the establishment of clear policy agendas for prisons, alongside reformatories, asylums and workhouses, directed by increasingly powerful central government inspectorates.[33] In the case of Ireland, Oliver MacDonagh locates the shift towards centralisation to the late eighteenth century, citing the establishment of the prison inspectorate in 1786.[34] It has also been argued that Ireland's colonial status prompted the curtailment of the powers of local administration in favour of central government at Dublin Castle. In terms of English and Irish prisons, centralisation was intended to embrace the convict prisons, where prisoners were held on 'probation' before transportation to the colonies, as well as local prisons administered by magistrates and local Boards of Superintendence, and attempts were also made to bring the latter in line with central policy.[35] Local prisons, meanwhile, served a number of

---

[31] Sir James Graham, Home Secretary, to J.T. Burt, Chaplain at Pentonville, 16 Dec. 1842, in Joshua Jebb, Second Report of the Surveyor-General of Prisons (1847) [867], p. 48.

[32] Ignatieff, A Just Measure of Pain.

[33] Bill Forsythe, 'Centralisation and Local Autonomy: The Experience of English Prisons 1820–1877', Journal of Historical Sociology, 4:3 (1991), 317–45, at p. 323.

[34] Oliver MacDonagh, The Inspector General: Sir Jeremiah Fitzpatrick and the Politics of Social Reform, 1783–1802 (London: Croom Helm, 1981).

[35] In Ireland, Boards of Superintendence, half of whom were magistrates, were responsible to county Grand Juries and municipal corporations. Grand Juries were the principal organs of local government. See Virginia Crossman, 'The Growth of the State in the Nineteenth Century', in James Kelly (ed.), The Cambridge History of Ireland, vol. 3, 1730–1880 (Cambridge: Cambridge University Press, 2018), 542–66. For the

functions: the detention of prisoners awaiting trial, debtors and those condemned to capital punishment, as well as being places of punishment for those sentenced to terms of up to two years.

English and Irish prison systems would come to rest on the foundations of rationality and beneficence, centring on the methodology of separate confinement that involved criminals in their own rehabilitation. Yet even as the system was being imported from the Eastern State Penitentiary in Philadelphia to England, these foundations were looking increasingly shaky.[36] By the late 1830s reports were implicating the 'Pennsylvania system' in the mental breakdown of inmates and reporting that cellular isolation was producing high rates of mortality and insanity.[37] Accompanied by mounting criticism, including a vigorous campaign in *The Times* newspaper, as discussed in Chapter 2, the separate system was applied initially and in its most severe form at Pentonville Model Prison in London in 1842, and a modified version was introduced in Ireland at its flagship prison, Mountjoy in Dublin, in 1850. By then the harmful impact of the separate system on prisoners' mental health had become increasingly evident.[38]

The new system of discipline centred on the architecture of the prison, with the prison cell the hub of operations. It was here, in a small space measuring around thirteen feet by seven by nine, that the convict was to experience the full force of separate confinement.[39] Though Jeremy

---

management of English prisons, see McConville, *A History of English Prison Administration*; McConville, *English Local Prisons 1860–1900*.

[36] For United States prisons, see David J. Rothman, 'Perfecting the Prison: United States, 1789–1865', in Norval Morris and David J. Rothman (eds), *The Oxford History of the Prison: The Practice of Punishment in Western Society* (New York and Oxford: Oxford University Press, 1998), pp. 100–16.

[37] *Thirteenth Report of the Board of Managers of the Prison Discipline Society* (Boston: The Society's Room, 1838), p. 236. See also David Wilson, 'Testing a Civilisation: Charles Dickens on the American Penitentiary System', *The Howard Journal of Criminal Justice*, 48:3 (2009), 280–96.

[38] U.R.Q. Henriques, 'The Rise and Decline of the Separate System of Prison Discipline', *Past & Present*, 54:1 (1972), 61–93, at p. 86. Despite aiming to exclude prisoners showing signs of mental weakness, Dr Forbes Winslow concluded in 1851 that 1.4% of Pentonville's inmates were suffering from mental illness compared with 0.25% of the general population: Forbes Winslow, 'Medical Society of London: Prison Discipline', *Lancet*, 57:1439 (29 Mar. 1851), 357–60. For Pentonville, see Catherine Cox and Hilary Marland, '"He Must Die or Go Mad in This Place": Prisoners, Insanity and the Pentonville Model Prison Experiment, 1842–1852', *Bulletin of the History of Medicine*, 92:1 (2018), 78–109.

[39] See Leslie Topp, 'Single Rooms, Seclusion and the Non-Restraint Movement in British Asylums, 1838–1844', *Social History of Medicine*, 31:4 (2018), 754–73, for seclusion in asylum practice.

Bentham's panopticon was never actually built in England or Ireland, it provided the inspiration for much prison design, particularly in its emphasis on surveillance. Pentonville, with its 500 inmates, was enclosed in an eighteen-foot perimeter wall, and, with three levels of solitary cells radiating from a central block, arranged so that the prison officers could not be seen by the prisoners, though they themselves could be watched at all times. It was created, as were the new generation of prisons that followed in England and Ireland, to produce isolation within the prison and from the outside world. Every detail was carefully worked out – from the thickness of the door and walls, the size of the windows, the plumbing, ventilation and heating – to ensure tight security and prevent prisoners from communicating with each other, while also maintaining the prisoners' health.[40]

The cell was intended to throw prisoners back on their own thoughts, recollections and regrets until they were ready to declare their repentance for past sins and crimes, clearing the path for their deep-seated reformation. The separate cellular system appealed to the prison authorities on punitive as well as reformatory grounds, and, while praising its potential for initiating real change in criminal behaviour, Reverend Joseph Kingsmill at Pentonville Prison affirmed that it was also 'calculated to strike more terror into the minds of the lowest and vilest class of criminals than any other [system] hitherto devised'.[41] Henry Hitchins, Inspector of Government Prisons in Ireland, argued that the strength of the separate system was its capacity to act as a deterrent, based on the 'dread' of the convict returning to the separate cell.[42] For the prisoners, however, 'there was in the first closing of the door behind them, a finality that betokened a dreadful new beginning'.[43] Why the authorities 'should leave a man alone with his thoughts for eight months I cannot possibly conceive', reflected prisoner John Lee of his experiences at the start of his sentence in Pentonville in 1885. 'I can think of nothing more calculated

[40] Robin Evans, *The Fabrication of Virtue: English Prison Architecture, 1750–1840* (Cambridge: Cambridge University Press, 1982), ch. 7; Heather Tomlinson, 'Design and Reform: The "Separate System" in the Nineteenth Century English Prison', in Anthony D. King (ed.), *Buildings and Society: Essays on the Social Development of the Built Environment* (London: Routledge, 1984), pp. 94–119; Butler, *Building the Irish Courthouse and Prison*, chs 5–7.
[41] Reverend Joseph Kingsmill, *Chapters on Prisons and Prisoners*, 3rd edn (London: Longman, Brown, Green, and Longmans, 1854), p. 116.
[42] National Archives of Ireland (NAI), Government Prison Office (GPO)/Letter Books (LB), Vol. 12, July 1849–Dec. 1851, p. 63.
[43] Priestley, *Victorian Prison Lives*, p. 39.

to drive a prisoner mad than eight months of solitude with nothing to think about but his own miseries, with no companion save despair.'[44]

Cases of mania, anxiety and depression, often attended by fearful delusions and hallucinations, became more widespread as new prisons were built and older ones adapted to impose the discipline of separate confinement. In effect it appeared not only to make prisoners who already had some form of pre-existing mental disorder worse, but also to be triggering mental breakdown. Yet, as shown in Chapters 2 and 3, the system of separate confinement endured and its implementation across the English and Irish prison estate, in both local and convict prisons, remained the aim of most prison administrators.[45] Adaptation to the separate system proceeded apace, and already by 1850 it was reported that some 11,000 purpose-built separate cells had been constructed or were nearing completion in England and fifty-five separate cellular prisons.[46] In Ireland the rate of building separate cells was slower owing to the disruption caused by the Great Famine (1845-52). Nonetheless in the 1860s provision for separate confinement was expanded as new wings were added to some local gaols and a small number of new prisons opened.

A number of local prisons were either rebuilt or, as in the case of Leicester Gaol, quickly adapted and expanded to meet the requirements of separation. Though largely admitting prisoners from Leicester and the agricultural county of Leicestershire, who were typically sentenced to short terms of imprisonment for offences against the game laws or vagrancy, in 1846 176 cells were certified as fit for separate confinement. Two years later, with surplus capacity, the magistrates began to lease cells for the confinement of government convicts.[47] Similarly Wakefield Prison built a new section constructed on the same plans as Pentonville in 1847, providing accommodation for 1,374 prisoners, much more than was required for the West Riding of Yorkshire area that it served, and over 400 cells were let to government convicts undergoing separate

---

[44] [John Lee], *The Man they Could Not Hang: The Life Story of John Lee*, Told by Himself (London: Mellifont Press, 1936), p. 53.
[45] See Miles Ogborn, 'Discipline, Government and Law: Separate Confinement in the Prisons of England and Wales, 1830–1877', *Transactions of the Institute of British Geographers*, 20:3 (1995), 295–311, for the persistence of the separate system and emphasis on imposing uniformity.
[46] Forsythe, *The Reform of Prisoners*, p. 45.
[47] Jacqueline L. Kane, 'Prison Palace or "Hell upon Earth": Leicester County Gaol under the Separate System, 1846–1865', *Transactions of the Leicestershire Archaeological and Historical Society*, 70 (1996), 128–46.

confinement, and later to the War Department for military prisoners.[48] There were efforts to implement similar structural changes to Irish local prisons; for example, the 'old' county Antrim Gaol was replaced in 1846 by the new Belfast House of Correction, which, modelled on Pentonville, had over 300 separate cells.[49]

The system that was initially designed to inspire reflection and produce reform among prisoners was radically reconsidered and modified in the 1860s and 1870s. Convict prisons, as discussed in Chapter 2, initially fulfilled the function of taking government prisoners in preparation for transportation to Australia or other colonies. However, after transportation was abandoned during the 1850s and 1860s, nine months of separate confinement in a convict prison was followed by an extended sentence of penal servitude in a public works prison and then release on licence if a period of remission had been earned.[50] Instead of being shipped to distant colonies after their initial probationary phase in separate confinement, convicts completed their terms of penal servitude in English and Irish prisons. This, in combination with 'the perceived threat of the "criminal class" or habitual offender' and the garrotting panics of the 1850s and 1860s, led to a more 'deterrence based approach', though in 1865 the minimum period of penal servitude was increased from three to five years rather than the seven years proposed by the 1863 Royal Commission on penal servitude.[51] After 1877 central government control extended to all prisons with the aim of introducing uniformity of conditions and punishment across the English and Irish prison estates.[52] This was expressed in a form of discipline that emphasised harsh punishment, hard labour, board and fare, and, as Chapter 3 argues, isolation in the separate cell was defined increasingly as a penal tool rather than as reformatory. This shift to a nationalised and more penal approach also produced many instances of mental breakdown, which were commented on in prisoners' own accounts of prison life, as inmates buckled under

---

[48] Wheatley, *Observations on the Treatment of Convicts in Ireland*, p. v; J. Horsfall Turner, *The Annals of Wakefield House of Correction* (Bingley: privately printed, 1904), pp. 233, 245.
[49] Report of the Inspectors General of Prisons in Ireland (RIGPI) 1845 (1846) [697], pp. 5, 20.
[50] Seán McConville, 'The Victorian Prison', in Morris and Rothman (eds), *The Oxford History of the Prison*, pp. 131–67, at pp. 131–8; Johnston, *Crime in England 1815–1880*, p. 112.
[51] Johnston, *Crime in England 1815–1880*, p. 96; Forsythe, *The Reform of Prisoners*, pp. 160–1.
[52] Ogborn, 'Discipline, Government and Law'; Forsythe, 'Centralisation and Local Autonomy'; McConville, 'The Victorian Prison'; Smith, 'The Irish General Prisons Board, 1877–1885'.

regimes that imposed brutal systems of hard labour and poor diet alongside cellular isolation.

Prisons and Their Prisoners

In 1835 a central government prison inspectorate was set up in Britain, a
body preceded in Ireland in the early 1820s. The inspectorates fed into
prison reform and, as Richard Butler has demonstrated, facilitated the
early exchange of ideas and knowledge between the two countries.[53]
After 1850 English prisons were administered by a Directorate that
managed convict prisons, and in 1877 the Prison Commission took over
the running of local prisons from county and borough magistrates.
Though distinct bodies, by the early 1890s membership was the same
and both were chaired by Sir Edmund du Cane, who had been appointed
Chairman of the Directors of Convict Prisons in 1869, and made chair of
the Prison Commission when it was established. A Convict Prison
Directorate was established for Ireland in 1854, which was superseded
by the General Prison Board in 1877. This took over the management of
county and borough prisons from Grand Juries and local Boards of
Superintendence, and also managed the convict prisons. The Board
was dominated by a small number of officials, notably Charles
F. Bourke who was chair from November 1878 until 1895.

Around ninety new prisons were built or extended in Britain between
1842 and 1877, while in Ireland there were thirty-eight local prisons and
four convict prisons in 1878.[54] After nationalisation, the English Prison
Commissioners and the Irish General Prison Board rationalised and
reconfigured the prison estates, closing down some institutions, while
expanding and renovating others. In Ireland, the Board pursued a policy
of congregating prisoners in fewer but larger prisons until the late nineteenth century as the size of prison population declined.[55] Across the
larger English prison estate there was significant variation in prison size,
levels of overcrowding, and individual prison environments and conditions, especially in London.[56] In the mid-1880s, new building works

---

[53] A government-salaried prison inspector, Sir Jeremiah Fitzpatrick, was appointed in
1786. See Richard Butler, 'Rethinking the Origins of the British Prisons Act of 1835:
Ireland and the Development of Central-Government Prison Inspection, 1820–35', *The
Historical Journal*, 59:3 (2016), 721–46.

[54] See Ogborn, 'Discipline, Government and Law'; Forsythe, *The Reform of Prisoners*,
pp. 93–4 for details on the number of prisons and the provision of cells for separate
confinement in England; Report of the General Prisons Board (Ireland) (RGPBI),
1879–80 (1880) [C.2689], pp. 3, 13.

[55] RGPBI, 1889–90 (1890) [C.6182], pp. 5–6.

[56] Report of the Commissioners of Prisons, 1880 (1880) [C.2733], pp. 7–8.

eased the pressure, though it continued to be an issue, particularly in the larger provincial cities of Birmingham, Manchester and Liverpool.[57]

In 1850 the British convict sector held around 6,000 convicts in five prisons, rented cells in local gaols and in five prison hulks; by 1865 it was holding 7,000 in eleven institutions. Around 17,500 prisoners were held by 1867 in English and Welsh local prisons, a small increase from the figure of 16,000 in 1844.[58] The Prison Commissioners for England commented later in the century on the 'remarkable decrease' in the prison population in the context of an increase in the size of the general population, from an estimated 19,818 on 31 March 1878 to 13,877 in 1890, a fall of 31.8 per cent.[59] There was also a decline in the number of persons charged with indictable offences, and in the number of 'criminals at large', which was estimated to be 31,000 in 1889–90.[60] In Ireland the number of convicts declined rapidly in the immediate post-Famine years, also in response to the huge reduction in population from death and migration, from 11,990 in 1847–51 to 1,826 in 1856–60 and to 1,114 in 1878.[61] The number in custody in local prisons totalled 2,663 in 1866 and, while there were fluctuations, thereafter it did not expand substantially. In 1891–92 the daily average number in Irish local prisons was 2,506 with an additional 443 male convicts and thirty-seven female convicts.[62] It was also estimated that the number of indictable offences and charges had declined by 11,123, or by 1.6 per 10,000 persons over the ten years from 1883 to 1892.[63] Yet despite declining prison numbers, in both England and Ireland the high rates of reoffending and committals for minor offences prompted extensive commentary among prison administrators and penologists. Of the 39,939 prison committals in Ireland in 1889–90, for example, nearly half, 17,820, were for 'drunkenness'.[64] Many habitual offenders were also mentally ill and weak-minded, and, as discussed in Chapter 3, while by the end of the nineteenth century prison medical officers and criminologists were insisting that criminality as well as insanity was 'treatable', they also asserted that prison served little purpose for weak-minded offenders.

[57] Report from the Departmental Committee on Prisons [Gladstone Committee] (1895) [C.7702] [C.7702–I], p. 78; Report of the Commissioners of Prisons, 1890 (1890) [C.6191], pp. 48–9.
[58] Forsythe, *The Reform of Prisoners*, p. 93.
[59] Report of the Commissioners of Prisons, 1890 (1890) [C.6191), p. 2.
[60] Wiener, *Reconstructing the Criminal*, pp. 216–17.
[61] RGPBI, 1879–80 (1880), pp. 9–10, 13.
[62] RGPBI, 1891–92 (1892) [C.6789], pp. 18, 20.
[63] Criminal and Judicial Statistics, Ireland, 1893 (1894) [C.7534], p. 17.
[64] RGPBI, 1889–90 (1890), p. 17.

Prison Medical Officers

While prison administrators pushed through policies intended to rational-ise and produce uniformity, exploration of a variety of English and Irish prison contexts reveals considerable divergence between them in the implementation of discipline. So too there was considerable variation in the way that mental illness among prisoners was dealt with, in the eager-ness of prison medical officers to impose regulations and in their skills, and in the processes of assessing whether prisoners were mentally ill, or, alternatively, poorly equipped to undertake the system of discipline, weak-minded or malingerers. As prison regimes shifted in the 1860s and 1870s towards an approach emphasising punishment and deterrence, so too did the role and remit of the doctors working within them adapt and alter. In the early years of the separate system, as shown in Chapter 2, chaplains were at least equal in their influence and power to prison doctors and claimed expertise in dealing with matters of the mind. However, several scandals and disputes prompted by the chaplains' overzealous commitment to this role eroded their influence, while new legislation in the mid-nineteenth century accorded more authority to prison medical officers, who began to envisage themselves as a discrete group of profes-sionals with their own skill sets and experience. As prison populations expanded, prison medical officers were compelled to deal with a large number of cases of mental disorder on a day-to-day basis, which put a strain on the management and governance of prisons as well as adding significantly to their workloads. Yet it also gave them practical experience in dealing with mental illness, and many prison medical officers began to envisage themselves as experts in psychiatry in criminal justice settings.

A focus on individual prisons and their archives has enabled us to test and nuance the conclusions of previous work on prison medical officers that has framed the challenges faced by them in terms of 'dual loyalty'. Wiener and Sim have emphasised the ways in which prison doctors were caught in a tension between supporting and enforcing the discipline of the prison, with regard to behaviour, diet and labour, as well as through their examinations of prisoners to deem them fit for punishment, and their role as arbiters of prisoners' health and wellbeing.[65] Meanwhile, Smith has highlighted the strain placed on some prison doctors in Ireland, who, during intense political campaigns, became 'men in the middle', caught between the various pressures of implementing discipline within prisons

---

[65] Sim, *Medical Power in Prisons*; Martin J. Wiener, 'The Health of Prisoners and the Two Faces of Benthanism', in Creese, Bynum and Bearn (eds), *The Health of Prisoners*, pp. 44–58.

during political crises, facing hostility from groups outside prisons, while also caring for their prisoner patients.[66] These tensions were certainly an important factor in prison settings, but can also be considered as typical of a range of institutional contexts during this period. Workhouses and asylums imposed budgetary and other limitations on the remit and scope of practice of the medical men who worked within them, and were governed, like prisons, by the directives of central government inspectorates. In these institutions too attitudes towards patients who were morally implicated in their plight, such as the workshy or drunkard, and thus in the circumstances that led to their institutional confinement, might be unsympathetic and severe, particularly as the number of admissions soared in many of these institutions. Provision of care in workhouses in particular was to a large extent dictated by the principle of less eligibility that might restrict the ability of medical officers to deliver care, enhance diet and treatment.[67]

Meanwhile, individual prison medical officers – working alongside and influenced by other prison officers – varied in their opinions, concerns and practices regarding mental illness, as well as in their talents and experience as medical practitioners. Many, as Wiener has suggested, appear to have framed prisoners' actions and responses to imprisonment in terms of moral responsibility and shared the codes, language and objectives of prison administrators more broadly, and, as some of our examples demonstrate, dealt harshly with prisoners who they suspected were feigning insanity.[68] Others appear to have taken a more humane or at least a more invested and active approach in taking care of their prisoner patients. Some were praised by prisoners in their accounts of prison life and in official inquiries, for their care and attention; others were described as ignorant, lazy, slipshod and poorly equipped for their position, and Oscar Wilde notably described prison medical officers 'as a class ignorant men', with 'no knowledge of mental disease of any kind'.[69] However, despite this variation in the talents and commitment of individual practitioners, many prison medical officers were eager to improve their professional standing, and to establish prison medicine as

[66] Smith, 'Irish Prison Doctors'.
[67] Jonathan Reinarz and Alistair Ritch, 'Exploring Medical Care in the Nineteenth-Century Provincial Workhouse: A View from Birmingham' and Virginia Crossman, 'Workhouse Medicine in Ireland: A Preliminary Analysis, 1850–1914', in Jonathan Reinarz and Leonard Schwarz (eds), *Medicine and the Workhouse* (Rochester, NY: University of Rochester Press, 2013), pp. 140–63, 123–39.
[68] Wiener, *Reconstructing the Criminal*, p. 122.
[69] Oscar Wilde, *Children in Prison and Other Cruelties of Prison Life* (London: Murdoch and Co., 1898), To the Editor of the *Daily Chronicle*, 27 May 1897, p. 14.

a specialist and skilled branch of practice. As demonstrated in Chapter 3, part of this process of striving for professional status – among doctors who normally had very little training in psychiatry – was to start to think about and emphasise what differentiated their work with mentally ill prisoners from those of psychiatrists working outside the prison system; what form did their expertise take, what did their experience tell them, and how did they perceive the relationship between criminality and mental disease and decline, and between the imposition of prison discipline and mental breakdown? Irish prison medical officers and asylum alienists drew heavily on the work of their English counterparts in the fields of prison and asylum psychiatry, consulting major publications by leading British experts, while English and Irish penal experts collaborated in official inquires and investigations in both contexts. Overall, this professional self-fashioning resulted in the production of a discrete taxonomy of mental illness, which, it is argued in Chapter 3, prompted a new form of psychiatry in the second half of the nineteenth century, paralleling but in many ways standing apart from the theories and practices of asylum doctors. At times, as shown in Chapters 4 and 5, this led to conflicts between prison doctors and asylum superintendents regarding the boundaries of their knowledge, insight and know-how, in the management and movement of patients between the two sets of institutions, and concerning decisions about whether prisoners were suffering from real or feigned insanity.

By examining mental disorder and responses to its manifestation in a diversity of nineteenth-century English and Irish prison settings, our book provides the first detailed analysis of the emergence of prison psychiatry and the experiences of prison medical officers treating the mentally ill as well as those of the incarcerated and mentally disturbed prisoner. Despite mounting evidence that mentally ill people were being committed to prison, and then subjected to regimes that caused further mental decline, and that prison regimes, particularly separate confinement, were causing insanity, the system was to endure until the turn of the twentieth century. The final chapter discusses the slow dismantling of the deterrent prison system and separate confinement as well as continuities with prisons today in terms of responses to the mentally ill within the prison estate and prisoners' experiences of mental illness. Time and again, we are reminded of this issue, as newspapers, public inquiries, reports and documentaries reveal shocking instances of suicide attempts, self-harm and homicide carried out by prison inmates suffering from mental health problems, as well as the devastating impact of solitary confinement on prisoners' mental wellbeing.[70]

---

[70] Shalev and Edgar, *Deep Custody*; Martynowicz and Moore, *Behind the Door*. See also Guenther, *Solitary Confinement*.

2 The Making of the Modern Prison System
Reformation, Separation and the Mind, 1840–1860

> The seclusion of the cell, depriving the prisoner of associations which divert the mind, leaves him to *reflect* upon his privations, and thus increases their severity. The Separate System at least satisfies, more than any other mode of imprisonment, this primary requirement of a sound penal discipline; – it is *severe*.[1]

In 1852 Reverend John Burt, Deputy Chaplain at Pentonville 'Model' Prison, London, published a vigorous and lengthy defence of the separate system of confinement, the disciplinary regime introduced to the prison when it opened in 1842. Inspired by the 'Philadelphia' system, Pentonville's 500 convicts worked, slept and ate in single cells, were separated from fellow convicts when at exercise and chapel, and were forbidden from communicating with each other at all times. The 'Model Prison' became emblematic of the most stringent and pure form of separate confinement and would be an inspiration to a future generation of prison architects and administrators, and the example for many prisons, including Ireland's model convict prison, Mountjoy, which opened in Dublin in 1850.

While Burt acknowledged that 'Pressure upon the mind under a Cellular System is a necessary concomitant of its characteristic excellence', his 1852 publication was largely a response to the mounting criticism and growing evidence that the regime at Pentonville was detrimental to the minds and mental wellbeing of prisoners.[2] By the 1850s, this criticism had resulted in modifications to the separate system at Pentonville though not the rejection of separate cellular confinement itself. Burt insisted that the minds of prisoners were protected at Pentonville through daily contact with prison personnel, notably prison chaplains and schoolmasters, contact largely absent in the disciplinary

[1] John T. Burt, *Results of the System of Separate Confinement as Administered at the Pentonville Prison, London* (London: Longman, Brown, Green and Longmans, 1852), p. 91 (emphasis in original).
[2] Ibid.

regimes devised at other prisons in America and England. 'Separation' at Pentonville, he asserted, 'was not solitude'.[3] Yet by 1852 Pentonville's engagement in a ten-year 'experiment' with the most rigorous form of separate confinement introduced to any of the 'modern' prisons of nineteenth-century England and Ireland was steadily being wound down. Some forty-four prisoners had been moved out of the separate system at the prison owing to concerns about their mental health, and seven were removed from Pentonville on 'mental grounds' as 'unfit for separate confinement'.[4] After 1847 Pentonville's Commissioners set about introducing a series of modifications to the disciplinary regime – principally by reducing the time spent in seclusion – in an attempt to alleviate its full rigour, and by the 1850s Pentonville was deemed a flawed experiment in prison discipline.

As Burt was pursuing his defence of separate confinement at Pentonville and of the system's key advocates, William Crawford and Reverend William Whitworth Russell, the regime was being introduced to prisons across England and Ireland and it would dominate prison regimes until the early twentieth century. Separation had been enshrined in the 1779 Penitentiary Act and was implemented in various forms by Sir George Onesiphorus Paul at Gloucester Prison in the 1790s, at Millbank Penitentiary in London, set up in 1816, and at Richmond General Penitentiary, Dublin, opened in 1820. The Prisons Acts of 1839 (England) and 1840 (Ireland) regularised its use in local gaols and houses of correction, enabling prison inspectors to certify prison cells fit for separate confinement. However, it was during the 1850s that the modified Pentonville version of the separate system would become embedded in prison regimes as a central tenet of discipline and organisation in convict prisons, gaols and houses of correction, as purpose-built and older institutions were adapted for its introduction.[5] This followed

---

[3] Ibid., p. 93.

[4] Report of the Directors of Convict Prisons (RDCP), 1851 (1852) [1524], Pentonville Prison: Medical Officer's Report, pp. 33, 37, 39.

[5] 2&3 Vict., c.56 (1839) and 3&4 Vict., c.44 (1840). These Acts supported but did not compel adoption of the separate system and they extended central government control over local prisons. See Seán McConville, *English Local Prisons 1860–1900: Next Only to Death* (London and New York: Routledge, 1995), p. 254 and Patrick Carroll-Burke, *Colonial Discipline: The Making of the Irish Convict System* (Dublin: Four Courts Press, 2000), p. 56. For regimes in local prisons, see Alyson Brown, *English Society and the Prison: Time, Culture and Politics in the Development of the Modern Prison, 1850–1920* (Woodbridge: Boydell, 2003); Richard Butler, *Building the Irish Courthouse and Prison: A Political History, 1750–1850* (Cork: Cork University Press, 2020) and Catherine Cox and Hilary Marland, '"Unfit for Reform or Punishment": Mental Disorder and Discipline in Liverpool Borough Prison in the Late Nineteenth Century', *Social History*, 44:2 (2019), 173–201.

the recommendations of several parliamentary inquiries into prison discipline in England and Ireland, and lobbying by prison inspectors, commissioners and penal reformers. Support for the modified version of the separate system was further reinforced and reinvigorated in the 1860s, as will be explored in Chapter 3, when there was a shift from the emphasis on reform to the discipline's penal benefits. Yet, time and again, reports of heightened instances of mental distress and disorder among prisoners accompanied the rolling out of the separate system across the two prison estates. In response, prison governors, chaplains and medical officers, as well as alienists working outside the criminal justice system, debated its impact on the mind, questioning how far separate confinement was implicated in the many cases of delusions, mania, self-harm and attempted suicide among prisoners.

The separate system, as implemented at Pentonville, emerged after decades of deliberation on the most effective means of punishing and reforming criminal behaviour through secondary punishment in houses of correction and gaols and transportation to the American colonies. From the late eighteenth century, coinciding with the disruption to transportation caused by the American Revolutionary War in the 1770s, penal and social reformers, including John Howard, Elizabeth Fry, James Neild and Sir Jeremiah Fitzpatrick, as well as bodies such as the Association for the Improvement of Prisons and Prison Discipline in Ireland, criticised the systematic abuse and the appalling hygiene and standard of medical care in gaols and bridewells throughout Britain and Ireland.[6] They sought the complete reform of prisons and of punishment regimes based on uniformity of treatment and well-ordered prison environments, an ambition that persisted beyond the revival of transportation in the late 1780s.[7]

---

[6] Roy Porter, 'Howard's Beginning: Prisons, Disease, Hygiene' and Anne Summers, 'Elizabeth Fry and Mid-Nineteenth Century Reform', in Richard Creese, W.F. Bynum and J. Bearn (eds), *The Health of Prisoners* (Amsterdam and Atlanta, GA: Rodopi, 1995), pp. 5–26, 83–101; James Neild, *State of the Prisons in England, Scotland and Wales* (London: John Nichols, 1812); Oliver MacDonagh, *The Inspector General: Sir Jeremiah Fitzpatrick and the Politics of Social Reform, 1783–1802* (London: Croom Helm, 1981); Butler, *Building the Irish Courthouse and Prison*, pp. 216–33; Maria Luddy, *Women and Philanthropy in Nineteenth-Century Ireland* (Cambridge: Cambridge University Press, 1995), p. 155.

[7] Randall McGowen, 'The Well-Ordered Prison: England, 1780–1865', in Norval Morris and David J. Rothman (eds), *The Oxford History of the Prison: The Practice of Punishment in Western Society* (New York and Oxford: Oxford University Press, 1998), pp. 71–99, at p. 76; Michael Ignatieff, *A Just Measure of Pain: The Penitentiary in the Industrial Revolution 1750–1850* (New York: Pantheon Books, 1978); Butler, *Building the Irish Courthouse and Prison*.

The plight of the insane in prisons was highlighted from the earliest stages of these campaigns; in 1777 Howard drew attention to the dire conditions in which 'lunatics' were held at bridewells, where they were denied treatment and languished in overcrowded and insanitary conditions, disturbing and alarming the other prisoners.[8] While advocating for prison reform in Ireland during the 1780s, Fitzpatrick, physician and first Inspector General of Prisons in Ireland, urged the removal of insane prisoners to hospitals.[9] Regarding the nature of the criminal mind, in 1830 Jeremy Bentham argued that criminal offenders were a race apart from other people – their 'minds are weak and disordered'.[10] In terms of the practicalities of their management, he suggested that they should not be left to themselves but needed close supervision, restraint and 'unremitted inspection'.[11]

Much has been written about the early history of prison reform in England, far less on Ireland. Nonetheless, historians have mapped the spiritual and philosophical roots of the separate system of confinement and of the 'rival' silent system, the most influential regimes of the early nineteenth century, identifying their transnational nature and the intellectual links between British, Irish and American penal reformers.[12] Throughout the eighteenth century, social commentators in England, including the novelist and dramatist Henry Fielding, promoted the introduction of different forms of separation to prisons for offenders awaiting trial, and Jonas Hanway, philanthropist and founder of the London Foundling Hospital, was among the first to propose separation for offenders under sentence in a purpose-built institution. His proposals strongly influenced John Howard's theories on prison discipline.[13] While the 1779 Penitentiary Act allowed for separation in purpose-built gaols

---

[8]   John Howard, *The State of the Prisons in England and Wales* (Warrington: William Eyres, 1780), p. 10.

[9]   His duties as Inspector General of Prisons included visiting lunatics confined in prisons and houses of correction. See MacDonagh, *The Inspector General*, p. 114.

[10] Jeremy Bentham, *The Rationale of Punishment* (London: Robert Heward, 1830), p. 354.

[11] Ibid., pp. 354–5, at p.354; and see Martin J. Wiener, 'The Health of Prisoners and the Two Faces of Benthamism', in Creese, Bynum and Bearn (eds), *The Health of Prisoners*, pp. 44–58, at p. 46.

[12] Ignatieff, *A Just Measure of Pain*; McGowen, 'The Well-Ordered Prison: England, 1780–1865'; David J. Rothman, 'Perfecting the Prison: United States, 1789–1865', in Norval and Rothman (eds), *The Oxford History of the Prison*, pp. 100–16; Miles Ogborn, 'Discipline, Government and Law: Separate Confinement in the Prisons of England and Wales, 1830–1877', *Transactions of the Institute of British Geographers*, 20:3 (1995), 295–311; MacDonagh, *The Inspector General*; Richard J. Butler, 'Rethinking the Origins of the British Prisons Act of 1835: Ireland and the Development of Central-Government Prison Inspection, 1820–35', *The Historical Journal*, 59:3 (2016), 721–46.

[13] Ignatieff, *A Just Measure of Pain*, p. 54.

and houses of correction, in practice it was rarely implemented, the most notable exception being the prison opened by Sir George Onesiphorus Paul in Gloucester, discussed below.

Despite early support among prison reformers for separation and cellular confinement, the most effective form of prison discipline was still being debated in the 1830s, shaped by new experiments with modes of imprisonment in America.[14] These exchanges largely focused on the 'Philadelphian' separate system, which attracted powerful support in Britain and Ireland over the rival silent system. Both systems supported the redeeming effects of solitude, yet while separation prevented communication and the spread of information among prisoners, largely through its architecture, the silent system enforced solitude and classification through punishment and discipline. Although the silent system was implemented in many prisons in America, by the 1840s separation had emerged as the clear winner in Britain and Ireland.[15]

A persistent feature of the debates among penologists and prison reformers, including vocal critics of the separate system, was the accusation that the new disciplinary regime of separate confinement was implicated in high incidences of mental disorder among prisoners. Michael Ignatieff and Ursula Henriques have examined concerns about outbreaks of mental distress at Pentonville when it first opened in 1842, implementing the purest and most rigorous form of separation.[16] Yet, there has been no sustained and detailed exploration of the relationship between the separate system as it was rolled out in local gaols, houses of correction and convict prison systems throughout the 1850s and 1860s and rates of mental breakdown among prisoners.[17]

This chapter explores this association, arguing that the incidence of mental distress and disorder in local gaols and convict prisons was much higher than was officially acknowledged and that the separate system was regarded by many commentators as a contributing factor, if not the primary cause, of high rates of mental illness. The 1850s and 1860s

---

[14] Robin Evans, *The Fabrication of Virtue: English Prison Architecture, 1750–1840* (Cambridge: Cambridge University Press, 1982), pp. 118–41.

[15] Ibid., pp. 318–45; Carroll-Burke, *Colonial Discipline*, p. 56. For a brief summary of the architecture of separate confinement, see ch. 1.

[16] Ignatieff, *A Just Measure of Pain*; U.R.Q. Henriques, 'The Rise and Decline of the Separate System of Prison Discipline', *Past & Present*, 54:1 (1972), 61–93. See also Catherine Cox and Hilary Marland, '"He Must Die or Go Mad in This Place": Prisoners, Insanity and the Pentonville Model Prison Experiment, 1842–1852', *Bulletin of the History of Medicine*, 92:1 (2018), 78–109.

[17] Forsythe reflects on the implications of these regimes for the minds of prisoners in William James Forsythe, *The Reform of Prisoners 1830–1900* (London and Sydney: Croom Helm, 1987).

saw vigorous debates on the question of how far disciplinary regimes in prisons prompted or exacerbated existing mental disorders among prisoners or whether criminals were inherently mentally weak and thus particularly vulnerable to mental collapse. Such exchanges took place in official reports and correspondence as well as in the books and articles produced by prison officials, including chaplains and doctors. The chapter also examines modifications to the system of separate confinement after the late 1840s that were shaped largely by this mounting criticism. As discussed below, the most rigorous forms of separation, introduced at Pentonville and adopted two years later in 1844 at Reading Gaol and in 1845 at Belfast House of Correction, were quickly modified. Yet the system endured and there was support for its introduction to local gaols in the 1850s. While local institutions did not always adhere to the separate system in full and its application in individual county gaols and houses of correction varied considerably, many, including larger city gaols, such Liverpool Borough Gaol, endeavoured to implement it as fully as possible.[18] As discussed in greater detail in Chapter 3, despite mounting evidence that the separate system damaged the minds of prisoners, support for the regime became even more entrenched in the 1860s and 1870s amid heightened anxieties triggered by reports of increased rates of criminality, recidivism and prison committals.

In addition to examining high-level debates and inquiries into penal policy, this chapter interrogates the ways in which mental disorder was reported, deliberated on and managed in Irish and English prisons, with Irish prisons and some English ones producing modifications to the system at a very early stage, intended to mitigate the impact of prison discipline on the mind. It explores how prison staff, medical and otherwise, assessed the mental health of prisoners and the management of mental breakdown for both male and female prisoners. While at Pentonville and several other prisons experimenting with separate confinement in the 1830s and 1840s the chaplain to a large extent assumed responsibility for managing the minds of prisoners, after the 1850s prison medical officers increasingly asserted their expertise in identifying cases of mental illness among prisoners, and, as discussed in Chapter 5, in distinguishing feigners and malingerers from 'true' cases of insanity. Permeating debates on how far the system of separate confinement provoked mental distress and discussions on how to manage this, was the issue of 'damage limitation', as criticism of disciplinary structures, philosophies and arrangements for the management of mental disorder

---

[18] Ibid., pp. 93–5; Cox and Marland, 'Unfit for Reform or Punishment'.

implied that there was something fundamentally wrong with the new system of prison discipline. Central prison administrators and prison officers had a vested interest in presenting the new system in a positive light, and those urging this particular brand of reform were keen to downplay the impact of separation on mental wellbeing. As this chapter demonstrates, some acknowledged the links between high rates of mental distress and the extreme rigour and taxing nature of the system of separate confinement, while others dismissed such connections and defended their institutional practices. Certain prisoners, as discussed in Chapter 4, were transferred to criminal or local lunatic asylums, often after long delays and lengthy deliberation among prison staff regarding their mental state. Others were sent to prison hospitals, confined to isolation cells, transferred to other institutions within the prison estate or discharged, and many were repeatedly punished for their disruptive behaviour in prison.

Rival Prison Regimes: The Silent and Separate Systems

Reflecting on the variety of prison disciplinary regimes, Hanway observed in 1776 that 'Everyone has a plan and a favourite system'.[19] Fundamental to debates on competing systems was the tension between the legitimate punishment of prisoners and imposition of the 'debt' owed to society, and the state's obligation to provide appropriate standards of care, even at a time when deprivation and poor living standards were the normal experience.[20] In his 1784 pamphlet, *An Essay on Gaol Abuses*, Sir Jeremiah Fitzpatrick observed:

the primary idea of prison is keeping the criminal in safe custody to answer to the state whose laws he has transgressed; humanity tells us the secondary idea is to harrow up his soul with the thoughts of future punishment and so render him penitent; and how can this be so effectively obtained as by keeping his body in good health on which depends the exquisiteness of that sensibility, which will awake in him the proper degree of alarm so necessary to his situation.[21]

Reformers, influenced by a combination of evangelicalism, Benthamite utilitarianism, and humane and practical concerns, sought to develop refined forms of punishment and work regimes. While evangelicals strove for the salvation of sinners by urging the spiritual and moral reform of prisoners, utilitarians looked for industrious convicts who could support

[19] Jonas Hanway, *Solitude in Prison* (London: J. Bew, 1776), p. 4. Cited in Henriques, 'The Rise and Decline of the Separate System', p. 65; James Stephen Taylor, 'Hanway, Jonas (*bap.* 1712, *d.* 1786)', *Dictionary of National Biography* (*DNB*), https://doi.org/10.1093/ref:odnb/12230 [accessed 23 Apr. 2018].

[20] Wiener, 'The Health of Prisoners', p. 46.

[21] Jeremiah Fitzpatrick, *An Essay on Gaol Abuses* (Dublin: Byrne and Brown, 1784), p. 73.

themselves and the prisons through work.[22] Nearly all agreed that unchecked association among prisoners promoted moral contamination, and various forms of separation of prisoners on the grounds of sex and longevity of criminal career were advocated. Each regime incorporated periods of spiritual reflection and religious exhortation. The Gloucestershire magistrate, Sir George Onesiphorus Paul, for example, introduced a regime of complete separation similar to separate confinement in his county gaol as early as 1791.[23] There, prisoners confined in single cells worked and reflected on religious tracts, benefited from the spiritual guidance provided by the chaplains, and endured punitive treadwheel exercise and a low diet. Preston Goal, even before the arrival of its influential chaplain, Reverend John Clay, took a prominent role in shaping national penal policy, its keeper James Liddell introducing a profitable labour system working with local textile firms.[24] The Inspector General of Prisons in Ireland, Fitzpatrick, favoured 'solitude, silence, labour and simple, cooling fare' as 'the effectual treatment'; although inspired by the work of Howard, he placed less emphasis on religious exhortations, and his pamphlet was largely shaped by medical and scientific principles.[25] While welcoming the contribution that convicts' industrial labour made to the cost of running gaols and prisons, Fitzpatrick opposed associated labour in prison, arguing that 'labour, with reflection on its useful consequences, would occupy the baneful vacuity of the mind'. 'Solitude would naturally soften the obdurate and lead to discoveries whilst corruption would from a want of evil communication naturally cease.'[26] He implemented a version of this regime at St James's Street Penitentiary, Dublin, when it opened for juveniles in 1790.[27]

By the early nineteenth century, spiritual reformers, who promoted complete separation and the centrality of reflection and prayer, had become influential, particularly within English government circles. Campaigners and prison officials who supported labour regimes were increasingly sidelined and their approach criticised for distracting

---

[22] Wiener, 'The Health of Prisoners', pp. 44–51.

[23] Forsythe, *The Reform of Prisoners*, pp. 15–29; Nicholas Herbert, 'Paul, Sir George Onesiphorus (1746–1820)', *DNB*, https://doi.org/10.1093/ref:odnb/21597 [accessed 23 Apr. 2018].

[24] Margaret DeLacy, *Prison Reform in Lancashire, 1700–1850: A Study in Local Administration* (Stanford, CA: Stanford University Press, 1986), pp. 205–6.

[25] Sir Jeremiah Fitzpatrick, *Thoughts on Penitentiaries* (Dublin: H. Fitzpatrick, 1790), p. 29.

[26] Ibid.

[27] MacDonagh, *The Inspector General*, pp. 138–41. Bentham was invited to submit plans for an Irish penitentiary, but they were rejected as too expensive and the commission withdrawn. See ibid., p. 140.

prisoners from the spiritual reflection essential for reform. The infamous treadwheel was installed in prisons across England and Ireland in the early nineteenth century.[28] While in the Lancashire prisons, the power it produced was used for manufacturing purposes, elsewhere the treadwheel was employed as a form of punishment, and it, along with other forms of futile work, replaced profitable and productive labour. An 1819 Select Committee praised Liddell's work at Preston that combined kindness with productive employment, but commented that 'religious care and instruction was wanting', opening the door to the appointment of John Clay as chaplain in 1823.[29]

In Ireland, support for profitable labour endured, notably among the two recently appointed Inspectors General of Prisons, James Palmer and Benjamin B. Woodward, who suggested linking the treadwheel 'to machinery connected with profitable manufacture' such as 'raising water and scotching flax'.[30] Hard labour, including stone breaking, they argued, was not only economical but also acted as a deterrent and guarded against 'making gaols too desirable'.[31] The Inspectors, however, insisted that profit from prisoners' labour was not the 'primary object' at the Richmond General Penitentiary, Dublin. Designed by the architect Francis Johnston, modelled on Millbank and centrally administrated, it was established as the 'flagship' experiment with the separate system of confinement and penitentiaries in Ireland. Richmond was intended for convicts aged between eighteen and thirty years, whose sentences for transportation were less than seven years, and reformation of the prisoners and training in a profitable trade was to be prioritised over punishment.[32] Richmond received its first convicts in 1820, and with the appointment of Governor William Rowan in 1823, the Inspectors were optimistic about its success. The penitentiary, however, soon became embroiled in a scandal over allegations of proselytism and conversions secured through torture, resulting in an official inquiry in 1826; its status as an exemplar of penal reform never recovered.[33]

---

[28] Report of the Inspectors General of Prisons in Ireland (RIGPI), 1824 (1824) [294], p. 16.

[29] Henriques, 'The Rise and Decline', pp. 67–8; DeLacy, *Prison Reform in Lancashire*, pp. 206–8. For Preston Gaol and the influence of Chaplain John Clay, see DeLacy, ch. 8.

[30] RIGPI, 1825 (1825) [493], p. 13. See Butler, 'Rethinking the Origins of the British Prisons Act of 1835' for details on the appointment of Palmer and Woodward.

[31] RIGPI, 1825 (1825), p. 33.   [32] RIGPI, 1824 (1824), p. 11.

[33] Henry Heaney, 'Ireland's Penitentiary 1820–1831: An Experiment that Failed', *Studia Hibernica*, 14 (1974), 28–39.

By the 1830s theorists of prison discipline fell into two main camps, advocating for the silent or the separate system.[34] The renewed interest in separation and the inspiration for the version of the separate system introduced to English and Irish prisons came from the Eastern State Penitentiary, Philadelphia, where it was first implemented in 1829. Shaped by the ideas of early reformists, such as Hanway, and in America by a group of, largely Quaker, social reformers, led by the influential physician, Benjamin Rush, the Philadelphian regime was meticulously planned and implemented. Designed to be challenging for prisoners, inmates had little or no contact with other prisoners or staff, were to reflect upon their crimes and be urged towards repentance and reform.[35] Prisoners on life sentences were confined in basic solitary cells, with provision for ventilation, heating and sanitation, for three years, sometimes more, emerging only for exercise in separate yards or for attendance at religious service in partitioned chapels.[36] While prisons designed for separation were more expensive to build – Jeremy Bentham's panopticon was the inspiration for John Haviland's radial plan for Eastern State Penitentiary – once opened they were less costly to run than the rival 'silent' system.[37] The silent system was associated with the Auburn and Sing Sing Penitentiaries in New York State where communication among prisoners was prohibited at all stages of their sentences. Though prisoners worked and dined in association, strict silence was rigorously enforced through harsh punishments. The system placed greater emphasis on instilling work habits among prisoners; advocates sought to bend prisoners to rules and regulations and were less optimistic as to their potential for reform.[38] The strengths and weaknesses of the two models were vigorously and publicly debated in the British and American press and in publications produced by their advocates. Visits to Eastern State, Auburn and Sing Sing also formed an essential part of the itinerary of early nineteenth-century European prison reformers interested in devising effective regimes for punishment and reformation. These regimes, they believed, would end the dreaded scourge of 'moral' contamination rife among prisoners confined in older

---

[34] A.T. Rubin, 'A Neo-Institutional Account of Prison Diffusion', *Law and Society Review*, 49:2 (2015), 365–99.

[35] Margaret Charleroy and Hilary Marland, 'Prisoners of Solitude: Bringing History to Bear on Prison Health Policy', *Endeavour*, 40:3 (2016), 141–7.

[36] Report of William Crawford, Esq., on the Penitentiaries of the United States (1834) [593], p. 10.

[37] Henriques, 'The Rise and Decline', p. 73.

[38] McGowen, 'The Well-Ordered Prison', p. 90; Rothman, 'Perfecting the Prison', p. 108.

gaols and bridewells, and provide the means for the true reformation of prisoners' minds and bodies in a suitably punitive environment.

Both systems attracted ardent and influential supporters among prison officials in England, though the silent system did not garner much official support in Ireland. George Laval Chesterton, Governor of Coldbath Fields House of Correction in Middlesex from 1829 to 1854, was a strong advocate of the silent system and a close friend of Charles Dickens, an equally outspoken critic of the separate system. Chesterton imposed the silent system comprehensively at Coldbath Fields, then the largest prison in Britain.[39] Convinced that most criminals were habitual, vicious and unreformable, he dismissed the separate system as 'doctrinaire sentimentality', which subjected prisoners to 'direful torture' and 'mental depression'.[40] Any signs of remorse or reformation among prisoners under that regime, he insisted, were temporary and once released, they would return to their previous habits.[41] Though the regime at Coldbath Fields was severe, Chesterton described the system at Eastern State as 'signally inhuman', lamenting the 'protracted sufferings of the miserable beings exposed to such refined torture'.[42] He also criticised its supporters for failing to acknowledge the 'mental depression' and agitation it caused prisoners whose mental states deteriorated while confined.[43] At Coldbath Fields, while prisoners were confined in separation in cells for long periods during the day, allowing for spiritual reflection, this was combined with associated labour, which permitted limited contact among prisoners. Despite the unheated cells and punishing work tasks, Chesterton's prisoners were reported to be healthier and rates of lunacy low compared with other prisons and even the national rate.[44]

The rival system of separate confinement, however, had persuasive advocates, and the most fervent of these were prison chaplains who envisaged for themselves an important role as spiritual guides and reformers. These included Reverend John Clay, a national authority on crime and punishment and prison chaplain at Preston Gaol from 1823. There he urged separation, though he permitted congregated schooling, worship and exercise. He also underlined the importance of religious

---

[39] Philip Collins, *Dickens and Crime* (New York: St Martin's Press, 1994), ch. 3.
[40] George Laval Chesterton, *Revelations of Prison Life* (London: Hurst and Blackett, 1856), vol. 2, pp. 14–15. Cited in Forsythe, *The Reform of Prisoners*, pp. 31–2.
[41] Chesterton, *Revelations of Prison Life*, vol. 2, pp. 247–8. Cited in Forsythe, *The Reform of Prisoners*, p. 32.
[42] Chesterton, *Revelations of Prison Life*, vol. 2, pp. 9–10.   [43] Ibid., p. 14.
[44] Henry Mayhew and John Binny, *The Criminal Prisons of London* (London: Griffin, Bohn & Co., 1862), p. 331.

services and spent upwards of six hours a day visiting prisoners in their cells. He saw crime as a moral failing and moral self-help, stimulated by religion and education, as a means of reform.[45] William Crawford and William Whitworth Russell were particularly influential in driving through the Pentonville experiment, with its forceful form of separation and key role for its chaplains. Crawford was a founder in 1815 of the Evangelical Society for the Improvement of Prison Discipline and the Reformation of Juvenile Offenders, an organisation that fostered connections with members of the political and social elites with the purpose of advancing a radical critique of prison conditions.[46] The Irish Inspectors General of Prisons quoted from the Society's reports while lobbying local governors and prison officials to implement prison reform in 1824, and the Association for the Improvement of Prisons and Prison Discipline in Ireland imitated its approach and principals.[47] Through his political links, Crawford obtained a commission from Home Secretary Sir James Graham to visit America in 1833 to report on the separate and the silent systems, with a view to recommending a suitable system for English prisons. Following his visit to Eastern State, Crawford became enthralled by the separate system, which combined a prolonged cellular system of separation with a limited number of cell visitations from reformatory prison personnel. Describing solitary imprisonment as 'exemplary' and remarking on the 'mild and subdued spirit' of the prisoners, during his visit Crawford also investigated four cases of insanity and one of idiocy at the prison. After consulting the prison surgeon, he concluded that the prisoners were suffering from mental disorders when committed, thereby excusing the regime from responsibility. He remarked too on the failure of Eastern State to appoint salaried chaplains and to instruct the convicts, 'vital defects which can alone be remedied by the appointment of a resident clergyman who shall not only regularly perform divine service on the Sunday but devote himself daily to the visiting of the prisoners from cell to cell'.[48] Crawford criticised other systems, including the silent system, for allowing criminals to associate, which, he claimed, made it impossible to prevent moral contamination. On Crawford's return to England, William Whitworth Russell, chaplain to Millbank Penitentiary, joined him in his support of separation.[49]

[45] Bill Forsythe, 'Clay, John (1796–1858)', *DNB*, https://doi.org/10.1093/ref:odnb/5561 [accessed 15 Dec. 2016].
[46] Forsythe, *The Reform of Prisoners*, p. 17; Bill Forsythe, 'Crawford, William (1788–1847)', *DNB*, https://doi.org/10.1093/ref:odnb/6646 [accessed 15 Dec. 2016].
[47] RIGPI, 1824 (1824), p. 13; Butler, *Building the Irish Courthouse and Prison*, p. 216.
[48] Report of William Crawford, Esq., on the Penitentiaries (1834), pp. 12–13, 414–15.
[49] Henriques, 'The Rise and Decline'.

Early experiments with separation, however, met with failure in both England and Ireland. Disquiet was expressed concerning the regime at Richmond General Penitentiary, Dublin soon after its establishment. Centrally governed, Richmond was intended for convicts sentenced to transportation or pardoned on condition that they emigrate to the colonies. The appointment of Governor William Rowan in 1823 resulted in a more rigorous implementation of separate confinement, based on a long 'course of industry, reflection, and instruction'.[50] Prisoners of both sexes were placed in separate confinement, and divided into three classes, progressing to first class with good behaviour. By 1826, however, ten recently released Roman Catholic convicts alleged that seventeen prisoners had been subjected to cruelties, punishments, deprivations and tortures to induce them to convert to Protestantism.[51] The subsequent inquiry into these allegations, conducted by the Inspectors General of Prisons and chaired by the law officer, John Sealy Townsend, was expanded to investigate other allegations of cruelty. While the commission of inquiry concluded in 1826 that torture had not been used, wholesale conversions to Protestantism were uncovered and many staff members, including the governor, were described as 'fanatical' evangelicals swept up in the Anglican 'second reformation' and the Methodist revival then sweeping across Ireland.[52] George Keppell, an ex-penitentiary officer, asserted that the 'irritation of the mind', experienced by the prisoners under punishment, had prompted their conversions.[53] The experiment with separation at Richmond was slowly abandoned. In the 1830s the prison was transferred to the city of Dublin and catered for untried prisoners, and by the early 1830s the building had been incorporated into Richmond Lunatic Asylum.[54]

Millbank Prison became the site of a further experiment in separate confinement when it opened in 1816. Based partly on Bentham's panoptical design, it housed up to 1,000 prisoners of both sexes, and, prior to the opening of Pentonville, was England's flagship penal institution. Costing £458,000 to build, it was the only prison administered by central government.[55] Concerns were soon expressed about the rigour of the

[50] Report of the Commissioners Directed by the Lord Lieutenant of Ireland to Inquire into the State of the Richmond Penitentiary in Dublin (1826–27) [335], p. 4.
[51] Heaney, 'Ireland's Penitentiary 1820–1831', p. 32.
[52] Report of the Commissioners into Richmond Penitentiary, Dublin (1826–27), p. 4; Heaney, 'Ireland's Penitentiary 1820–1831'.
[53] Report of the Commissioners into Richmond Penitentiary, Dublin (1826–27), p. 82.
[54] RIGPI, 1834 (1834) [63], p. 18; Heaney, 'Ireland's Penitentiary 1820–1831', p. 32.
[55] David Wilson, 'Millbank, the Panopticon and Their Victorian Audiences', *The Howard Journal of Criminal Justice*, 41:4 (2002), 364–81.

prison regime, and the 1823 Select Committee into conditions at the penitentiary recommended modifications to prevent physical and mental illnesses among prisoners.[56] However, William Whitworth Russell, who became chaplain at Millbank in 1830, moved the prison's discipline further towards the cellular system of separation and was noted for his enthusiasm for religious sermons and exhortations as a means of prompting reflection and reformation.[57] Russell was highly influential at Millbank and his authority was second only to the governor. During his tenure there, Russell provided persuasive evidence on the benefits of cellular confinement to Select Committees on prison reform in 1831 and, along with Crawford, was appointed Prison Inspector for London in 1835. As Inspectors, though their powers of enforcement were limited, they wielded considerable influence – essentially devising national prison policy – until their deaths in 1847.[58]

The support of Russell and Crawford for separation met with fierce criticism, much of which focused on the damage to the minds of prisoners. Two Lord Chancellors, Lord Brougham and Lord Lyndhurst, opposed separation, Lyndhurst describing it as 'harsh, unnecessary and severe'.[59] In his travelogue *American Notes*, published in 1842 following a trip to North America, Charles Dickens famously condemned the separate system at the Eastern State Penitentiary. He wrote of the 'immense amount of torture and agony which this dreadful punishment prolonged for years inflicts upon the sufferers'. 'No man has a right to inflict upon his fellow creature … this slow and daily tampering with the mysteries of the brain,' which Dickens held to be 'immeasurably worse than any torture of the body'.[60] The American Prison Discipline Society was also vocal in its criticism of the Eastern State Penitentiary and separate system for causing mental breakdown among prisoners. In the Society's 1838 report they described the effects of the Pennsylvania system on the minds of inmates, arguing that isolation increased rates of mortality and insanity at the institution. They continued to criticise the system in *The Journal of Prison Discipline and Philanthropy* throughout the 1830s.[61]

---

[56] Report from the Select Committee on the Penitentiary at Millbank (1824) [408], pp. 3–6.
[57] Bill Forsythe, 'Russell, William Whitworth (1795–1847)', *DNB*, https://doi.org/10.1093/ref:odnb/73632 [accessed 15 Dec. 2016].
[58] Butler, 'Rethinking the Origins of the British Prisons Act of 1835', pp. 744–5.
[59] Cited in Forsythe, *The Reform of Prisoners*, p. 36.
[60] Charles Dickens, *American Notes for General Circulation, Vol. 1* (London: Chapman and Hall, 1842) (with an Introduction and Notes by Patricia Ingram, London: Penguin Classics, 2002), p. 111.
[61] Charleroy and Marland, 'Prisoners of Solitude', p. 142. The 'Philadelphia' system continued to receive adverse publicity; in 1848, Francis Gray published a comparative study of its implementation in American and British prisons. He concluded that 'the

In England, *The Times* took up the cause against the introduction of the separate system, publishing a number of critical editorials and in 1841 Peter Laurie, President of Bethlem Hospital, cautioned:

Immure such a being for a lengthened period in solitary confinement, isolate him ... and you will find him the most helpless and resourceless wretch within himself that ever crawled, without energy to look forward, or courage to look back; with no mind to reason, or head or heart to support him, seeing only in the recesses of his own guilty mind and heart a dreary and dreadful void ... Misery will follow the want of excitement, melancholy will give place to despair, and if not relieved by contact with living beings, madness or idiocy must follow.[62]

Before Pentonville opened in 1842, specific allegations were also levelled at the regime at Millbank. Following the departure of Russell from Millbank, his successor, Reverend Daniel Nihil, who acted as both governor and chaplain, had strictly enforced a system of separation and intense spiritual reflection at the prison, which antagonised prison staff who were required to transform themselves into 'religious missionaries'. When he introduced stricter regulations to prevent communication between inmates, reports of prisoners presenting with delusions, mania and insanity increased. Nihil's regime was investigated and consequently relaxed; by 1840 the period in separation was reduced to the first three months of each sentence. The governor and managing committee resigned in the following year and the prison was converted into a depot for transportation to Australia.[63]

Such evidence had little impact on Russell and Crawford whose commitment to the separate system was unshakeable. After their appointment as prison inspectors, they continued to attack 'unsuitable' practices in penal institutions and to publicly criticise local officials. They became instruments of a more decisive intervention from the Home Office in local prison affairs, shaping national penal policy and new prison rules, as well as the 1839 Prisons Act, which provided the statutory basis for the separate system of confinement in England.[64] From this position, they were decisive in shaping the 'Model Prison' and disciplinary regime introduced at Pentonville.

The isolation of the prisoner, 'to force him to reflection, and thereby to produce a beneficial effect upon his mind', had been the aim of the Irish

system of constant separation ... even when administered with the utmost humanity, produces so many cases of insanity and death as to indicate most clearly, that its general tendency is to enfeeble the body and the mind'. See Francis Gray, *Prison Discipline in America* (London: John Murray, 1848), p. 181 and Rubin, 'A Neo-Institutional Account', p. 388.
[62] *The Times*, 20 May 1841.   [63] Henriques, 'The Rise and Decline', pp. 75–6.
[64] Forsythe, *The Reform of Prisoners*, pp. 36–7.

Inspectors General of Prisons for several decades, and the movement towards the 'new era of prison discipline' of separate confinement gained fresh momentum in the 1840s.[65] Reflecting on separate confinement and the silent system in 1839, while dismissing other regimes, Majors Palmer and Woodward concluded 'the advantages of the "Separate," above any other system of Prison discipline, is clearly Proved'.[66] In 1840, legislation was passed which permitted confining prisoners in separation, for whole or part of their sentence, in cells approved as suitable. This was followed, in 1841, by the appointment as Prison Inspector of Dr Francis White who replaced the recently deceased Woodward.[67] White also took on responsibility for inspecting lunatic asylums, and later became the first Inspector of Lunacy in 1843. In their first joint report on prisons, White and Palmer reflected on the progress of separate confinement in Irish prisons, noting some earlier ambivalence about the regime:

the then Inspectors General of Prisons, had some doubts as to the expediency of the system being adopted at once, without some checks and protection being first established against the possibility of its degenerating into anything like cruelty, from the want of sufficient guards and inspection, or into injury to the health of individuals, from too continued a confinement, unless accompanied by constant employment, the use of books, and frequent intercourse with officers or visitors, not Prisoners.[68]

Lacking statutory powers to compel local Grand Juries and prison boards of superintendence to implement separation, they invoked 'soft power' to encourage its introduction as a form of 'experiment' to try 'its effects, previous to recommending so large an outlay as altering the entire Prison would cost'.[69] While White and Palmer reported favourably on new purpose-built prisons, such as that in Belfast, County Antrim, designed by the architect Charles Lanyon on the Pentonville model and containing over 300 cells, and on a small number of county gaols that had been adapted for separation, including the County Gaol at Wicklow, in most prisons separation was not provided for.[70] Dublin's city and county prisons, including Newgate and Kilmainham, were robustly criticised for their poor conditions.[71] During his visit to Newgate in 1841, White found:

a wretched maniac, who was locked up in one of these vaults every night, and left to lie by himself, without light or fire, on a miserable bed upon the floor.... Humanity

---

[65] RIGPI 1825 (1825), p. 19.   [66] RIGPI, 1839 (1840) [240], pp. 6–7.
[67] 3&4 Vict., c.44, s.IV (1840); RIGPI, 1841 (1842) [377], p. 1.
[68] RIGPI, 1841 (1842), p. 5.   [69] Ibid.
[70] Ibid.; RIGPI, 1845 (1846) [697], pp. 5, 20; Butler, *Building the Irish Court House and Prison*, p. 292.
[71] RIGPI, 1841 (1842), pp. 7, 16.

shudders at the contemplation of such suffering, and a state of things so much opposed to the principles of reason and religion ought to be immediately altered. Upon my representation this poor lunatic was allowed to sleep in a better description of cell.[72]

Describing the 'progress of prison discipline' as 'a science of slow growth', in their report for 1842 White and Palmer recorded little advance in their experiment with separate confinement in Irish prisons. They blamed this on the Grand Juries' reluctance to incur the costs of adapting existing prisons or constructing purpose-built institutions for the implementation of separation.[73]

The Belfast Grand Jury, however, was accorded lavish praise by White and Palmer for their support for the construction of a new House of Correction at Belfast, which they anticipated would become a 'Model Prison for Ireland'.[74] White, much more so than Palmer, was a strong advocate of separate confinement in prisons and keen to differentiate the regime from the 'continuous solitary confinement that led to such disastrous results when first tried in America'.[75] Lanyon, the county surveyor and architect, visited Pentonville when planning Belfast House of Correction, which received its first prisoners in 1845.[76] The prison had 320 single cells over four wings, two for males with three stories and two for the female prisoners with two stories.[77] Separation was implemented throughout, including in the chapel, which was divided into stalls, and at exercise and outdoor labour. Prisoners wore peaked caps to disguise their features while moving through the building.[78] There were three chaplains appointed to the prison: the Episcopalian Chaplain, Allen; Presbyterian Chaplain, Shaw; and the Roman Catholic Chaplain, McLoghlen.[79]

Meanwhile, in 1843, the Inspectors sought financial support for building in Dublin 'a Model Convict Prison, as in London, such as would permanently improve the habits of the convicts, and be an example to our county gaols, on a better site with ample accommodation'.[80] They repeated these pleas for a *national model* prison' in subsequent annual reports and, while praising the Grand Jury and Board of Superintendence at Belfast Gaol, in 1845 they concluded that a 'perfect trial' of the system had yet to be completed.[81] Despite the Inspectors'

[72] Ibid., p. 18.   [73] RIGPI, 1842 (1843) [462], p. 1.
[74] Ibid., p. 26; see ch. 1, n. 35 for an explanation of the role of Grand Juries.
[75] RIGPI, 1843 (1844) [535], p. 29.
[76] RIGPI, 1842 (1843), p. 26; RIGPI, 1843 (1844), p. 29.
[77] RIGPI, 1843 (1844), p. 29.   [78] RIGPI, 1845 (1846), p. 20.
[79] RIGPI, 1849 (1850) [1229], p. 38.   [80] RIGPI, 1843 (1844), p. 8.
[81] RIGPI, 1844 (1845) [620], pp. vi–vii; RIGPI, 1845 (1846), p. 5.

commitment, the establishment of a system of convict prisons in Ireland with a model prison based on the separate system at its heart was delayed for some years. The catastrophic impact of the Great Famine (1845–52) swelled the populations of local gaols and convict prisons, and, even though the numbers transported rose during the crisis, government convicts awaiting transportation steadily accumulated, placing the prison system under severe pressure. In 1845 there were 627 government convicts in custody; by 1849 the number had reached nearly 4,000.[82] Home Secretary Sir James Graham was apprised of the accommodation crisis, and the Board of Works in Ireland entered negotiations for the purchase of a site for a new prison. However, by July 1846 building work had not commenced.[83] Instead, the existing prison infrastructure was expanded and repurposed; in 1847 Spike Island barracks in Cork was converted into a convict prison for 600 inmates and Philipstown barracks in King's County was fitted up in 1845, while older gaols in Dublin were converted into convict depots in the 1840s.[84] A 'Model Prison' in Dublin, underpinned by an ideological commitment to separation, was belatedly opened in 1850.

Model Prisons and the Mind

It was above all Pentonville Model Prison, admitting its first prisoners in 1842, that embodied a decisive shift towards the separate system. Crawford and Russell, along with Pentonville's Board of eleven Commissioners, including two physician members, Dr Benjamin Brodie and Dr Robert Ferguson, and Joshua Jebb, Surveyor-General of Prisons and Pentonville's architect, closely supervised the construction and management of the prison and the appointment of senior staff, the governor, chaplains, schoolmasters and medical officers. In his role as Surveyor-General of Prisons, Jebb became very influential in the design and oversight of prisons on the separate system, though he would also develop reservations about the regime. Remarking in 1850 that 'separation is the only basis on which the discipline of a prison can exist', Jebb also expressed concern that any improvement among prisoners under separation would dissipate when their period of separate confinement ended, and he remained committed to emphasising the role of labour as

---

[82] Carroll-Burke, *Colonial Discipline*, p. 58.
[83] National Archives of Ireland (NAI), Government Prison Office (GPO)/Letter Books (LB), Vol. 1, May 1846–Aug. 1849, 16 July 1846, np.
[84] RIGPI, 1847 (1847–48) [952], p. 5.

crucial aspect of prison discipline that promoted the wellbeing of prisoners.[85]

The Pentonville 'experiment' was intended to be exacting and punitive, to break the prisoner down through complete solitude in the prison cell where 'he will be disposed to self communication, for he has no companion but his own thoughts'.[86] At the same time, it was designed to produce thoroughgoing penitence and reform in a process led by the chaplains, chiefly through their individual cell visitations. Crawford and Russell carefully identified convicts suitable for the regime, which after eighteen months' probation would conclude in transportation and a new life in Australia; they were to be first offenders, physically and mentally healthy, and aged between eighteen and thirty-five years, able to withstand the taxing regime and benefit from reform. As Sir James Graham commented, 'Pentonville shall be for adults what Parkhurst now is for juvenile offenders – a prison of instruction and of probation, rather than a gaol of oppressive punishment.'[87] Parkhurst, a project also led by Crawford and Russell, had opened in 1838, with solitary confinement for a period of four months forming the cornerstone of its discipline, 'affording', as Jebb reflected in 1858, 'time for reflection, and securing much amelioration in the feelings and disposition of the boys'.[88]

Incarceration at Pentonville and the period of probation, was to be first in a system of staged punishments decreasing in rigour with each consecutive step, with future conditions following transportation to Australia contingent on convicts' behaviour at Pentonville; an exemplary record could culminate in a complete pardon.[89] Solitude and separation was rigorously imposed at Pentonville; convicts worked, ate and slept while confined to their cells for twenty-three hours per day. All communication was forbidden. They were moved through the prison hooded in masks, exercised in separation in specially designed yards, and were placed in separate stalls, referred to as coffins by the prisoners, at chapel (Figure 2.1). Prisoners were trained in a trade and taught by

---

[85] Forsythe, *The Reform of Prisoners*, pp. 45, 63. Jebb's significance has been covered extensively in the secondary literature. See ibid.; Evans, *The Fabrication of Virtue*; Clive Emsley, 'Jebb, Sir Joshua (1793–1863)', *DNB*, doi.org/10.1093/ref:odnb/14683 [accessed 4 Oct. 2018].

[86] Report of Inspectors of Prisons of Great Britain, Part 1 (1837–38), p. 28. See also Cox and Marland, 'He Must Die or Go Mad in This Place'.

[87] Report of the Commissioners for the Government of the Pentonville Prison (RCGPP) (1843) [449], p. 5.

[88] Cited in John A. Stack, 'Deterrence and Reformation in Early Victorian Social Policy: The Case of Parkhurst Prison, 1838–1864', *Historical Reflections/Réflections Historiques*, 6:2 (1979), 387–404, at p. 394.

[89] RCGPP (1843), pp. 7–8; Forsythe, *The Reform of Prisoners*, p. 71.

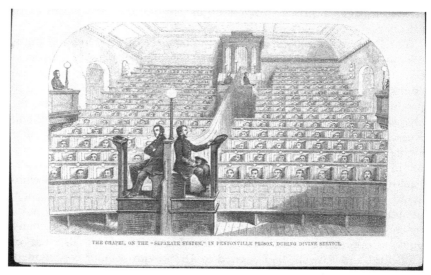

Figure 2.1 The chapel, on the 'separate system', in Pentonville Prison
during divine service
Source: Henry Mayhew and John Binny, *The Criminal Prisons of London*
(London: Griffin, Bohn & Co., 1862). Credit: British Library

schoolmasters, preparing them for their new lives in the colonies. The
moral and spiritual reformation of the convicts fell mainly to the chaplains who also directed the work of the schoolmasters and selected books
for the library. Prisoners attended daily religious services and the prison
chaplains devoted many hours each day to visiting convicts in their cells,
discussing their past lives and exhorting them to repent and reform.
Chaplains gained detailed knowledge of each convict, his character,
disposition and habits, which was minutely recorded in journals and
general registers. The chaplains also assumed a central role in directing
the separate system.[90] At Pentonville Reverend James Ralph and his
successor, Reverend Joseph Kingsmill were second only to the governor
in terms of authority.

During the 1840s, Pentonville's formative years, the chaplains
affirmed their expertise and close knowledge of the minds of convicts,
gained through their cellular visitations and observations, which afforded
them the 'best opportunity of knowing their [convicts'] feelings'.[91] The
prison's regulations underlined the importance of vigilant observation by

[90] RCGPP (1844) [536], pp. 8–10, 11.   [91] RCGPP (1845) [613], p. 11.

the chaplain, with the assistance of the surgeon, of the '*state of mind* of every prisoner'.[92] Reverend Kingsmill's report for 1845 provided a detailed assessment of convicts' responses to the separate system, commenting on the determination of some, unable to withstand the degradation and isolation, to break prison rules and secure removal from the prison. The 'well educated and intelligent men', those who were 'always thinking', he claimed, benefited from the regime. While these convicts reportedly found separation a 'severe punishment', they were 'grateful' for 'the religious and moral advantages which a paternal Government afforded to them'.[93] Kingsmill, who linked mental wellbeing to prisoners' capacity to be reformed and their minds reanimated through education, would later moderate his support for separation.

While Crawford, Russell and Kingsmill publicly defended Pentonville and the separate system, with Crawford and Russell insisting that the availability of the officers and regular visitations from prison personnel distinguished it from the system at Eastern State Penitentiary and protected the convicts' minds, inside the prison there were regular consultations and exchanges between chaplains, medical officers, schoolmasters, warders and Pentonville's Commissioners regarding the prisoners' mental and physical health.[94] The risk to the mind of convicts and the danger of mental breakdown was acknowledged in the Pentonville Prison Act (1842), which specified that convicts who showed signs of mental illness were to be reported to the Secretary of State and transferred to an asylum.[95] In practice, as will be demonstrated below, this happened infrequently and usually only after extensive deliberation. Evidence of growing concern about prisoners' mental wellbeing, however, occurred in 1843, when Chaplain Ralph was forced to resign following a spike in cases of 'morbid religious symptoms'. Convicts were reported to be suffering from insanity, mania, depression and hallucinations, many with religious overtones, which Rees and the Pentonville Commissioners linked to Ralph's excessive religious teachings.[96] In December 1843, for example, Rees reported 'That Prisoner Wm. Cowle Reg. No. 385 is decidedly hallucinated, said, that Christ pervades him, & gives him sensations' and 'That the Devil visits him & converses with him in a flame of fire'. Cowle was removed to the infirmary but his condition steadily deteriorated; he became violent, talked only about religion and refused food. In January 1844 Rees recommended he be

---

[92] *The Times*, 1 May 1843, 24 Nov. 1843.   [93] RCGPP (1845), p. 11.
[94] Burt, *Results of the System of Separate Confinement*, p. 93.
[95] 5&6 Vict., c.29, s.XXIII (1842).
[96] The National Archives (TNA), PCOM 2/84, Pentonville Prison, Middlesex: Minute Books, 1842–44, Special Meeting, 16 Dec. 1843, pp. 238–9.

removed to an asylum.[97] Faced with several disturbing cases, Rees suggested 'Prisoners, R. Henshaw Reg. No. 210 and Wm. Johnson Reg. No. 222 should not go to the chapel service for a few days' and that bibles, prayer books and hymn books be removed from some prisoners' cells.[98]

By the end of 1843, Ralph had been replaced by the Assistant Chaplain, Kingsmill, but Medical Officer Rees and Chaplain Kingsmill continued to report on convicts who were 'strongly affected by religious impressions', threatened to self-harm or commit suicide and were 'suffering much from mental depression'.[99] Kingsmill and Rees disagreed on individual cases, such as that of convict James Graham [convict no. 635], who described his delusions relating to death and his mother's health to Kingsmill in July 1845. Kingsmill concluded there was 'nothing in Reg. 635 … indicating the presence of any delusions'. However, Rees, who also called upon the advice of physician Commissioners Brodie and Ferguson, resolved he was insane and should be removed to an asylum. This decision was subsequently amended when Dr Seymour visited the prison to advise and concluded that Graham would recover. Graham continued to experience attacks of mania and was eventually removed to Bethlem in November 1845.[100]

Many of these protracted and time-consuming exchanges were concerned with identifying whether convicts' behaviour denoted 'real' cases of insanity, requiring removal to Bethlem, or were cases of malingering, weak-mindedness, or evidence of convicts' inability to withstand the severity of the regime. In dealing with them, the Pentonville officers and Commissioners were keen to protect the reputation of the prison and the separate system against accusations of cruelty, inhumanity, and provocation of mental breakdown. Transfers to lunatic asylums, as in the case of Graham, were resisted and delayed, in order to 'test' or verify diagnosis of insanity and to downplay the incidence of mental disorder among convicts. Pentonville's official publications limited their reporting of mental illness largely to those convicts transferred to asylums and cases of suicide.[101] The chaplains' and medical officers' detailed

[97] Ibid., 9 Dec. 1843, pp. 231–2, 3 Jan. 1844, p. 251.
[98] Ibid., 9 Dec. 1843, pp. 230–1.   [99] Ibid., 23 Sept. 1843, p. 187.
[100] TNA, PCOM 2/353, Pentonville Prison, Middlesex: Chaplain's Journal, May 1846–Mar. 1851, 5 July 1845, pp. 31–4; 14 Nov. 1845, p. 111. See ch. 4 for the transfer of prisoners between prisons and asylums.
[101] Our conclusions differ from those of Ian O'Donnell, whose study of mental breakdown at Pentonville in the 1840s draws largely on official reports and suggests that in some instances separation might have proved beneficial. See Ian O'Donnell, *Prisoners, Solitude, and Time* (New York and Oxford: Oxford University Press, 2014).

investigations into convicts presenting with hallucinations, anxiety, self-harm, mania, depression, morbid feelings and irritability, recorded in minute books and the chaplain's journal, were not replicated in annual reports. Rather, these public documents insisted that the minds of the prisoners were improved through seclusion, teaching, and preaching and that the mental condition of the prisoners was 'most satisfactory'.[102]

The dangers of the system were, however, becoming increasingly evident. Already in the 1840s, the Home Office recommended pardons and medical discharges for Pentonville convicts deemed unfit for transportation or whose life would be endangered by further imprisonment.[103] Of those pardoned on medical grounds, the majority suffered from physical illnesses such as convict G.M. (no. 9640), who was discharged in December 1846 with pulmonary consumption.[104] Medical pardons were included in Pentonville's mortality statistics suggesting convicts were released in anticipation of their deaths.[105] There were few medical discharges of prisoners with symptoms of mental distress or insanity, although in June 1849 convict Clewett (no. 1860) was 'discharged with a free pardon, on medical grounds, suffering under chronic disease of the brain'.[106]

The factors informing a decision to organise medical releases were not recorded in great detail, and it is unclear how such decisions were reached and whether the advice of prison medical officers concerning the health of the prisoner was a decisive consideration. The potential danger to the public posed by prisoners experiencing mental distress, however, may explain prison officials' reluctance to authorise medical releases on these grounds. For example, Sir George Grey rejected a request from Pentonville's Commissioners to pardon convict Beckett, who had served only fifteen months of his sentence for a 'serious' offence. Beckett was reported to be labouring under hallucinations.[107] In November 1848, he had attracted the attention of Pentonville's Governor and Medical Officer Rees when he was noted to be 'strange in manner' – he 'fancies he hears his name called, and sees it written upon the walls' – and was recommended for transfer to the garden

---

[102] RCGPP (1845), p. 19. For more detail of individual cases and disputes between the prison officers concerning their veracity, see Cox and Marland, 'He Must Die or Go Mad in This Place'.
[103] TNA, PCOM 2/86, Pentonville Prison, Middlesex: Minute Books, 1846, 2 Jan. 1847, p. 146. The dates given for Pentonville's Minute Books do not always tally with their content.
[104] RCGPP (1847) [818], p. 49.   [105] Ibid., p. 52.
[106] TNA, PCOM 2/88, Pentonville Prison, Middlesex: Minute Books, 1848, 21 Apr. 1849, p. 186, 2 June 1849, p. 228.
[107] Ibid., 21 Apr. 1849, pp. 186–7.

class.[108] On 23 December 1848, Rees noted that Beckett was still hallucinating and removed him to the prison infirmary where he remained until 31 December before he was returned to normal prison discipline.[109] Within four days Beckett was back in Pentonville's infirmary where he continued to experience delusions, hearing noises and voices speaking to him.[110] His condition deteriorated further, prompting the Pentonville Commissioners to submit their unsuccessful request for his medical release in March 1849.[111] While it is uncertain whether Becket was eventually discharged, his case highlights the selective use of medical releases in cases when convicts exhibited signs of mental distress or insanity, and the cautious approach of the Home Office when dealing with such cases.

Further emphasising the risks of separation, between 1845 and 1848, a series of damming reports highlighted the poor mental condition of convicts removed from Pentonville and transferred onto ships destined for transportation to Van Dieman's Land. On boarding ship, the 'Pentonville graduates' exhibited alarming symptoms, variously described as epileptic, convulsive fits and hysteria. Surgeon-superintendent to the *Stratheden*, Henry Baker, described how within forty-eight hours of arrival on the ship, nineteen Pentonville convicts were affected with 'Epileptic Fits', many suffering three or four. Convicts sent from other prisons were free from such attacks, which Baker related to the eighteen to twenty months Pentonville prisoners had spent in separate confinement.[112] To diminish the outbreaks of 'mental imbecility' on board ship and prepare convicts for the 'ordinary habits of life', convicts destined for a transport colony were placed in association at Millbank prison for short periods prior to embarkation or in associated work in Pentonville, carrying out tasks such as wood cutting or garden work. These attempts to prevent the transition from the separate system to association being 'too sudden and overwhelming' largely failed.[113]

Though removals to Bethlem were resisted, the number of convicts transferred there began to build up, confirming fears about the negative impact of the regime on prisoners' mental wellbeing, and prompting public commentary. Elizabeth Fry was concerned that the separate

---

[108] Ibid., 25 Nov. 1848, pp. 71–2.   [109] Ibid., 23 Dec. 1848, p. 97, 13 Jan. 1849, p. 106.
[110] Ibid., 27 Jan. 1849, p. 120, 24 Feb. 1849, p. 151.   [111] Ibid., 24 Mar. 1849, p. 168.
[112] TNA, Admiralty Papers (ADM) 101 69/6, Medical Journal of the *Stratheden*, Convict Ship, from 22 July 1845 to 7 Jan. 1846 by Henry Baker, Surgeon and Superintendent, 1845–46. See also examples cited by Katherine Foxhall, *Health, Medicine and the Sea: Australian Voyages c. 1815–1860* (Manchester and New York: Manchester University Press, 2012), p. 35.
[113] RCGPP (1847), p. 5; RCGPP (1847–48) [972], p. 7.

system would cause a decline in bodily and mental health, and a number of widely read periodicals pitched into the debate, with the *Illustrated London News* denouncing the Pentonville regime as destructive of human individuality.[114] In 1847 Peter Laurie, President of Bethlem Hospital, condemned Pentonville's system of discipline in *The Times*, commenting on the steady flow of 'lunatic' prisoners from Pentonville to Bethlem that he attributed to the damaging effects of the separate system on the minds of prisoners.[115] Laurie had been an opponent of the separate system since its introduction at Millbank and in 1846 he published a comprehensive critique of its impact on prisoners in Britain and America, providing figures on rates of mental breakdown in individual prisons to uphold his argument.[116]

After the sudden deaths of Crawford and Russell in 1847, the regime at Pentonville was toned down, and Jebb and other Pentonville Commissioners reasserted their influence over the management of the prison. In 1848, the length of separation was reduced to twelve months and to nine months by 1853. Also in that year, Portland Prison was opened to allow for associated labour among convicts in public works prisons prior to transportation.[117] The link between Pentonville and transportation diminished further in 1853 with the replacement of sentences of less than fourteen years' transportation with penal servitude.[118] By the late 1840s, even Chaplain Kingsmill, formerly a staunch advocate of the separate system, was expressing ambivalence about the regime. Initially confining his concerns to his journal, his daily observations of cases of mental breakdown and the undermining of the physical and mental energy of the prisoners prompted a more public expression of doubt in his annual reports. In 1849 he declared in his report to the Pentonville Commissioners, that 'Its value in a moral point of view has been greatly over-rated', though he believed the separate system still offered the opportunity for reflection, to awaken the conscience of prisoners and was the best deterrent against the repetition of crime.[119] Reflecting on his own experiences in 1852, Kingsmill repeated the observations of a physician employed at a New Jersey Penitentiary:

---

[114] Elizabeth Fry, *Memoirs of the Life of Elizabeth Fry* (London: John Hatchard, 1847), vol. 2, p. 396; *Illustrated London News*, 6 Dec. 1845, p. 358. See also Ernest Teagarden, 'A Victorian Prison Experiment', *Journal of Social History*, 2:4 (1969), 357–65.

[115] Peter Laurie to the Editor, *The Times*, 11 Jan. 1847.

[116] Peter Laurie, *"Killing no Murder;" or the Effects of Separate Confinement on the Bodily and Mental Condition of Prisoners in the Government Prisons and Other Gaols in Great Britain and America* (London: John Murray, 1846).

[117] Forsythe, *The Reform of Prisoners*, p. 72.   [118] Ibid.

[119] RCGPP (1850) [1192], p. 16.

A little more intercourse with each other, a little more air in the yard, has the effect upon the mind and the body that warmth has on the thermometer; almost every degree of indulgence showing a corresponding rise in the health of the individual. That an opinion to the contrary should be advocated at this time seems like a determination to disregard science in support of a mistaken but favourite policy.[120]

The Dogma of Separation

Despite increasing evidence that the Pentonville regime could inflict harm on the minds of prisoners, both central and local-level prison administrators retained a strong commitment to the separate system. In his report on Belfast House of Correction for 1849, Inspector Frederick Long acknowledged there were 'evils' as well as benefits to the separate system of confinement. In terms of the 'injury caused to the health of the prisoners' and the effect 'frequently produced in causing aberration of mind', drawing on the opinions of Dr Purdon, surgeon for the House of Correction, he noted that 'in no one instance has the mind of any individual become affected in the prison'.[121] Purdon claimed young prisoners seldom suffered and that there was 'not a single record of a female suffering in any respect from the system'.[122] Long also noted it had never been 'necessary to relax the discipline on medical grounds' and that some prisoners had endured separation for two years without any adverse consequences. He concluded there was 'nothing in the discipline of the prison that is the least injurious to the mental or bodily health of its inmates'.[123]

Although Kingsmill's support became more muted, driven by his experiences at Pentonville, most chaplains were enthusiastic. They published influential texts on the system and its benefit to the mind, and in so doing shored up their own influence. In 1846, Reverend John Field, chaplain at Reading Gaol, dismissed concerns about the injurious effect of separation on prisoners' physical health, claiming mortality rates at Eastern State Penitentiary and at Reading had improved following its introduction.[124] Field drew on a series of reports by the Inspectors of State Prisons in America, Pentonville's Commissioners, and several official inquiries into prison discipline in England, which downplayed claims that separation prompted insanity among prisoners. Rather than

[120] RDCP, 1852 (1852–53) [1656], Pentonville Prison: Chaplain's Report, p. 27.
[121] RIGPI, 1849 (1850) [1229], p. 37.   [122] Ibid.   [123] Ibid.
[124] John Field, *The Advantages of the Separate System of Imprisonment* (London: Longman, 1846), pp. 210–18.

blaming the separate system, cases of insanity were, he insisted, a product of hereditary predisposition and largely attributable to the admission of prisoners with existing mental disorders that re-emerged while in confinement.[125] His book was published in the same year as Laurie's denouncement of the separate system, and Laurie mocked Field's eulogising of his own exertions in his annual report on Reading Gaol, as well as his efforts to glean information respecting the sanity of the 'scattered relations' of some twenty-seven prisoners: 'proof that these twenty-seven were breaking down – that their minds were giving way; and then this evidence was hunted up to prop a falling case'.[126]

The 'exemplar of the reformist chaplains' was Clay of Preston.[127] Under his influence, the county's newly appointed visiting justices introduced separation at Preston and Kirkdale prisons after 1846.[128] Reverend Richard Appleton, Field's predecessor at Reading and an ardent supporter of separation, was appointed chaplain at Kirkdale Prison. In his 1848 annual report, he insisted that 'I do not see any tendency in it [separation] to overthrow, or even enfeeble, the mind'.[129] In his 1852 defence of the system, Reverend John Burt asserted that it was the modifications introduced to the system after the deaths of Russell and Crawford, relaxing the 'rigour' of separation, that had rendered it 'inoperative or unsafe'. In its most extreme manifestation, Burt claimed, there had been few cases of mental breakdown, and these were attributable to existing mental weakness in the convicts effected.[130] Burt not only persisted in his support of separate confinement, he sought exposure of the prisoners to the purest, 'Pentonville', form.

Despite this enthusiasm, some experiments with the regime, including versions implemented at Birmingham Borough Gaol and at Leicester Gaol, were excessively cruel, and there were allegations of abuse of power by prison officials, severe punishments and deaths among prisoners. Birmingham had opened in 1849, and was designed for the separate system, with Captain Alexander Maconochie as the first Governor. Although Maconochie was soon replaced by Lieutenant William Austin, a modified version of Maconochie's 'mark system' was implemented for prisoners aged under seventeen. In the early 1850s, a wave of suicides and suicide attempts among juvenile prisoners, rumours of 'alleged cruelties' to prisoners, including the weak-minded, and an

---

[125] Ibid., pp. 219–25.   [126] Laurie, *"Killing no Murder"*, pp. 13–14.
[127] Forsythe, *The Reform of Prisoners*, p. 49.
[128] Forsythe, 'Clay, John (1796–1858)'; DeLacy, *Prison Reform in Lancashire*, p. 220.
[129] Liverpool Record Office (LRO), H365.3 ANN, *Kirkdale Gaol Chaplain's Annual Report* (Preston, 1848), p. 9.
[130] Burt, *Results of the System of Separate Confinement*, p. 4.

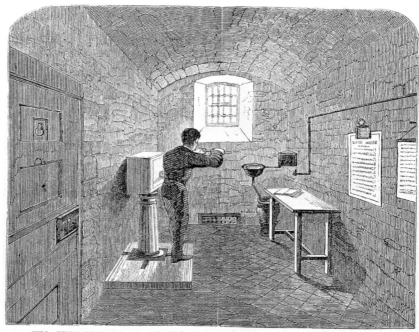

CELL, WITH PRISONER AT "CRANKLABOUR," IN THE SURREY HOUSE OF CORRECTION.

Figure 2.2 Cell with prisoner at 'crank labour' in the Surrey House of Correction
Source: Henry Mayhew, *London Labour and the London Poor* (London: Charles Griffin & Co., 1851). Credit: Wellcome Collection. Attribution 4.0 International (CC BY 4.0)

inquest into the suicide of a fifteen-year-old prisoner, Edward Andrews, prompted an inquiry into the management of the gaol.[131] The subsequent 1853 Royal Commission found that prisoners had been cruelly and inhumanly treated and revealed instances of excessive and punitive infliction of 'crank work', repeated and prolonged flogging, and dangerous restriction of prisoners' diets leading to severe physical deterioration and repeated suicide attempts among prisoners.[132] One juvenile, Richard

[131] Wolfson Centre for Archival Research (WCAR), Birmingham Central Library (BCL), Birmingham Vol. 16 [pamphlets], 64872 System of Discipline in Borough Gaol: J. Allday, *True Account of the Proceedings Leading to, and a Full & Authentic Report of, The Searching Inquiry, by Her Majesty's Commissioners, into the Horrible System of Discipline Practised at the Borough Gaol of Birmingham* [1853].

[132] Royal Commission of Inquiry into the Condition and Treatment of the Prisoners Confined in Birmingham Borough Prison (1854) [1809], pp. 3–5.

Scott, whom the chaplain described as being 'nearly an imbecile', had made three separate attempts at self-destruction.[133] Emphasising the illegality of the actions of prison staff, especially the surgeon, Mr Blount, and Austin, and clearly anxious to disassociate the separate system from such actions, the Commissioners noted Blount had omitted to provide proper care

in the treatment of some classes of prisoners for whose safety special arrangements were needed: the epileptic, those of unsound mind, and those who had manifested a disposition to commit or attempt suicide. To leave men thus afflicted in separate cells, without any attendant, was at the least a grave error of judgement.[134]

The events at Birmingham Gaol gained extensive local and national press coverage, and were the basis of the Charles Reade's novel, *Its Never too Late to Mend*, published in 1856. However, the scandal, and a similar outrage at Leicester Gaol, which also resulted in an official inquiry into allegations that prisoners were excessively punished for failing to complete task work at the crank, did not undermine support for the separate system or the authority of prison officers.[135]

Meanwhile, in 1850, the long-awaited model convict prison, designed for 450 single occupancy cells for male convicts, opened at Mountjoy in Dublin. The responsibility for overseeing the implementation of separate confinement in the prison fell to Henry Martin Hitchins, the Inspector General of Government Prisons in Ireland.[136] He had visited Pentonville Prison in January 1850, three years after the deaths of Crawford and Russell, to observe the prison 'at all hours, and in all stages of its discipline'. In his subsequent report, he commented on the modifications being introduced at Pentonville, in particular the almost universal rejection of the prolonged period of probation 'as too severe, affecting both the mental and physical condition of the convict and tending to stupefy'. Hitchins was especially critical of the promotion of religious instruction at the prison, dismissing it as a 'dead failure'. The chapel seats at Pentonville, he noted, 'disfigured by grotesque carving and gross inscription, attest the diligence if not the piety of the inmates'.[137]

---

[133] Ibid., p. 19.   [134] Ibid., p. 31.
[135] Helen Johnston, *Crime in England 1815–1880: Experiencing the Criminal Justice System* (London and New York: Routledge, 2015), pp. 95–6; Forsythe, *The Reform of Prisoners*, pp. 118–19.
[136] Hitchins was employed at the Chief Secretary's Office from 1826 and had little prison experience prior to his appointment as Inspector General of Government Prisons in 1847. See Tim Carey, *Mountjoy: The Story of a Prison* (Dublin: Collins Press, 2000), p. 52.
[137] NAI, GPO/LB, Vol. 12, July 1849–Dec. 1851, p. 53 (emphasis in original).

At Mountjoy, the role of the chaplains – Roman Catholic, Church of Ireland and Presbyterian – was to be less influential than in England. They were 'to visit convicts in cells for conversation every day and visit school classes' but were forbidden from exercising 'direct control over the School master', who, in turn, was to confine his work to secular education. Concerns over allegations of proselytism, especially in relation to educational and religious instructions, persisted in prisons, and in other nineteenth-century institutions, including workhouses and asylums. To guard against these allegations, and protect the minds of prisoners, Hitchins selected chaplains who were of a 'high character' and less ardent in their ministry.[138] He also insisted that the 'disturbance' of chaplains' visitations to cells should not interfere with convict labour, especially at convict depots such as Smithfield.[139] For Hitchins, separation was to be the 'principle' upon which Mountjoy prison would be conducted, but 'many details of Pentonville which being extreme are necessarily futile, may be safely avoided'.[140] The strengths of the regime were its capacity to act as a deterrent – the 'dread' of the convict returning to the separate cell – and as a mechanism for enforcing education and industrious habits, either through convict labour or reading. Its success depended on the 'minds of the prisoners being fully occupied'.[141] 'The great object ... to be attained', Hitchins asserted, was 'to deter from further infraction of the law.'[142]

Aware of the links being made between the separate system and insanity, Hitchins warned Mountjoy's first Medical Officer, Dr Francis Rynd, who had previously worked at Smithfield Convict Depot, to carefully assess the mental as well as the physical condition of incoming convicts.[143] As he noted, the criticisms of the regime were 'principally directed to the injurious tendency of [a] long period of separate confinement to produce a general debility of mind and body'. Echoing the concerns of Pentonville's Chaplain Kingsmill on the endangerment of the mind resulting from separate confinement, Hitchins outlined three groups of prisoners most at risk of succumbing to 'utter prostration of the

---

[138] Ibid., pp. 53, 63, 64 (emphasis in original).   [139] Ibid., p. 63.
[140] Ibid., p. 53 (emphasis in original).   [141] Ibid., p. 63.
[142] Report of the Inspector of Government Prisons in Ireland, 1851 (1852–53) [1634], p. 43.
[143] NAI, GPO/LB, Vol. 12, July 1849–Dec. 1851, p. 35. Francis Rynd (1801–67) was educated at Trinity College, Dublin and the Meath Hospital. He was surgeon to the Meath Hospital from 1836, had a lucrative private practice in Dublin and was medical surgeon for Smithfield Prison in the late 1840s and Kilmainham in the 1850s, as well as medical superintendent at Mountjoy Male Prison until 1857. L.H. Ormsby, *Medical History of the Meath Hospital and County Dublin Infirmary* (Dublin: Fannin and Co., 1888), pp. 206–9; Davis Coakley, *Irish Masters of Medicine* (Dublin: Town House, 1992), pp. 99–105.

mental powers' or 'imbecility'.[144] These were prisoners whose 'prevailing character ... is that of sullenness' or in whom 'insanity is hereditary'; those unable to acquire a trade, or benefit from instruction or education; and prisoners who demonstrated a 'tendency ... to dwell unhealthily on any one subject, to the exclusion of all others'.[145] Rynd had previously expressed doubts about the effectiveness of the separate system, observing in 1846 that

Men who from low moral principles, confinement, fear of punishment, grief at their separation from family and friends, and perhaps from remorse from crimes have lost vigour and elasticity of life so protective of sound health, and sunk into the torpid depression of mind and body that renders them so susceptible of disease and above all of fever.[146]

In selecting convicts suitable for the regime at Mountjoy, Rynd and Hitchins also adapted the 'Pentonville' criteria. Initially, it was proposed to transfer prisoners directly from county gaols to Mountjoy 'so that separation might be in Ireland, as in England, the first stage in convict discipline'. However, the poor physical condition of convicts, many still suffering the effects of the Great Famine, rendered large numbers unsuitable for the severe regime at Mountjoy.[147] Rather than admit convicts 'notoriously unsuited to the discipline', Hitchins and Rynd concluded the 'sturdy criminal' was more suited to the regime:

The expectations which may be formed of a beneficial change from youth, previous character, or inexperience in vice, are thus practically set aside, while the sturdy criminal is pronounced as a suitable subject for its moral and industrial advantages, and the indulgence of tickets-of-leave, because he alone is physically fit to undergo the restrictions of the system.[148]

The Governor at Mountjoy, Robert Netterville, implemented Hitchins' modified system. However, following an inspection in July 1850, Hitchins criticised Netterville for permitting the rule of silence to break down while prisoners were at work. He also maintained that the prison officers were too lenient and reminded the governor that

prisoners committed to your charge have been convicted of grave offences against God and man, that they have forfeited their civil rights and are confined as much, to say the least, to protect society against their evil practices as to afford them an opportunity of repentance and reformation. It is therefore of primary importance

[144] RCGPP (1847), p. 41; NAI, GPO/LB, Vol. 12, July 1849–Dec. 1851, p. 36.
[145] NAI, GPO/LB, Vol. 12, July 1849–Dec. 1851, p. 36.
[146] NAI, GPO/Miscellaneous (XB)/3, Convict Prisons Minute Book, 1846–48, Surgeon Rynd's Report on Proposed Enlargement of Smithfield, 17 Nov. 1846.
[147] Report of the Inspector of Government Prisons in Ireland, 1851 (1852–53), pp. 37, 43.
[148] Ibid., p. 38.

that the prisoners should be brought to a proper sense of their condition and after the religious exhortations of the chaplains nothing so directly tends to effect this object as a firm and steady exercise of a severe discipline.[149]

Rynd continued to reject large numbers of prisoners; in June 1854, the Prison Commissioners reported that he had excluded 35 per cent of the prisoners sent to him as 'unfit to undergo separate imprisonment of 12 months' duration, or incapacitated for employment at the trades'.[150]

While the authority of the chaplains and their significance within the separate system had diminished following Pentonville's experiences, they remained significant actors in implementing separation at Mountjoy and were 'implicitly confided in by the convicts, the depositary of his secret thoughts and wishes'.[151] Some, such as the Protestant Chaplain, Reverend Gibson Black, were strong advocates of the regime. Assessing the progress of the prison after its first full year in operation, Black observed in 1851:

Under the system of complete isolation, strictly adhered to for so long as the convicts' health can endure it, I would not despair of the most hardened offender being raised from degradation, and made susceptible to the sanctifying influences of the Gospel of Christ. The Word of Truth addressed to the most guilty in the solitude of the cell, where all disturbing circumstances of an external character are shut out, is often reflected on with an intensity of interest which exemplifies the meaning of that pointed inquiry – 'Is not my word like as a fire! saith the Lord; and like a hammer that breaketh the rock in pieces?'[152]

Despite Hitchins' instructions aimed at restricting the chaplains' interference with the educational system at the prison, Neal McCabe, the Roman Catholic chaplain, provided a detailed assessment of the quality of school instruction, and, according to his account, he was deeply involved in the prison school. In contrast, Gibson confined his comments to religious instruction at the prison. McCabe's report for 1851 also included a detailed exposition on the relationship between crime rates, criminality and poverty in which he demonstrated some ambivalence about separate confinement, characterising it as a regime that encouraged dishonesty and dissimulation:

I could not venture to offer any opinion on the merits of the silent and separate system, as compared with other systems of prison discipline.... I would prefer

[149] NAI, GPO/LB, Vol. 12, July 1849–Dec. 1851, p. 130.
[150] Convict Prisons (Ireland). Copies of Correspondence Relative to the Management and Discipline of Convict Prisons, and the Extension of Prison Accommodation, with Reports of Commissioners (1854) [344], p. 17.
[151] NAI, GPO/LB, Vol. 12, July 1849–Dec. 1851, p. 63.
[152] Report of the Inspector of Government Prisons in Ireland, 1851 (1852–53), p. 58.

association to a system under which they are incessantly endeavouring to communicate with each other, and with success, whilst pretending the strictest regularity. Now, such a system of dissimulation is most injurious to their moral training; for sincerity and openness of character are virtues which convicts, in general, require to learn.[153]

Hitchins and Rynd were confident of the modifications implemented at Mountjoy and reported with satisfaction on the absence of mental disease in the prison during 1851. They attributed this to the careful selection of convicts, the close vigilance and attention paid to prisoners by the officers, and the provision of trade and employment to occupy the minds of prisoners.[154] In his own report for the year, Rynd went further, stressing that the success was due to the 'almost unrestricted power' conceded to him as medical superintendent of the prison, which permitted him to introduce 'relaxations of strict prison discipline' essential for the management of the convicts.[155] He did not refer in his report to the attempted suicide of convict Brennan, who cut his throat with a knife in his cell in January 1851. In his initial assessment of Brennan, Rynd had been unprepared to state whether the suicide attempt was caused by mental debility or was a feigned attempt. The prisoner had previously self-harmed while confined at County of Down Gaol, wounding himself several times with sharpened pieces of tin and glass and evading restraints. The medical officer at the Down Gaol, Dr Brabazon, also alleged that Brennan did not intend to seriously injure himself and had previously simulated dysentery by adding blood to his stool. After his suicide attempt at Mountjoy, Rynd ordered Brennan to be placed in secure restraint.[156]

Convicts diverted from Mountjoy as unsuitable for the regime were transferred to Spike Island Public Works Prison and to Philipstown Government Prison. Spike had operated for several years 'as the place of last resource to the invalid convict, or an asylum to the incurable'. In the annual report for 1851 it was reported that 20 per cent of prisoners at Spike were chronic patients of 'one kind or another' and that 600 prisoners were either in hospital or convalescent wards, at a time when there was accommodation for 2,300 prisoners.[157] Mountjoy convicts, who had undergone the full rigour of separation, were then removed to Spike but maintained in 'distinct wards and separate working parties' away from

[153] Ibid., p. 63.   [154] Ibid., pp. 41, 53.   [155] Ibid., p. 54.
[156] NAI, GPO/Incoming Correspondence (CORR)/1851/Mountjoy/Item no. 74, Correspondence relating to the attempted suicide by Convict Brennan in Mountjoy, 23 Jan. 1851.
[157] Report of the Inspector of Government Prisons in Ireland, 1851 (1852–53), pp. 19, 20, 21.

other prisoners to avoid contamination while awaiting transportation.[158] A group of seventy-five convicts sent by steam ship from Mountjoy to Spike in May 1851 had been in separation for periods varying from ten to fourteen months.[159] While Mountjoy was claimed to be relatively free of 'mental disease', incidences of mental distress and disorder were reported at the other convict depots and prisons where Mountjoy convicts were transferred. Alongside numerous 'weak-minded' convicts removed from Mountjoy to Spike Island, other Spike prisoners, such as Michael Hayes and Thomas Kehoe, were diagnosed as insane. Kehoe, a convict under sentence of ten years' transportation, was transferred from Spike to Dundrum Lunatic Asylum in March 1851.[160]

Women held at Grangegorman Convict Depot also showed signs of insanity. Mary Kelly, committed to Grangegorman in August 1845, had allegedly feigned insanity on hearing she was to be transported. When finally placed on board the convict ship, *The Tasmania*, with 136 other women and thirty-seven children, she 'exhibited symptoms of violent insanity, or assumed them', scaring other prisoners, by tearing their 'clothes, caps and hair ... striking the commander, surgeon, and sailors'.[161] Reverend Bernard Kirby, chaplain to the Grangegorman Depot, failed to calm her and she was eventually removed back to Grangegorman, and in March 1846 transferred to Richmond Lunatic Asylum.[162] By 1849, Grangegorman had forty cells for prisoners in separate confinement, and held sixty-six female lunatics in different wings of the prison.[163] Again, in July 1850 two women were declared unfit for embarkation on a transport ship on grounds of insanity and recommended by the medical attendant for removal to an asylum or for commutation of their sentences.[164] Such was the concern about conditions at Grangegorman, in October there were calls to abandon it as a convict depot and instead establish a distinct institution that fully

[158] NAI, GPO/LB, Vol. 2, Jan. 1849–Dec. 1852, H. Hitchins to Major T. Reddington, 28 Apr. 1851, p. 248.
[159] NAI, GPO/LB, Vol. 12, July 1849–Dec. 1851, H. Hitchins to the Governor of Spike Island, 10 May 1851, p. 235.
[160] NAI, GPO/LB, Vol. 2, Jan. 1849–Dec. 1852, Case of Michael Hayes, p. 84; ibid., H. Hitchins to Major T. Reddington, 11 Mar. 1851, p. 229.
[161] 'Scene on Board The Tasmania Convict Ship', *The Hobart Town Courier and Government Gazette*, 13 Dec. 1845. We are grateful to Joan Kavanagh for the original newspaper reports.
[162] Joan Kavanagh and Dianne Snowden, *Van Diemen's Women: A History of Transportation to Tasmania* (Dublin: The History Press, 2015), pp. 112–13.
[163] RIGPI, 1849 (1850), p. 31.
[164] NAI, GPO/LB, Vol. 2, Jan. 1849–Dec. 1852, Letter from H. Hitchins, 27 July 1850, p. 113.

implemented the separate system or for female convicts to be sent directly to the colonies.[165] Meanwhile, Dr Francis White, in his role as the Inspector of Lunacy, encountered insane convicts from Spike Island when visiting Dundrum Criminal Lunatic Asylum. Noting that these convicts were allowed 'free intercourse' while at Spike, he asserted that his experience of Mountjoy and other prisons did not support claims that separate confinement generated insanity.[166]

Over the next few years, the incidence of feigned and 'true' suicide attempts at Mountjoy increased and Rynd continued to reject large numbers of prisoners as unfit for the regime. Correspondence between Hitchins and Governor Netterville suggests that in 1854, a batch of 13 prisoners were removed from Mountjoy on Rynd's orders in February and a further 12 in April, 88 in June and 126 in October.[167] In the same year, two suicide attempts and a third incident described as a feigned suicide attempt were reported to Hitchins.[168] The length of time prisoners spent in separation had also been extended beyond Hitchins' original recommendations. In April 1854, Rynd submitted his third application requesting the removal of convicts who been in separation in Mountjoy from twelve to sixteen months, informing Hitchins that one had died and a further eleven were in hospital.[169] In 1855, Rynd commented on the prison hospital being full of these 'patients broken down by ... confinement'.[170] Observing the impact on convicts of being kept for prolonged periods in separation – 'from nine months to eighteen, frequently, from various causes, prolonged to twenty, and even to twenty-two months' – Rynd noted that every convict:

not only experienced all the depressing influence of confinement (generally twenty-two consecutive hours in the cell at a time), but was exposed to the effects of trade labour in the cell, which, every where, and under every circumstance, has been found so injurious. All convicts could scarcely be supposed to possess mental and physical strength sufficient to sustain them under trials so protracted and severe.[171]

In that year there were four suicide attempts and one case of 'feigned' insanity at Mountjoy, yet in his official report Rynd noted there were no cases of mental disease.[172]

---

[165] Ibid., 7 Oct. 1850, p. 150.
[166] Report on the District, Criminal and Private Lunatic Asylums in Ireland, 1853 (1852–53) [1653], p. 16.
[167] NAI, GPO/CORR/1854/Mountjoy/Item nos 13, 32, 41, 134.
[168] Ibid., Item nos 110, 149, 156.   [169] Ibid., Index.
[170] Report of the Directors of Convict Prisons in Ireland (RDCPI), 1855 (1856) [2068], p. 52.
[171] Ibid., p. 51.   [172] Ibid., p. 53.

Apparently undeterred by evidence of the danger that separate confinement posed to prisoners' minds, by 1850 ten prisons had been built on the Pentonville design in England, and ten more had been converted for separate confinement.[173] The Select Committee on Prison Discipline, chaired by Home Secretary Sir George Grey, published its recommendations in 1850, which supported the introduction of 'entire separation' throughout English local gaols and houses of correction, and convict prisons with some modifications introduced to convicts' routine at labour and religious worship, though they were still prohibited from breaking the rule of silence. In his evidence, J.G. Perry, Inspector of Prisons for the Southern and Western Districts of England from 1843 and Medical Inspector of Prisons, advocated for its application across all prisons in Ireland. He also asserted that instances of mental disorder among prisoners were a consequence of improper implementation of separation.[174] There were some critical voices. Dr William Baly, medical officer at Millbank Prison since 1840, expressed his concerns to Grey's Select Committee, noting that prisoners who had undergone separate confinement and were sent to Millbank had suffered in their mental and physical health, and he was especially opposed to placing young prisoners in separation as they were particularly vulnerable to mental breakdown.[175] Support for the regime, however, dominated the proceedings and the tone of the evidence.

Such espousal of the separate system in penal policy, Miles Ogborn argues, reflected the Victorian quest for 'uniformity' and disciplinary rationality that would satisfy ratepayers and prisoners that punishment was applied equally and fairly in prison, a rationale that became more enthrenched in the 1860s and 1870s.[176] Modified forms of separate confinement were systematically introduced throughout the 1850s, in both older prisons and the new generation of 'modern' purpose-built institutions. It remained the preferred disciplinary regime in England and Ireland as transportation was steadily wound down and replaced with penal servitude after 1853. With its decline, prisons were no longer temporary holding places and portals for convicts awaiting transportation, but now had assumed a more fundamental position in the criminal

---

[173] Ignatieff, *A Just Measure of Pain*, pp. 197, 207.

[174] Report from the Select Committee on Prison Discipline together with the Proceedings of the Committee, Minutes of Evidence, Appendix and Index [Grey Committee] (1850) [632], p. 126. For Perry, see McConville, *English Local Prisons*, p. 105, n. 26.

[175] Grey Committee (1850), pp. 176–86.

[176] Ogborn, 'Discipline, Government and Law', p. 304; Bill Forsythe, 'Centralisation and Autonomy: The Experience of English Prisons 1820–1877', *Journal of Historical Sociology*, 4:3 (1991), 317–45.

justice system and in the quest for punishment and reformation.[177] By 1856, among just under 130 local gaols, houses of correction and convict prisons, forty-six across England reported separate confinement to be 'fully carried out'. Among the forty-two places of confinement across Ireland, by 1856 only six fully implemented separation.[178] Though relatively few gaols were built in Ireland in the post-Famine decade, new facilities expanded provision for separation, including substantial additional wings opened at the Armagh County Gaol in 1855 and at Kilmainham in 1863 (Figure 2.3).[179]

Prison policy was largely preoccupied with convict prisons, even though local goals and houses of correction housed the vast majority of English and Irish prisoners and in some ways were of greater significance.[180] Convict prisons held those convicted of felonies or serious misdemeanours who had been sentenced to transportation and after the 1850s penal servitude. Local gaols, in contrast, had mixed populations of government prisoners alongside those convicted of minor misdeamours and serving shorter sentences, as well as prisoners held on remand. The government prisoners held in local goals might be awaiting transfer to the convict system, though some rented cells to the government and housed convicts during their probationary period.[181] Though there were fluctuations in the size of local gaol populations, with a rapid turnover of often substantial numbers of prisoners, they were more likely to be subject to overcrowding.[182] Conditions were often poor and imposing separate confinement difficult. In some, only a portion of the prison made provision for separation, or it broke down as the prison became overcrowded.[183] While there was variation between local gaols with regard to diet, labour and punishment, they were typified by harsh

[177] Forsythe, *The Reform of Prisoners*, p. 72.
[178] In Ireland, these were Cork Female Convict Depot, the county and town gaols in Antrim, Armagh, Kilkenny county and Louth in addition to Mountjoy. See Prisons (Separate Confinement) (1856) [163], pp. 1–7, 8.
[179] Butler, *Building the Irish Courthouse and Prison*, pp. 315–35.
[180] McConville, *English Local Prisons*, p. 98.
[181] Seán McConville, *A History of English Prison Administration, Vol. 1, 1750–1877* (London, Boston and Henley: Routledge & Kegan Paul, 1981), p. 429.
[182] At the start of 1859, there were 17,920 prisoners confined in local prisons in England and Wales. See *Judicial Statistics*, 1859 (1860) [2692], p. xxvi. The figures for Ireland are complicated by the large numbers committed during the Famine. In 1846 there were 43,311 confined in Irish local gaols, 115,871 in 1850 and 73,733 in 1854. See RIGPI, 1853 (1854) [1803], p. viii.
[183] Report from the Select Committee of the House of Lords on the Present State of Discipline in Gaols and Houses of Correction [Carnarvon Committee] (1863) [499], pp. iii–vi.

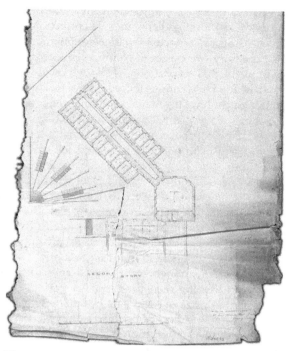

Figure 2.3 First floor plans of additions, Armagh Jail, William Murray, Architect, January 1846
Source: RIAI Murray Collection, Irish Architectural Archive, Dublin

conditions and disciplinary regimes that imperilled the physical and mental health of their prisoners. By the mid-1850s, however, the Inspectors General of Prisons claimed that conditions in Irish prisons had improved somewhat as the longer-term effects of the Great Famine eased inside and outside the prison environment.[184]

Chaplains and Medical Officers

As exemplified at Mountjoy, modifications were introduced to separate confinement as it was implemented across the two prison estates, and by

---

[184] See, for example, RIGPI, 1854 (1854–55) [1856], p. xiii.

the late 1850s the prison medical officer was assigned more responsibility and greater authority within the prison, although the chaplain continued to advise on matters relating to the minds of prisoners. From the eighteenth century onwards, legislation provided for the appointment of surgeons to English and Irish gaols, houses of correction and bridewells, although this was not always fully implemented. During the 1850s and 1860s prison medical appointments were more tightly regulated, and, particularly in convict prisons, medical officers began to establish themselves as a distinct professional group.[185] These changes were in part prompted by concerns about the excessive religious exhortations pursued by chaplains such as Nihil and Ralph, which, it was believed, contributed to high rates of mental disorder at Millbank and Pentonville in the 1840s. The first medical officers to English convict prisons were appointed in the 1840s, and provisions for their appointment firmed up by the Act for the Better Government of Convict Prisons of 1850, which brought convict prisons under central government control. Birmingham Borough Gaol, for example, instructed the surgeon to attend the prison twice weekly in 1849, though he was to check on sick prisoners as well as those in separate confinement on a daily basis. In 1860 he was expected to be in attendance each day at the prison, and oftener if necessary. There was much more detail about his role in the rules for 1860, which also included supervision of an infirmary warder.[186] At Liverpool Borough Gaol, after it opened in 1855 as one of the largest prisons in England designed for separate confinement, prison regulations charged doctors with visiting every prisoner twice a week, while prisoners in solitary confinement or close confinement were to be visited daily. Prisons drew attention to the observation of prisoners' mental state, as at Liverpool Gaol where the rules stipulated, if the doctor believed 'the mind or body of a prisoner is likely to be injuriously affected by the discipline or treatment', he was to alert the chaplain who was to 'pay attention to the state of mind of prisoners'.[187] The 1865 Prisons Act, discussed in detail in Chapter 3, made provision for the appointment of surgeons to local

---

[185] See Chapters 3–5 for prison medical officers' attempts to establish their expertise in terms of specialist knowledge of prisoners' mental status with regard to taxonomy, transfers to asylums and the detection of feigning.

[186] WCAR, BCL, LS11/2/5/13, *Regulations for the Government of the Prison, Provided and Established at Birmingham, in and for the Borough of Birmingham, 1849*, p. 33; LS11/2/5/12, *Rules and Regulations for the Government of the Common Gaol and House of Correction of the Borough of Birmingham, 1860*, p. 32.

[187] *Liverpool Mercury*, 7 Sept. 1857; Prisons (Separate Confinement), 1856, pp. 1–7, 8; LRO, 347 JUS/4/2/1, *Rules and Regulations for the Government of the Liverpool Borough Gaol and House of Correction at Walton-on-the-Hill, Near Liverpool* (1855), pp. 31–6, at pp. 31, 34.

prisons in England, with a proper schedule of responsibilities, replacing the previous situation where local general practitioners attended prisons occasionally or in some cases only in emergencies.[188]

In Irish prisons, medical officers were appointed under the 1786 Prison Act, and the requirement for regular visitations was firmed up under the 1826 Act for Consolidating and Amending the Law relating to prisons in Ireland.[189] Under that Act, Grand Jury-appointed prison surgeons were required to visit all sick prisoners in local gaols at least twice a week, and to inspect the hospital and healthy inmates. They were also charged with examining all prisoners on admission and before discharge.[190] The 1856 Prisons (Ireland) Act, amended earlier legislation for local prisons and required Boards of Superintendence to devise prison rules and regulations.[191] By 1862 the Board of Superintendence for the City of Dublin prisons, which included the Richmond Bridewell and the Grangegorman Female Penitentiary, required the medical officer to visit each prison daily, examine all prisoners who were ill, and inspect prisoners in separate confinement at least every second day.[192] The medical officer was charged with paying close attention to the mental and bodily health of prisoners in separate confinement, and if any ill effects from the discipline were observed, he was to 'authorize the Governor to carry out such relaxation of discipline'.[193] While the Roman Catholic chaplain was to visit daily, the Church of Ireland and Presbyterian chaplains attended three days a week, including Sundays.[194] There were similar rules for local gaols outside Dublin. At County of Londonderry Gaol, where all the cells for female prisoners, and some of those for male prisoners, were approved for separate confinement, the Board of Superintendence charged the non-resident surgeon with visiting at least twice weekly. He was to see each male and female prisoner in their cells, and to pay particular attention to prisoners in separate confinement. Any concerns relating to the detrimental effects of separate confinement on the minds or bodies of prisoners were to be

---

[188] Anne Hardy traces the roots of the English Prison Medical Service up to the late nineteenth century in 'Development of the Prison Medical Service, 1774–1895', in Creese, Bynum and Bearn (eds), *The Health of Prisoners*, pp. 59–82, at pp. 59–61.
[189] MacDonagh, *The Inspector General*, p. 80; 7 Geo. IV, c.74, s.LXXII (1826).
[190] 7 Geo. IV, c.74, s.LXXII (1826).
[191] 19&20 Vict., c.68, s.XIX (1856); 'The Corporation', *The Irish Times*, 2 Nov. 1861.
[192] Dublin City Archives, Dublin City Council, Board of Superintendence of the City of Dublin Prisons, BSP/mins/03, Minute Book, 14 Dec. 1853–23 Dec. 1856, 19 Nov. 1856, p. 311; *Bye-laws for the City of Dublin Prisons by the Board of Superintendence* (Dublin, 1862), pp. 27–8.
[193] *Bye-laws for the City of Dublin Prisons*, pp. 28–9.   [194] Ibid., p. 21.

reported to the Governor.[195] The rules for County of Kildare Gaol at Naas, approved for the separate system of confinement in the male and female prison, required that 'individual separation' be 'strictly enforced with all criminal prisoners, whether tried or untried'.[196]

At convict prisons, the 1854 Act for the Formation, Regulation and Government of Convict Prisons confirmed the authority of the Lord Lieutenant in relation to the appointment of medical staff.[197] At Mountjoy Prison the medical officer was to examine all 'complaining sick' every morning, and attend at any time in the case of serious illness of prisoners or officers. He was required to play close attention to the mental and bodily health of prisoners in separate confinement, and advise the governor on the effects of the discipline on prisoners, suggesting, when necessary, the relaxation of the discipline.[198] As discussed in Chapter 3, in 1867 a single full-time post of resident medical officer was approved, replacing two non-resident medical officer positions at Mountjoy Male and Female Prisons, following an acrimonious dispute with Dr Robert McDonnell, who served as Mountjoy's medical officer after 1857.[199] By the 1860s, at both convict and local prisons in Ireland, and in contrast with England, the avenue of communication, on matters relating to the minds of prisoners, usually by-passed chaplains, and instead went directly from the medical officer to the governor.

Prison medical officers also became more forceful in asserting their expertise in the management of the minds of prisoners and their workloads increased with their investigations and observations into individual cases, consultations with other doctors, and, in some cases, organisation of removals to other prisons or to asylums. In January 1854, Surgeon Francis Bulley at Reading Gaol reported on three prisoners whose mental states had become a matter of concern. One, John Clarke, had been in an asylum in Kent on two or three occasions prior to his prison committal and was again removed to an asylum. Another prisoner,

[195] *Bye-laws, Rules and Regulations of the County of Londonderry Gaol* (Londonderry, 1862), pp. 9–10.
[196] *Bye-laws, Rules and Regulations of the County of Kildare Gaol* (Naas, 1861), p. 9.
[197] 17&18 Vict., c.76, s.VII (1854).
[198] Correspondence Relative to Change in Medical Management of Mountjoy Convict Prison 1868 (1867–68) [502], p. 21. Also see *Rules to be Observed in Mountjoy Male Prison* (Dublin, 1867).
[199] Correspondence Relative to Change in Medical Management of Mountjoy Convict Prison 1868 (1867–68), p. lvii; 'Mountjoy Prison', *The Irish Times*, 30 Mar. 1868; RDCPI, 1867 (1867–68) [4084], p. 7; C.A. Cameron, *History of the Royal College of Surgeons in Ireland* (Dublin: Fanin and Company, 1916), pp. 496–9; D'A. Power and J.B. Lyons, 'McDonnell, Robert (1828–1889), Surgeon', *DNB*, https://doi.org/10.1093/ref:odnb/17464 [accessed 23 Apr. 2017].

William Ship, was admitted to the prison infirmary experiencing delusions, though 'it is hoped that by care and attention confirmed Insanity may be prevented'. Thomas Ford, reported on admission to be of unsound mind, was diagnosed as having a 'weakened' intellect related to a head injury; 'it has not been considered necessary to treat him altogether as an insane person altho' orders have been given that his conduct should be carefully watched'. William Ship was later removed to Bethlem.[200]

At Clerkenwell House of Detention, which functioned as a remand prison after 1847, Surgeon Henry Wakefield saw large numbers of mentally disturbed offenders. He was overwhelmed by the burden of assessing every prisoner on admission for signs of mental disorder and by the high number of attempted suicides, especially among women, who revealed evidence of excessive drinking, destitution and abuse.[201] Wakefield was obliged to enlist the assistance of Chaplain George Jepson in monitoring these cases, who worked tirelessly with prisoners committed on charges of suicide, removing them to asylums, workhouses or to friends and family to be cared for.[202] In October 1859 two suicide attempts were reported, of a woman who had attempted to throw herself over a balustrade of the upper gallery and a male prisoner who, after attempting to drown himself in a basin of water, was removed to a padded cell, where he tried to strangle himself with his shirt sleeves. Wakefield complained about the number of magistrates' requests to report on the state of mind of prisoners, a task not specified as part of his duty. Such requests had increased from nine in 1858 to twenty-seven in the first three-quarters of 1859. The Visiting Justices to the prison, acknowledging the level of concern about cases of mental breakdown, suggested that in any future appointment of a surgeon it be made part of his ordinary duties to certify as to the state of mind of prisoners in all cases where required.[203]

The alterations to penal policy and slow decline of transportation in the late 1850s prompted changes to the staged format of penal discipline. The probationary period in separate confinement remained at its core, but, alongside this, a ticket-of-leave system, which allowed prisoners to

---

[200] Berkshire Record Office (BRO), Q/SO/24, County of Berkshire Sessions Order Book, Apr. 1853–July 1855, General Quarter Sessions, Surgeon's Reports, 2 Jan. 1854, p. 218, 3 Apr. 1854, p. 281.
[201] London Metropolitan Archives (LMA), MA/G/CLE/114–177/ Item no. 156, *Annual Report of the Governor, and of the Surgeon and Chaplain*, 1859, p. 10.
[202] Ibid., pp. 9–10.
[203] LMA, MA/G/CLE/190/Item no. 184, *Report of the Visiting Justices of the House of Correction*, 1859.

be released on licence subject to good behaviour in prison, was introduced. In some quarters, enthusiasm for such modifications was muted by scepticism about the effectiveness of the system of separate confinement for the reformation of prisoners as well as their mental wellbeing. William Milner, surgeon to Wakefield Prison, expressed his doubts about separation in 1847, pointing out that, while infirmary admissions had declined, more prisoners were being treated in their cells; 'there appeared little doubt that the cases of mental delusion might be attributed to the separate system ... shewing that the system of total separation was not universally applicable'.[204] In January 1849 Joshua Jebb highlighted a further issue when a group of convicts transferred from Wakefield to Portland Prison, appeared, according to Jebb, to be in a 'very low condition'. One was found to be 'insane but quiet and harmless, another in an advanced state of consumption', seven others had scorbutic swellings and a large number suffered spongy gums.[205] Jebb concluded that the convicts had been given insufficient diet and that their impaired health was also attributable to the long periods of separate confinement they had undergone, notably those held for six months at Millbank and then a further twelve at Wakefield. He stressed that the question of diet should be concerned with 'how much is necessary to enable them [convicts] to bear the discipline without greater depression to their physical and mental powers'.[206] Modifications to the dietary and exercise regimes were introduced at Wakefield in the late 1840s, resulting in a decline in reported incidences of insanity at the prison, which was by this time praised over Pentonville for its successful governance, while Pentonville continued to be associated with high rates of mental breakdown.[207] By the late 1850s, however, the magistrates at Wakefield Prison, which had been significantly enlarged in 1847, had become alarmed at the high rates of reoffending among its prisoners, noting a rise from 7 per cent in 1854 to nearly 31 per cent in 1861. Among inmates returned to prison between 1854 and 1861, over 53 per cent were admitted within one year of discharge. Acknowledging that the

---

[204] Wakefield County Record Office, QS 10/56, Quarter Sessions Order Book, Oct. 1846–Apr. 1850, Wakefield Adjourned Sessions, Surgeon's Report, 9 Dec. 1847, p. 98 (emphasis in original).

[205] TNA, HO 45/1451, Lunacy; Poor Law and Paupers; Prisons and Prisoners, Sept. 1846–Jan. 1849, Convict Department at Wakefield, J. Jebb to Home Office, 6 Jan. 1849, Memo by Lieut Colonel Jebb in Reply to Sir George Grey's Queries on Mr Hill's Letter of 18 Dec. 1848.

[206] Ibid. (emphasis in original).

[207] Cox and Marland, 'He Must Die or Go Mad in This Place', p. 106. See ch. 3 for an extended discussion of the relationship of diet with mental breakdown.

increase was partially linked to the decline in transportation, the magistrates contended that the figures pointed to a defect in the disciplinary system and its failure to prepare prisoners for release.[208]

Meanwhile Hitchins at Mountjoy was forced to retire owing to a scandal concerning his inept management of the transportation of a group of women convicts. He had permitted the women be sent directly from Mountjoy, where they were held in separate confinement, to the ships bound for Australia. On arrival in Western Australia the female convicts, some of whom had been in prison since the Great Famine, were found to be 'reduced to the condition of mere machines ... debilitated by protracted imprisonment, diseased to an alarming extent, indolent to a degree by long habit, and noticeably ill-trained'.[209] There were complaints about the 'filthy' state of the female convicts and the embarkation of insane convicts during 'lucid intervals'.[210] By 1854, the Irish Prison Commissioners had also concluded that the implementation of the separate system at Mountjoy under Hitchins' tenure was seriously flawed and insisted the primary purpose of the discipline, 'moral and religious improvement', be reasserted.[211] There were also complaints about prison conditions; owing to overcrowding in convict prisons, three to four prisoners shared one cell, and there was indiscriminate association during work. At Grangegorman women's prison up to five prisoners shared one cell.[212]

Sir Walter Crofton, appointed chair of the newly established Directors of Convict Prisons for Ireland in 1854, promptly set about introducing his 'mark' system to Irish convict prisons.[213] Under Crofton's system, convicts were kept in separate confinement at Mountjoy for the first or

---

[208] Edward Balme Wheatley, *Observations on the Treatment of Convicts in Ireland with Some Remarks on the Same in England by Four Visiting Justices of the West Riding Prison at Wakefield* (London: Simpkin, Marshall, and Co., 1862), pp. vi, viii, xix.

[209] Reverend Orby Shipley, *The Purgatory of Prisoners: or, An Intermediate Stage between the Prison and the Public, Being Some Account of the New System of Penal Reformation Introduced by the Board of Directors of Convict Prisons in Ireland* (London: John Henry and James Parker, 1857), p. 35. See also Carey, *Mountjoy*, p. 60; *Freeman's Journal*, 2 Feb. 1855.

[210] NAI, GPO/LB, Vol. 2, Jan. 1849–Dec. 1852, Letter from H. Hitchins, 19 June 1852.

[211] Convict Prisons (Ireland). Copies of Correspondence Relative to the Management and Discipline of Convict Prisons (1854), p. 18; Carroll-Burke, *Colonial Discipline*, pp. 95–8.

[212] Shipley, *The Purgatory of Prisoners*, pp. 35–6.

[213] Sir Walter Frederick Crofton (1815–97) was an influential authority on prisons and penal reform, and developed a version of Alexander Maconochie's progressive or staged system of penal discipline. As well as serving as Chair of the Directors of Convict Prisons for Ireland, he was special commissioner in Ireland for prisons, reformatories and industrial schools (1868–69). He was appointed to the Irish Privy Council in 1869 and was Chairman of the General Prisons Board in Ireland (1877–78). He was

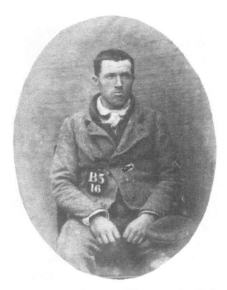

Figure 2.4 Thomas A. Larcom, Photographs Collection, Volume 1,
'Some of the More Serious Offenders Confined Under Penal and
Reformatory Discipline in Mountjoy Government Cellular Prison in
Dublin', August 1857
Source: 'Photograph #51 [John Byrne]', *The New York Public Library Digital
Collections*, Manuscripts and Archives Division, The New York Public
Library, 1857. https://digitalcollections.nypl.org/items/510d47dc-9623-a3d9-
e040-e00a18064a99

probationary stage. The period in separation could last from eight to
twelve months depending on the men's conduct and for the first three
months of this period, they were forbidden work except for picking
oakum in cells. Prisoners then progressed to the second stage; those with
a trade remained at Mountjoy, others were sent to the public works
associated prison at Spike Island while 'weak' convicts were sent to
Philipstown Prison prior to its closure in 1862. At the final stage convicts
were sent to the intermediate prisons at Smithfield or at Lusk, County
Dublin. In preparation for release, Smithfield convicts attended lectures
by James Organ on a range of practical and moral topics intended to

Commissioner of County and Borough Gaols in England (1865–68) and involved in the
National Association for the Promotion of Social Science. See Martin McElroy,
'Crofton, Sir Walter Frederick', in James McGuire and James Quinn (eds), *Dictionary
of Irish Biography* (Cambridge: Cambridge University Press, 2009), https://doi.org/10
.3318/dib.002189.v1 [accessed 23 Apr. 2019].

instill personal responsibility, self-control and 'mental training'.[214] Throughout the various stages of Crofton's system, labour was treated as a privilege, which prisoners strove towards, rather than a punishment as in Wakefield and other English prisons. Crofton's system stressed reformation through religious and spiritual teachings combined with individualistic self-interest promoted by systems of rewards, gratuities, marks and badges for good behaviour.[215]

Following an inspection of the Irish system, a group of Wakefield magistrates claimed 75 per cent of men progressed to the intermediate prisons and exhibited a 'remarkable improvement' in physical and mental health.[216] Wakefield's medical officer, Dr Brady, went on to claim 'No real or feigned insanity, no attempt at suicide, no assaults on officers, no malingering, no scheming even to get into hospital, or to remain there after recovery' occurred in the intermediate prisons of Lusk and Smithfield.[217] There was great enthusiasm for Crofton's system within the National Association for the Promotion of Social Sciences, notably on the part of penal reformers Matthew Davenport Hill and Mary Carpenter, the German jurist Franz Von Holtzendorff and the Reverend Orby Shipley, which prompted intense debate on the merits of the system.[218] The Irish system was strongly resisted by Sir Joshua Jebb and John Burt, among others, who dismissed it as one of '*Disposal*' rather than '*Discipline*', while advocates of Crofton's regime pitted it against Jebb's version of penal servitude, which emphasised the role of labour as an aspect of punishment.[219]

Despite various modifications to separate confinement as implemented in English and Irish local and convict prisons after the late 1850s, incidences of mental disorder continued to manifest themselves among prisoners. Standing in contrast to the conclusions of the Wakefield magistrates, surviving prison character books and official

---

[214] Carroll-Burke, *Colonial Discipline*, pp. 171–5.   [215] Ibid., p. 191.
[216] Wheatley, *Observations on the Treatment of Convicts in Ireland*, p. 56.   [217] Ibid., p. 55.
[218] *The Reader*, 18 Apr. 1863; P.W.J. Bartrip, 'Hill, Matthew Davenport (1792–1872)', *DNB*, https://doi.org/10.1093/ref:odnb/13286 [accessed 23 Apr. 2018]; Mary Carpenter, *Our Convicts*, vol. II (London: Longman, Green, Longman, Roberts & Green, 1864); Baron Von Holtzendorff, *Reflections and Observations on the Present Condition of the Irish Convict System translated by Mrs Lentaigne* (Dublin: J.M. O'Toole and Son, 1863); Shipley, *The Purgatory of Prisoners*.
[219] *Reports and Observations on the Discipline and Management of Convict Prisons, by the Late Major-General Sir Joshua Jebb, K.C.B., Surveyor General of Prisons, &c., &c.* (London: Hatchard and Co., 1863), p. 17; John. T. Burt, *Irish Facts and Wakefield Figures in Relation to Convict Discipline in Ireland* (London: Longman and Co., 1863) (emphasis in original); McConville, *English Local Prisons*, pp. 87–8. See also Lawrence Goldman, *Science, Reform and Politics in Victorian Britain: The Social Science Association, 1857–1886* (Cambridge: Cambridge University Press, 2002).

correspondence highlight harsh responses to cases of mental distress and disorder before and after the introduction of Crofton's mark system to the convict prison system. Some incidences culminated in the removal of convicts to Dundrum Criminal Lunatic Asylum after it opened in 1850 or to other local asylums. One such case was James alias Thomas Carthy, convicted in March 1851 and sentenced to seven years' transportation. While his previous conduct in the county gaol – he had three convictions – was described as good, he deteriorated when placed in separate confinement at Mountjoy. He spent two periods in separation, one lasting sixteen months and a second for over ten months, and for both terms he was reported to be 'very bad'. Between November 1855 and January 1857, he was punished for misconduct over twenty times, repeatedly confined in dark cells, and placed on a bread and water diet in his own cell. He was transferred between Spike, Phillipstown and Mountjoy prisons on several occasions and when discharged, in March 1858, removed to Cork District Lunatic Asylum.[220]

Women under the Separate System

The extension of separate confinement across both prison estates included the construction of 'model' prisons for women, intended to replace older penitentiaries, such as Millbank in London and Grangegorman in Dublin, where women had been subject to separate confinement for short periods prior to transportation.[221] With the announcement that Van Dieman's Land would no longer accept female transportees after 1852, and the end of female transportation in 1853, Sir Joshua Jebb, Chair of the Directorate of Convict Prisons, reorganised provision for female convicts. The first purpose-built female convict prisons, designed for separate confinement, were opened in Brixton in 1853 and at Mountjoy Female Prison in 1858.[222] Brixton, catering for up to 650 prisoners, soon became overcrowded and after 1855, a pentagon

---

[220] NAI, GPO/PN/5, Philipstown Character Book, 1851–59, Reg. no. 1185, Thomas or James Carthy.

[221] For details on Millbank Prison, see Neil Davie, '"Business as Usual?" Britain's First Women's Convict Prison, Brixton 1853–1869', *Crimes and Misdemeanours*, 4:1 (2010), 37–52. For details on Grangegorman Female Penitentiary, Dublin, see Elaine Farrell, *Women, Crime and Punishment in Ireland: Life in the Nineteenth-Century Convict Prison* (Cambridge: Cambridge University Press, 2020), p. 12; Beverly A. Smith, 'The Female Prisoner in Ireland, 1855–1878', *Federal Probation*, 54:4 (1990), 69–81. After 1837 Grangegorman received all female prisoners for Dublin and all female convicts awaiting transportation. Of the 259 available cells in 1839, 94 were used to hold women in separate confinement. By 1849 conditions at the prison had deteriorated significantly owing to overcrowding and the effects of the Great Famine, and in March the prison was hit by the cholera epidemic. See RIGPI, 1839 (1840), pp. 7, 20.

[222] Davie, 'Business as Usual?'; Smith, 'The Female Prisoner in Ireland', p. 75.

at Millbank was reallocated for the separate confinement of women.[223] By the time Mountjoy opened, with individual cells for well over 400 women, it was part of Crofton's remodelled Irish convict prison system.[224]

Separate confinement as devised for male convict prisons was regarded as unsuitable for female convicts, and women, described as unable to withstand prolonged periods in isolation and more susceptible to mental anxieties than male prisoners, were placed in separation for four rather than twelve months. Hard labour, an important component of the reformative process for male prisoners, was not extended to female-only convict prisons. In keeping with mid-nineteenth-century ideas of gender, women's prison labour focused on the domestic and the restoration of female and maternal qualities; women required saving twice, from their criminality and their upturning of expected female behaviour.[225] Some governors sought a severe prison regime for women. Chesterton, Governor at Coldbath Fields, insisted that through their immoral and criminal behaviour, women had forfeited prospects for sympathetic treatment and should be subjected to the full rigours of the prison regime.[226] Irish female convicts were described as being more tainted than their English counterparts; 'wholly debased, such debasement being mainly a result of ignorance'.[227] Inspector Hitchins considered the 'abandonment of the strictest Separation unadvisable' in the case of Irish women prisoners and, prior to the opening of Mountjoy Female Prison, he lobbied for a harsher regime than that devised for Brixton. In 1853, he resisted Jebb's proposal that the prison be built on the cellular construction used at Dartmoor – a less expensive building – on the grounds it would allow association by 'day in large rooms or the dispersion of the prisoners on out-door labour'.[228]

Liverpool Borough Gaol provides an outstanding example of the challenges provoked by a large female prison population.[229] Many of its huge number of female committals were repeat offenders, admitted for being

---

[223] Lucia Zedner, *Women, Crime and Custody in Victorian England* (Oxford: Clarendon Press, 1991), p. 179.

[224] RDCPI 1858 (1859) [2531], pp. 89–90.

[225] See Rachel Bennett, '"Bad for the Health of the Body, Worse for the Health of the Mind": Female Responses to Imprisonment in England, 1853–1869', *Social History of Medicine*, 34:2 (2021), 532–52; Davie, 'Business as Usual?', p. 41; Zedner, *Women, Crime and Custody*, p. 185.

[226] Zedner, *Women, Crime and Custody*, p. 140.

[227] NAI, GPO/LB, Vol. 3, Jan. 1853–Dec. 1854, H. Hitchins to Thomas Larcom, 10 Dec. 1853.

[228] Ibid.

[229] Liverpool Borough Gaol, known as 'Liverpool Borough Prison' from the late 1860s, is discussed in greater detail in Chapters 3 and 4. See also Cox and Marland, 'Unfit for Reform or Punishment'.

drunk and disorderly or on charges of prostitution. The female wing was almost consistently overcrowded, and as a result, women prisoners doubled up in cells and the separate system was periodically abandoned. For example, in October 1855, a month after the prison opened, the Liverpool Visiting Justices observed there were only 407 cells for between 416 and 429 female prisoners. In October, the governor allowed women to sleep in association while in May 1857 straw beds were supplied for 'doubling-up' in cells.[230] In June 1857 some 621 female prisoners were confined in the prison.[231]

With the continuing use of Millbank to confine women, most female convicts in England underwent the probationary stage of sentences in separation at Millbank, while in Ireland they served it at Mountjoy Female Prison. On completion of the probationary period, women in both systems were then permitted a less punitive regime, yet they were not moved to associated labour prisons, as was the case with men. In Ireland, after separation, convict women were retained at Mountjoy, while in England they were moved to Brixton. They were then permitted to associate while at school, chapel and taking exercise, though the range of work available to them was mainly domestic, revolving around cooking, cleaning, sewing and laundry.[232]

Women whose behaviour improved further could then be transferred to 'refuges', also female-only institutions intended to provide a period of 'lighter' prison discipline, prepare women for release and provide additional domestic training. Jebb believed the taint of criminality made it harder for women convicts, especially younger women, to secure employment and argued time spent in refuges enhanced their prospects on release and would have a 'softening' effect on them.[233] From 1856 Fulham operated as the main refuge for convict women in England, where they were allowed to associate with the 'aim of encouraging responsibility and restoring self-respect'.[234] At Mountjoy women who had earned marks for discipline, industry and schooling under Crofton's system could be removed to one of two Dublin refuges – the Catholic Goldenbridge refuge run by the Sisters of Mercy and the

[230] LRO, 347 MAG/1/2/1, Minutes of the Quarterly and Annual Meetings of the Visiting Justices of the Borough Gaol and House of Correction, also Special Gaol Sessions, 1852–64, 27 Oct. 1855, p. 50; ibid., 20 May 1857, p. 82.
[231] LRO, 347 JUS 4/1/2, Minutes of Justices Sessions Gaol and House of Correction, Oct. 1864–Jan. 1870, *Reports of the Governor, Chaplain, Prison Minister and Surgeon for 1864*, p. 5.
[232] Zedner, *Women, Crime and Custody*, p. 180.   [233] Ibid., p. 181.
[234] Davie, 'Business as Usual?', p. 41.

Protestant one at Heytesbury Street – or released on licence or ticket on leave.[235]

Women, whether in convict prisons or local gaols, were regarded as troublesome, volatile, disruptive and prone to depression of spirits, suicide attempts and unable to withstand long prison sentences. In his second report on Brixton, Surgeon J.D. Rendle noted: 'female prisoners, as a body, do not bear imprisonment so well as the male prisoners; they get anxious, restless, more irritable in temper, and are more readily excited'.[236] In addition to this tendency to 'break out', a phrase repeatedly used to describe women's behaviour, Rendle referred to women's low spirits, frequent crying and repeated suicide attempts.[237] The 1862 rules laid down for Grangegorman Female Penitentiary required the prison matron, not the governor, to inquire into charges of misconduct against women, as the indelicate nature of the language, and the 'equally objectionable' evidence, should not be heard by male officers.[238] At Clerkenwell, Surgeon Wakefield reported that of the 107 suicide attempts in 1859, 84 were made by women: 'The majority were more or less in a state of intoxication, when the attempt was made; but, in several of the females cases, sad histories of cruel treatment and destitution were elicited from them. They were all placed under close observation.'[239]

Similar remarks were made about female convicts in Mountjoy, who Prison Superintendent, Delia Lidwell or Lidwill, described in 1859 as losing 'all control of reason', breaking windows, destroying bedding and tearing 'clothing with their teeth'.[240] In that year, four women were removed to asylums, while an unspecified number were retained at Mountjoy under medical observation. One was convict Mary Murray, who was especially troublesome; aged twenty-four, Dr Awly Banon described her as one of the 'worst and most incorrigible cases' he had ever seen. Prior to her arrival in Mountjoy, she had been held in 1858 at Cork Gaol and at Grangegorman Female Penitentiary where she had been violent, assaulting officers and other prisoners, and had been repeatedly placed in iron handcuffs and on the punishment diet.[241]

---

[235] Smith, 'The Female Prisoner in Ireland', p. 75.
[236] RDCP, 1854 (1854–55) [1986], Brixton Prison: Medical Officer's Report, p. 393.
[237] RDCP, 1855 (1856) [2126], Brixton Prison: Medical Officer's Report, 1855, p. 297.
[238] Bye-laws for the City of Dublin Prisons, p. 173.
[239] LMA, MA/G/CLE/114–177/Item no. 156, Annual Report of the Governor, and of the Surgeon and Chaplain, 1859, p. 10.
[240] For Lidwill, see Farrell, Women, Crime and Punishment in Ireland, pp. 175–9.
[241] NAI, GPO/CORR/1859/Mountjoy (Female) Prison/Item nos 223, 257, 265, 283. Dr A.P. Banon was a Licentiate of the Royal College of Surgeons in Ireland and Surgeon to

Described as 'ferocious and dangerous' by Banon, at Mountjoy she repeatedly tore up her cell and the furniture. Her removal to Dundrum was decided in June 1859 when she was discovered lodged between the mason work of the cell window and the glass. She had torn up the cell skirting with her hands, unscrewed the bolt that secured the iron grating at the window, and had loosened blocks from the wall. She then got inside the iron bars and broke the windowpanes. When discovered her hands were cut and bloody and her arm was badly hurt; nonetheless, she was very abusive to the prison officers. Drs McDonnell and Banon promptly certified her removal to Dundrum, from where she made her escape in January 1864.[242] Commenting on Murray, and the three other convicts transferred to asylums, Banon noted that 'from the peculiarity of their symptoms, I had some difficulty in coming to the conclusion that they were actually insane in the usual acceptation [sic] of the word'. He had, however, resolved they were 'fit subjects for a lunatic asylum, at least more so than for a prison'. Following a detailed description of the cases, a catalogue of their destructive and volatile behaviour in prison, Banon concluded that prison tended to aggregate the 'morbid condition' of their minds and called for an 'intermediate institution between a prison and a lunatic asylum'.[243]

Repeat offenders, especially women on sentences for prostitution and drunk and disorderly behaviour, many of whom were young, were particularly vexing for prison officials, and the responses of medical officers, chaplains and governors to these women, including those experiencing mental distress and disorder, was harsh. One woman found to be insane while in Reading Gaol in 1849 was described by Chaplain Field as a 'wandering prostitute. Her mind evidently enfeebled when she was first committed, and her temper uncontrollable. The loss of reason in her case was the result of debauchery and of a brutalizing vice.'[244] Among the convicts transferred from Mountjoy to lunatic asylums in 1859 was a twenty-six-year-old woman who had been convicted twenty-four times for larceny and disorderly conduct, and had led an 'abandoned life'. While Banon did not believe her to be as 'vile and vicious' as other women, she would stand naked when her cell door was opened, laugh

---

Jervis Street Hospital, Dublin. See *The Irish Medical Directory for 1843* (Dublin: W. Curry Jr and Co., 1843).

[242] NAI, GPO/CORR/1859/Mountjoy (Female) Prison/Item nos 223, 257, 265, 283; RDCPI, 1859 (1860) [2655], p. 69.

[243] RDCPI, 1859 (1860), pp. 65, 68–9.

[244] BRO, Q/SO/22, County of Berkshire Sessions Order Book, 1849–50, Chaplain's Annual Report, 15 Oct. 1849, p. 238.

in a 'silly manner' and talk to herself.[245] The scale of the issue was especially acute at Liverpool. In 1855 4,820 women were convicted on drunk and disorderly charges; 642 of these were between fifteen and eighteen years of age.[246] It was estimated that there were '695 brothels, 81 houses of accommodation and 102 houses where prostitutes lodge' in Liverpool, with over 2,000 women and girls 'known as professed prostitutes'.[247] Some prison officials at Liverpool despaired of reforming female prisoners in this environment. As Governor Jackson observed in 1859:

No system of prison discipline will have the greatly desired effect of either deterring or reforming these immoral and depraved women, so as to prevent them returning to their dissolute and intemperate habits, while there are so many receptacles ready for them, and so many inducements and facilities afforded to them in Liverpool.[248]

Conclusion

Many other prisoners attracted similar judgement as being unfit for reform and for the discipline of separate confinement owing to their weak mental state and their inability to withstand the rigour of the regime. If they became insane, then it was claimed that was due to their existing mental instability or weakness, hereditary madness, or their reprehensible behaviour and life of vice.[249] Alongside the woman cited above, Chaplain Field at Reading contended that of the four further cases of insanity occurring in 1849, 'I cannot think that with any of them the development of insanity was assignable to any peculiarity of separate confinement.' The first prisoner, a government convict, showed symptoms of mental aberration so quickly that Field claimed it was 'incipient' when he was committed. The second, who had been a soldier in the West Indies, became deranged after an attack of fever and never recovered his mental faculties; he had been court martialled numerous times. Another had been of unsound mind long before her committal, her grandmother was insane and her father had been treated for disease of the brain. And in the last case, the prisoner had been wounded in the head by a pickaxe while working on a railway, had lost part of his skull and since then had

[245] RDCPI, 1859 (1860), p. 69.
[246] Report of the Inspectors of Prisons of Great Britain, Northern and Eastern Districts (1857–58) [2373], p. 22.
[247] Ibid., p. 23.
[248] Report of the Inspectors of Prisons of Great Britain, Northern District (1860), [2645], p. 31; See Cox and Marland, 'Unfit for Reform or Punishment' for a detailed discussion of responses to mental disorder among male and female prisoners at Liverpool Prison.
[249] See Cox and Marland, 'He Must Die or Go Mad in This Place' for further examples.

been ungovernable whenever provoked.[250] At Mountjoy, convicts who showed signs of mental collapse while in separation were said to be weak-minded prior to entering the prison. Convict Patrick Ryan, a disruptive prisoner admitted in February 1854, was transferred from Mountjoy to Philipstown and described by Rynd as having the 'appearance of [weak intellect] ever since his first admission here'.[251] In his defence of the regime at Mountjoy, Rynd insisted that rigorous inspection and diversion of such prisoners on admission, the exact implementation of the period of separation and careful medical oversight of the regime would protect convicts and ensure there were fewer cases 'whose complaints, if not occasioned, were enhanced and aggravated by the prison discipline'.[252]

In these instances, continued confinement in separation or punishments for unruly behaviour was dismissed as pointless by medical officers who argued such prisoners were not only incapable of reform but that longer periods in separation would produce 'real' insanity. These prisoners were often removed from separation to the prison hospital or allowed association in cells or at work and processed across the prison estate to associated labour prisons, and, as exemplified earlier in this chapter, some were medically discharged.[253] Others were eventually admitted to lunatic asylums, as will be explored in more detail in Chapter 4. Though managed in different ways, increasingly the mental and moral weakness of these prisoners was linked to their criminality, a view that became more entrenched among prison staff, including medical officers, by the late nineteenth century and explored in Chapters 3 and 5.

It is likely that some of the prisoners admitted to convict and local prisons had experienced previous instances of mental breakdown, were 'weak-minded' or particularly vulnerable to mental collapse. Yet the eagerness of prisons to defend the system – as Laurie pointed out in his critique – was exemplified by the efforts of prison officers to preempt accusations concerning the ill effects of separation through their investigations and the presentation of evidence showing insanity prefaced rather than resulted from imprisonment. As the regime was toned down, its severity reduced, this only served to prompt claims that it was the failure to implement it rigorously and in full that resulted in the mental collapse of prisoners. Yet, as Mayhew and Binny concluded in their overview of London prisons in 1862, the regime appeared to have resulted in

[250] BRO, Q/SO/22, County of Berkshire Sessions Order Book, 1849-50, Chaplain's Annual Report, 15 Oct. 1849, p.238.
[251] NAI, GPO/CORR/1854/Mountjoy/Item no. 14.
[252] RDCPI, 1855 (1856), pp. 51-2.
[253] RDCP, 1852 (1852–53), Pentonville Prison, pp. 33, 37, 39.

excessively high rates of insanity. Between 1842 and 1849 the number of cases of lunacy occurring in Pentonville was ten times the national figure: twenty-two cases or 62 per 10,000 compared with 5.8 for prisons across England and Wales. In Millbank the rate was even higher, with sixty-five cases of insanity or 87.5 per 10,000 between 1844 and 1851. 'These figures', they added, 'tell awful tales of long suffering and deep mental affliction.'[254] They were also likely to represent, as cases of insanity declared in official reports, only a small proportion of the prisoners suffering from delusions, anxiety, depression of spirits or morbid feelings who appeared regularly in the prisons' institutional records. It was this day-to-day revelation of the harm imposed by separation that caused Kingsmill to lose faith in the efficacy of separate confinement after being one of its keenest advocates and Hitchins to moderate the system as it was introduced to Ireland.

Yet despite observing the damage that the prison environment and system of discipline inflicted on prisoners, many other prison officials, such as Inspector of English Prisons Herbert P. Voules, and the Inspectors of Prisons in Ireland, maintained an enduring faith in the overall efficacy of the separate system. While critical of the severe conditions in some prisons, the Irish Inspectors insisted on the safety of the separate system, 'once correctly and humanely implemented'.[255] That the regime caused mental distress among a minority of prisoners was regarded as a minimal disadvantage when balanced against the apparent benefits of the system. For many penologists and officials it presented the most viable opportunity to reform and save criminals while also reducing criminality. The latter concern, the reduction of 'criminality', came increasingly to the fore in the late 1860s as crime rates and repeat offending continued to rise, and, with the ending of transportation, the expanding prison population became a more visible and persistent problem. The official response to criticisms of the expensive 'modern' prison system for failing to reform was to develop a more punitive prison regime, still based on separation but with less emphasis on reformation. The chaplains who had so dominated the early years of the separate system, and who were strongly associated with the initial optimism surrounding moral and spiritual reform, were pushed increasingly towards the periphery. The new penal approach that had deep implications for prisoners' mental wellbeing and for the prison staff enforcing it, especially the medical officers, will be explored in the next chapter.

---

[254] Mayhew and Binny, *The Criminal Prisons of London*, pp. 103–4.
[255] RIGPI 1858 (1859 Session 2) [2557], p. xxiv; Report of the Inspectors of Prisons of Great Britain, Northern and Eastern Districts (1857–58), pp. 13, 27.

3   The Prison Medical Officer
Deterrence, Dual Loyalty and the Production
of Psychiatric Expertise, 1860–1895

Some display a marked degree of dullness or stupor; others sharpness
and cunning more allied to the tricks of monkeys than the acts of
reasonable men.[1]

When John Campbell published his reminiscences of thirty years' experience as a prison medical officer in 1884, his comments on the traits of
prisoners, quoted here, encapsulated the change in attitude towards
prisoners that dominated penal policy in the late nineteenth century.
Prisoners, once perceived as redeemable, were now regarded as unreformable, incorrigible, and of poor mental and physical stock. From the
late 1850s onwards, fuelled by accusations that prisons were not deterring repeat offenders and that crime was increasing and becoming more
brutal, British and Irish legislatures and publics expressed increased
disquiet about the effectiveness of their prison systems. The flagship
convict prisons, Mountjoy and Pentonville, lost their 'model status',
and their significance as emblems of rehabilitation diminished, while
the aims of spiritual reformists were dismissed as naïve and ineffectual.[2]
Prison policy shifted away from disciplinary regimes emphasising reform
towards the rigorous enforcement of expressly punitive regimes, including the separate system of confinement. This involved all prison officers,
but placed prison medical officers in a particularly challenging position.
As they strove to recreate themselves as experts in prison medicine and to
enhance their professional status, they were also implicated in imposing
new and severe systems of discipline, which proved detrimental to the
physical and mental health of many prisoners, and 'debasing to the
mental faculties'.[3]

[1] John Campbell, *Thirty Years' Experience of a Medical Officer in the English Convict Service*
(London, Edinburgh and New York: T. Nelson and Sons, 1884), p. 73.
[2] Report of the Directors of Convict Prisons (RDCP), 1885–86 (1886) [C.4833], p. viii;
Report of the General Prisons Board (Ireland) (RGPBI), 1879 (1878–79) [C.2447], p. 6.
[3] Report from the Departmental Committee on Prisons [Gladstone Committee] (1895)
[C.7702] [C.7702–I], p. 19.

The hardening of attitudes towards prisoners was evident in two influential commissions of inquiry into convict and local prison systems. The 1863 Royal Commission established to Enquire into the Operation of Transportation and Penal Servitude in Convict Prisons in Britain and Ireland and the 1863 House of Lords Select Committee on Prison Discipline in England (Lord Carnarvon's Committee) collated detailed evidence from prison governors, medical officers, chaplains and inspectors, and made wide-reaching recommendations for changes in penal policy. The Carnarvon Committee was particularly important; its recommendations shaped legislation, including the 1865 English Prison Act, while the outlook of the witnesses exemplified the tone of late nineteenth-century penal policy and the direction of subsequent legislation. Under new rules introduced from the 1860s onwards, separate confinement remained intrinsic to the English prison system, but became more penal with greater emphasis on the uniform enforcement of hard labour and strict adherence to meagre dietary scales.[4] To incentivise good behaviour, a version of the mark or 'stage' system, which had been a feature of convict prison discipline in Ireland from the 1850s, was introduced to English convict and local prisons allowing for 'the possibility of [prisoners'] promotion to a less arduous stage by obedience and docility'.[5] Following the death of Joshua Jebb, Chairman of the Directorate of Convict Prisons, in 1863, Sir Walter Crofton, former Director of the Irish Convict Prisons (1854–62), worked with the Home Office on the 1865 Prison Act, developing a version of the progressive system for English prisons.[6] There was support for a similarly punitive penal policy in Ireland, although it was not always implemented in the form of legislative changes. The 1865 English Prison Act, for example, was not extended to Irish local prisons. However, from the 1860s, a shift towards a more penal approach characterised the work of the Inspectors General of Prisons, Dr John Lentaigne and J. Corry Connellan, and their successors.[7]

---

[4] Seán McConville, *English Local Prisons 1860–1900: Next Only to Death* (London and New York: Routledge, 1995), pp. 97–148.

[5] William James Forsythe, *The Reform of Prisoners 1830–1900* (London and Sydney: Croom Helm, 1987), p. 160.

[6] National Library of Ireland (NLI), Mayo Papers, MS 43,817/1, Letter from Walter Crofton to Lord Naas, 8 Oct. 1866.

[7] Report of the Inspectors General of Prisons in Ireland (RIGPI), 1865 (1866) [3690], pp. xlviii–xlix. Hoppen has argued that by the mid-1860s the 'assimilation doctrine', which characterised British policy in Ireland from the 1830s, gave way to an approach that emphasised Irish differences and distinct legislation. See K. Theodore Hoppen, *Governing Hibernia: British Politicians and Ireland 1800–1921* (Oxford: Oxford University Press, 2016), p. 175.

Alarming statistics on recidivism fuelled the growing dissatisfaction with reformist penal policy and advocates of rehabilitation. Increasingly, prison administrators became preoccupied with halting the growth of the prison population and deterring reoffending.[8] The Habitual Criminals Acts of 1869, shaped by Crofton, introduced harsher sentencing for repeat offenders and extended police supervision of released prisoners in England and Ireland.

There was also a push from senior government and prison officials, notably Sir Edmund Du Cane, Chairman of the Directorate of Convict Prisons, and Crofton, for greater levels of centralisation and uniformity in implementing penal policy and regulations, and this underpinned the reconfiguration of administrative structures and the drive for nationalisation.[9] The 1877 Prison Acts centralised the English and Irish prison systems, further eroding the autonomy of local bodies, including the Justices of the Peace and Grand Juries responsible for managing local prisons.[10] In England nationalisation resulted in the establishment of the Prison Commission under Du Cane. Holding the post of chair until 1895, his term was associated with the implementation of strict prison policies and harsh prison conditions, an approach extensively criticised during Gladstone's 1895 Departmental Committee on Prisons. In Ireland, the 1877 Act created the General Prisons Board, initially chaired by Crofton, who was succeeded in October 1878 by Charles F. Bourke, one of two Inspectors General of Prisons. Bourke's brother, Richard Southwell Bourke (Lord Naas), was Chief Secretary for Ireland from July 1866 to September 1868, and an influential voice in shaping penal policy.[11] Among other aims, nationalisation was intended to rationalise

---

[8] Martin J. Wiener, *Reconstructing the Criminal: Culture, Law, and Policy in England, 1830–1914* (Cambridge: Cambridge University Press, 1990), p. 149. For Crofton's influence, see Lawrence Goldman, *Science, Reform, and Politics in Victorian Britain: The Social Science Association, 1857–1886* (Cambridge: Cambridge University Press, 2002), Part II, 'Reform'.

[9] McConville, *English Local Prisons*, pp. 188–234; Beverly A. Smith, 'The Irish General Prisons Board, 1877–1885: Efficient Deterrence or Bureaucratic Ineptitude?', *Irish Jurist*, 15:1 (1980), 122–36; Miles Ogborn, 'Discipline, Government and Law: Separate Confinement in the Prisons of England and Wales, 1830–1877', *Transactions of the Institute of British Geographers*, 20:3 (1995), 295–311. For Du Cane, see Bill Forsythe, 'Du Cane, Sir Edmund Frederick (1830–1903)', *Dictionary of National Biography (DNB)*, https://doi.org/10.1093/ref:odnb/32910 [accessed 3 Feb. 2015].

[10] Smith, 'The Irish General Prisons Board'; Ogborn, 'Discipline, Government and Law'.

[11] Smith, 'The Irish General Prisons Board', p. 123; James Quinn, 'Bourke, Richard Southwell 6th earl of Mayo', in James McGuire and James Quinn (eds), *Dictionary of Irish Biography (DIB)* (Cambridge: Cambridge University Press, 2009), http://dib.cambridge.org/viewReadPage.do?articleId=a0804 [accessed 24 Apr. 2020].

prison estates and produce significant economies, and soon after its introduction, several local prisons were closed and staff dispensed with.[12]

Increasingly prison medical officers became more fully occupied in providing medical attention to prisoners and more directly involved in imposing prison discipline. Prison rules outlining the roles of prison surgeons, developed in the late eighteenth and early nineteenth centuries, were tightened in the 1860s and 1870s, as legislation and prison regulations expanded the duties and responsibilities of prison medical officers. As discussed in Chapter 2, the first sets of regulations charged doctors with regularly visiting prisoners and convicts, especially those placed in separate confinement, to watch out for the adverse effects of the regime. The 1865 English Prison Act, directives from the Home Office and the Chief Secretary's Office, and published rules and regulations for individual prisons, required doctors to attend prisons at least twice a week and to examine each prisoner during these visits.[13] At Mountjoy Convict Prison, a single full-time resident medical officer, Dr James W. Young, was appointed in 1867 to replace two non-resident medical officers, the high-profile Dr Robert McDonnell at the main prison and Dr Awly Banon at Mountjoy Female Prison.[14] The status of some appointees became more prestigious. Dr David Nicolson, who worked as Medical Officer at Woking, Portland, Millbank and Portsmouth Prisons before moving to Broadmoor Criminal Lunatic Asylum in 1876, became a leading authority on prison medicine and criminal

[12] Rosalind Crone with Lesley Hoskins and Rebecca Preston, *Guide to the Criminal Prisons of Nineteenth-Century England*, vol. 1 (London: London Publishing Partnership, 2018), p. 25; McConville, *English Local Prisons*, pp. 149–87; Forsythe, *The Reform of Prisoners*, p. 195; Smith, 'The Irish General Prisons Board', pp. 122–3.

[13] Anne Hardy, 'Development of the Prison Medical Service, 1774–1895', in Richard Creese, W.F. Bynum and J. Bearn (eds), *The Health of Prisoners* (Amsterdam and Atlanta, GA: Rodopi, 1995), pp. 59–82, at pp. 59–61; *Bye-laws for the City of Dublin Prisons by the Board of Superintendence* (Dublin, 1862); *Bye-Laws, Rules and Regulations of the County of Londonderry Gaol* (Londonderry, 1862); *Bye-Laws, Rules and Regulations of the County of Kildare Gaol* (Naas, 1861); *Rules to Be Observed in Mountjoy Male Prison* (Dublin, 1867).

[14] 17&18 Vict., c.76, s.VII (1854); Correspondence Relative to Change in Medical Management of Mountjoy Convict Prison 1868 (1867–68) [502]; 'Mountjoy Prison', *The Irish Times*, 30 Mar. 1868; Report of Directors of Convict Prisons in Ireland (RDCPI), 1867 (1867–68) [4084], p. 7. On his departure from Mountjoy, McDonnell and his supporters claimed the prison authorities orchestrated his removal for being 'too kind' to the prisoners, especially the untried Fenian prisoners held at Mountjoy: Beverly Smith, 'Irish Prison Doctors – Men in the Middle, 1865–90', *Medical History*, 26:4 (1982), 371–94; Banon died suddenly in May 1867. At the time he was physician to Mountjoy Female Convict Prison and Dublin City Prisons, and a surgeon to Jervis Street Hospital. See TPCK/5, Kirkpatrick Medical Biographies, Royal College of Physicians of Ireland.

psychology.[15] Although there was no direct equivalent to Nicolson in Ireland in terms of his professional profile, after his departure from Mountjoy, McDonnell served on the 1884 Royal Commission on Prisons in Ireland, while Dr Hercules MacDonnell, Medical Officer at Dundalk Prison, published on penal policy and, as discussed below, was a vocal critic of the 1877 General Prisons (Ireland) Act.

More generally, by the second half of the century, prison medical officers were emerging as a discrete professional group, notably in convict prisons, where 'they had common professional interests, served a common authority, participated in a recognizable career structure, and evolved for themselves a distinct professional ethos'.[16] Many, like John Campbell and Robert McDonnell, had transferred to prison service following careers in the army and navy, but increasing numbers devoted their entire professional careers, particularly in the convict service, to prison medicine.[17] In line with an increased emphasis in dealing with mental disorder as an aspect of their workload, a small number moved between employment in criminal lunatic or public asylums and prisons. A prison appointment provided a reliable salary and in some cases accommodation, for some in the locales where they had been raised.[18] Dr William Ralph Milner, the son of a local surgeon, who qualified in 1838, was employed as apothecary to Wakefield Dispensary before being appointed resident surgeon to the convict department of Wakefield Prison in 1847 at a salary of £200.[19] The surgeons and doctors employed by local prisons in Ireland had typically served as town dispensary doctors; in 1852 the physician to County Donegal Gaol, Dr Robert Little, had been employed as doctor to the Letterkenny Dispensary, while Dr Thomas Dillon, the magistrate for County Mayo, was the

---

[15] See James Crichton-Browne, 'David Nicolson', *Journal of Mental Science*, 79:324 (Jan. 1933), 1–3.

[16] Hardy, 'Development of the Prison Medical Service', p. 60.

[17] See, for prison surgeons' status and training in early nineteenth-century England, Peter McRorie Higgins, *Punish or Treat?: Medical Care in English Prisons 1770–1850* (Victoria, BC and Oxford: Trafford, 2007), ch. 3.

[18] Crowther and Dupree's expansive survey of doctors entering medical careers in late nineteenth-century Britain concluded that the three members of their cohort taking up full-time prison service were from impoverished backgrounds. One of the three, William Simpson Frew, son of a tilemaker, spent ten years employed in short-term posts before becoming a prison medical officer, first and briefly at Woking and then at Dartmoor, where he spent the rest of his career. M. Anne Crowther and Marguerite W. Dupree, *Medical Lives in the Age of Surgical Revolution* (Cambridge: Cambridge University Press, 2007), pp. 218–19.

[19] Hilary Marland, *Medicine and Society in Wakefield and Huddersfield 1780–1870* (Cambridge: Cambridge University Press, 1987), pp. 263, 413–14.

physician for the County Gaol, surgeon to the County Infirmary and former surgeon to Westport Dispensary.[20]

The career of Dr William Augustus Guy, an authority on prison medicine and prison diet, has been summarised in detail by Anne Hardy, who explains that, unlike many of his contemporaries, he came to the prison service with a set of deeply embedded views and principles. He was an established sanitarian, who had served as Professor of Forensic Medicine and then Dean at King's College London, before taking up the post of Superintending Medical Officer at Millbank Prison between 1859 and 1865.[21] Guy was responsible for introducing a new dietary to English prisons in 1864, directed at reducing food allowances, and held 'unyielding views on the discipline required to achieve social justice', forged by his loathing of idleness and waste.[22] According to Hardy, the contrast with Dr Robert Gover, who succeeded Guy at Millbank and served as Medical Inspector of Local Prisons and Superintending Medical Officer of Convict Prisons after 1877, was stark.[23] Commencing as assistant surgeon at Portsmouth in 1857, and then resident surgeon under Guy at Millbank, Gover spent his entire career in the prison service, and was noted for his pragmatic and humane approach.[24] According to ex-convict Henry Harcourt, who provided detailed evidence to the 1878 Penal Servitude Commission, including details of prison medical officers' cruelties, 'a more humane and better man does not exist than Dr Gover'.[25] Nonetheless, Gover advocated the use of the treadwheel, not least as a guard against shirking, and was vigorous, as shown in Chapter 5, in his efforts to root out the feigning of mental disorder. Dr Patrick O'Keefe, Medical Officer at Spike Island and Mountjoy Convict Prisons from the 1870s, was less popular among prisoners. Prior to his appointment, Inspector Murray had expressed a preference for 'an Irishman, and one if possible who has had some

---

[20] *Irish Medical Directory for 1852* (London: John Churchill, 1853).
[21] Hardy, 'Development of the Prison Medical Service', p. 62; G.T. Bettany, 'Guy, William Augustus (1810–1885)', *DNB*, https://doi.org/10.1093/ref:odnb/11801 [accessed 17 Dec. 2020].
[22] Hardy, 'Development of the Prison Medical Service', p. 63.
[23] Dr Robert Mundy Gover studied medicine at St Bartholomew's London and in Paris, qualifying in 1856. He spent his entire professional life in the prison service, working at Portsmouth Prison, then Millbank, where he was appointed Chief Medical Officer in 1865. He became a Medical Inspector of Prisons in 1878. Royal College of Physicians Munk's Roll: http://munksroll.rcplondon.ac.uk/Biography/Details/1843 [accessed 9 Jan. 2018].
[24] Hardy, 'Development of the Prison Medical Service', pp. 61, 69.
[25] Ibid., p. 69. See also Philip Priestley, *Victorian Prison Lives: English Prison Biography, 1830–1914* (London: Pimlico, 1985), ch. 8 for prisoners' views on prison doctors.

experience in the practical working of a Poor Law rural district'.[26] Citing the positive results derived from the employment of Dr James Young, Resident Medical Officer at the Mountjoy Convict Prison, Murray cautioned against a 'naval or military practitioner'.

These gentlemen … rarely if ever possess that faculty of individualization which should distinguish the medical officer of a convict prison, and they are not habituated to exhibit, whether through feeling or from assumption, the soothing, interested manner which acts so powerfully upon the temperament of the great body of Irish Convicts, whether male or female.[27]

While Young was praised for his kindness, O'Keefe was criticised by Convict E.F. for 'inhuman cruelty' in keeping 'poor maniacs in perpetual cells until reason had become undermined from hunger, flogging, and deprivation of the air of heaven'.[28]

Prison medical officers varied in terms of their commitment to prison work, evidenced by the frequent complaints about their neglect of paperwork, poor record keeping and failure to attend the prison regularly or to absent themselves, noted by magistrates and prison administrators. At Spike Island, Dr Jeremiah Kelly was severely reprimanded by Crofton following the death of a convict who was treated by a hospital attendant in Kelly's absence. On further investigation, Crofton discovered that Kelly was in the habit of leaving the prison for several hours during the night.[29] In turn, prison surgeons grumbled about their expanding workloads and inadequate recompense. F.A. Bulley, surgeon to Reading Gaol, complained in 1853 that his quadrupled workload following the introduction of the separate system had not been matched by a salary increase. Caring for 187 prisoners and 22 officers, he received only £80 per annum compared with the surgeon at York who had a similar number of prisoners but was paid £300. In response to Bulley's request, the magistrates argued that he devolved too much work to his assistant to warrant a salary increase, noted that there were complaints about his tardiness and failure to complete registers and reports, and threatened

---

[26] National Archives Ireland (NAI), Government Prison Office (GPO)/Letter Books (LB), Vol. 9, Jan. 1871–Dec. 1874, Letter from Patrick Murray, 19 Oct. 1872.

[27] Ibid.

[28] Royal Commission into Penal Servitude Acts, Minutes of Evidence [Kimberley Commission] (1878–79) [C.2368] [C.2368–I] [C.2368–II], p. 838.

[29] NAI, GPO/LB, Vol. 15, Jan. 1856–Dec. 1856, Walter Crofton to Dr Kelly, Spike Island, 21 July 1856. For allegations of medical negligence against Kelly at Spike Island Convict Prison, see Cal McCarthy and Barra O'Donnabhain, *Too Beautiful for Thieves and Pickpockets: A History of the Victorian Convict Prison on Spike Island* (Cork: Cork County Library, 2016), pp. 249–78.

him with dismissal.[30] In 1882, the salaries of Irish prison doctors ranged widely from £60 for medical officers at smaller local prison like Castlebar, County Mayo, to £200 for the medical officer at Cork Male and Female prisons, while Young, who served Mountjoy Male and Female Prisons, had a salary of £360.[31]

In the years after nationalisation, new and detailed schedules of responsibilities for prison medical doctors were developed, although positions at local prisons remained part-time and non-residential.[32] By mid-century epidemic diseases had largely vanished from prisons, but the space this created in terms of prison medical officers' workloads was amply filled with cases of mental breakdown. Increasingly, doctors were also required to implement and support the prison's disciplinary practices, to make judgements on the amount of food prisoners required, and determine whether prisoners were mentally and physically fit for labour and punishment.[33] Dr Quinton claimed in his autobiography outlining his career as a prison medical officer that by the late nineteenth century detailed medical examinations were made on reception and great care taken in assessing prisoners' ability to undergo hard labour; this, Quinton suggested, represented a sea change and commitment that many long-serving prison surgeons were not willing to accommodate.[34] Prison regulations also charged prison staff with guarding against the unnecessary infliction of cruelty on physically and mentally 'weak' prisoners and with maintaining the health of prisoners within the testing prison environment. Joe Sim contends that the constraints these regulations placed on prison medical officers, often referred to as 'dual loyalty', hampered the ability of prison medicine to work either independently or benevolently. It produced tensions between doctors' status as employees of the

[30] Berkshire Record Office (BRO), Q/SO/24, County of Berkshire Sessions Order Book, Apr. 1853–July 1855, General Quarter Sessions, Surgeon's Report, 4 Apr. 1853, pp. 4, 6, General Quarter Sessions, Report Visiting Justices, 17 Oct. 1853, p. 156.

[31] *Irish Medical Directory for 1882*. In 1920 the *British Medical Journal* concluded that smaller prisons still provided employment for local medical practitioners, while only larger prisons warranted full-time posts. Salaries for Medical Officer Class II were £300–£500 and for Class I £550–£700, plus unfurnished accommodation or an allowance in lieu. By 1920 there were 15 medical officers Class II, 10 Class I and 33 part-time medical officers. *British Medical Journal* (*BMJ*), 2:3114 (4 Sept. 1920), 377.

[32] Hardy, 'Development of the Prison Medical Service', p. 60; Rules for Local Prisons, Ireland (1878–79) [261], p. lxiii; Copies of Two Orders in Council Approving of Rules and Special Rules made by the General Prisons Board for Ireland, 1885 (1884–85) [132], p. 2; Smith, 'The Irish General Prisons Board'.

[33] Correspondence Relative to Change in Medical Management of Mountjoy Convict Prison 1868 (1867–68), pp. 21–2.

[34] R.F. Quinton, *Crime and Criminals 1876–1910* (London: Longmans, Green and Co., 1910), pp. 55–7.

prison system and their roles in monitoring and approving the disciplinary aspects of the prison regime, and the obligation to care and lobby for the health of their prisoner patients.[35] Martin J. Wiener has also highlighted the 'disciplinary face of Victorian public medicine', arguing that there was an affinity between Victorian punishment and medicine.[36] In this chapter, we consider the repercussions of these regulations for medical officers' management of the mental health of their charges, and ask whether and how deeply medical officers were implicated in the imposition of disciplinary regimes that resulted in or exacerbated mental breakdown. Our research demonstrates significant variation in the ways individual prison medical officers working in England and Ireland implemented discipline and responded to mental breakdown among prisoners, a topic examined in detail in the second section of this chapter.

Simultaneously, medical and psychiatric opinion on the nature and cause of criminality became more penal in the late nineteenth century, as faith in the potential for reform began to evaporate. Penologists and social commentators were disheartened by failed efforts to reform and rehabilitate, and they were, like prison administrators, alarmed about the high level of reconviction. By the late nineteenth century, seeking explanations for past failures and new 'remedies', penologists and psychiatrists researched and published on scientific criminology and the relationship between crime, degeneracy and mental unfitness. Rejecting the theories of Caesar Lombroso and other continental criminologists on the 'born criminal', they emphasised the ways in which criminology in the British Isles varied in approach.[37] Criminologists and psychiatrists in England and Ireland did not, as Forsythe has shown, 'begin to search around for human apes or tribal types for they did not apply a rigid theoretical framework to their descriptions'.[38] Rather, as Campbell's comments at

---

[35] Joe Sim, *Medical Power in Prisons: The Prison Medical Service in England 1774–1989* (Milton Keynes and Philadelphia, PA: Open University Press, 1990), pp. 42–3.

[36] Wiener, *Reconstructing the Criminal*, p. 129; see also Neil Davie, *Tracing the Criminal: The Rise of Scientific Criminology in Britain, 1860–1918* (Oxford: Bardwell Press, 2006), p. 272; Peter Becker and Richard F. Wetzell (eds), *Criminals and Their Scientists: The History of Criminology in International Perspective* (Cambridge: Cambridge University Press, 2006).

[37] Stephen Watson, 'Malingerers, the "Weakminded" Criminal and the "Moral Imbecile": How the English Prison Officer Became an Expert in Mental Deficiency, 1880–1930', in Michael Clark and Catherine Crawford (eds), *Legal Medicine in History* (Cambridge: Cambridge University Press, 1994), pp. 223–41; Davie, *Tracing the Criminal*. For debates on the relationship between criminality and eugenics in the US, see Nicole Hahn Rafter, *Creating Born Criminals* (Champaign, IL: University of Illinois Press, 1997).

[38] Forsythe, *The Reform of Prisoners*, p. 182.

the opening of this chapter demonstrate, they imperfectly absorbed a version of positivist science and evolutionary theories as they became disillusioned with reform. By the 1880s they, along with other social commentators, began to argue that criminality and mental capacities were 'relative constitutional fixedness'.[39]

This chapter also assesses the implications of the altered medical and penal landscape for the mental condition of prisoners in local and convict prisons in late nineteenth-century England and Ireland. While McConville has acknowledged that concerns about the relationship between disciplinary regimes and mental distress in local prisons influenced penal policy, there has been limited analysis of the implications of the refashioning of prison discipline on the minds of prisoners.[40] Wiener has argued that after the debates on the relationship between the separate system of confinement and mental breakdown in the 1830s and 1840s, interest in and commentary on the issue dissipated until the 1870s.[41] Yet disquieting rates of mental disorder continued to be reported in local and convict prisons and were discussed in various official inquiries examining prisons and penal policy as discipline was strictly enforced after the 1860s.

This chapter examines the changing role of the prison medical officer and considers whether the constraints of dual loyalty, alongside overwhelming workloads in environments ill-suited to medical and psychiatric care, overpowered the potential of medical officers to pursue regimes mindful of prisoners' wellbeing, instead becoming 'integral to the control and disciplinary apparatus of the modern prison'.[42] The first section examines the debates around the implementation of changes to penal policy in the late nineteenth century, with a particular focus on the contributions of influential prison medical officers as well as senior prison officials and reformers. It investigates whether those charged by the state with responsibility for prisons and for the minds of prisoners were troubled by the gap between the stated aim of penal policy – that the 'ordinary condition' of prisoners did not allow gratuitous suffering or danger to life and health – and the reality of the institutions they managed. It also considers whether, as penal policy evolved, there was debate and conflict among prison administrators regarding their responsibilities for prisoners' mental wellbeing.

---

[39] Ibid., pp. 183, 187.   [40] McConville, *English Local Prisons*, pp. 291–2.
[41] Wiener, *Reconstructing the Criminal*, p. 125.
[42] Joe Sim, 'The Future of Prison Health Care: A Critical Analysis', *Critical Social Policy*, 22:2 (2002), 300–23, at p. 301.

The second section of the chapter focuses on medical expertise and knowledge production, and assesses the responses of English and Irish prison doctors to the positivist turn in the field of criminal justice and the specific problem of the habitual criminal in terms of their day-to-day practices. Assessments of English criminology by Neil Davie, Stephen Watson and others have focused on debates on the theories of the criminal mind, and the feeble-minded, and how they could be traced, observed and defined.[43] Our sources, which, alongside official reports, include the archives of individual prisons, underline the challenges presented to medical officers by the 'lunatic criminal', in a context shaped increasingly by anxiety about the rise in recidivism, high prison populations and failure to reform. Medical officers became ever more assertive in identifying themselves as experts in prison medicine, and, as Chapters 4 and 5 also explore, in understanding and dealing with mental illness in prison. As Hardy has pointed out, this was challenging work. 'I am completely at the mercy of these men,' Brixton Prison's Medical Officer noted in 1882, alluding to the lack of cell accommodation for 'troublesome mental cases'.[44] Most prison medical officers received little formal or practical training in psychiatry and few had experience of working in lunatic asylums.[45] Yet, as the second section of this chapter demonstrates, prison medical officers formulated a specific taxonomy and classification of mental illness related to lunatics who were also criminals. Local and convict prisons became sites of knowledge production, as prison medical officers developed distinct medical categorisations, which embedded prisoners' criminality and 'criminal natures' in their mental conditions and states. We draw on prison medical officers' descriptions and correspondence about their prisoner patients, and on what became an extensive medical journal literature, which oftentimes dealt deftly and dismissively with continental criminal anthropology, before moving on to the practicalities of management, and to individual cases and examples to explore the everyday management of mental health in prison.

---

[43] Watson, 'Malingerers, the 'Weakminded" Criminal and the "Moral Imbecile'; Davie, *Tracing the Criminal*, pp. 269–81. See also Daniel Pick, *Faces of Degeneration: A European Disorder, c.1848–1918* (Cambridge: Cambridge University Press, 1989).

[44] Hardy, 'Development of the Prison Medical Service', p. 73.

[45] McConville, *English Local Prisons*, pp. 300–1. For the training of English prison officers, see Helen Johnston, '"Reclaiming the Criminal": The Role and Training of Prison Officers in England, 1877 to 1914', *The Howard Journal of Criminal Justice*, 47:3 (2008), 297–312; Helen Johnston, 'Moral Guardians? Prison Medical Officers, Prison Practice and Ambiguity in the Nineteenth Century', in Helen Johnston (ed.), *Punishment and Control in Historical Perspective* (Houndmills: Palgrave Macmillan, 2008), pp. 77–94.

I THE HARDENING OF PENAL POLICY AND PRACTICES

Diet, Labour and the Separate System of Confinement

The two major parliamentary commissions of 1863, reviewing prison regimes in local and convict prisons, encapsulated the shift in tone and approach to late nineteenth-century penal policy. Throughout the 1850s the rigour of the separate system as implemented in convict prisons had been toned down under Jebb's chairmanship of the Directors of Convict Prisons, and prisoners' mental and physical health was reported to have improved under this modified regime.[46] Some early adaptations of the separate system had aroused criticism, not least an experiment at Reading Gaol, implemented by Chaplain Field and aimed at enhancing prisoners' reading and comprehension skills. It was fiercely criticised by the Visiting Justices and Prison Inspectors, and in 1854 penal labour was reasserted at the gaol.[47]

In 1857 and 1864 amendments to the Penal Servitude Acts sought to reinforce the disciplinary regimes in convict prisons. With the death of Jebb in 1863, an influential barrier to the assertion of punitive and deterrent disciplinary ethos in convict prisons was removed.[48] More stringent implementation of the separate system of confinement was advocated, with the 1863 Royal Commission on Transportation and Penal Servitude concluding that penal servitude was not 'sufficiently' dreaded. Witnesses noted, for example, that the average convict spent less than nine months in separate confinement and insisted that the period of separation be implemented fully and ameliorated only when there was a threat of physical or mental injury to convicts.[49] The Commission recommended reversing many of the modifications introduced in the 1850s and advocated for the introduction of separation for able-bodied convicts at the public works prisons at Chatham, Portsmouth, Portland and Gibraltar, and Dartmoor and Woking Invalid Prisons.[50] The system of granting marks or credit for good

---

[46] Seán McConville, *A History of English Prison Administration, Vol. 1, 1750–1877* (London, Boston and Henley: Routledge & Kegan Paul, 1981), p. 405.

[47] Rosalind Crone, 'The Great "Reading" Experiment: An Examination of the Role of Education in the Nineteenth-Century Gaol', *Crime, History & Societies*, 16:1 (2012), 47–74.

[48] McConville, *English Local Prisons*, p. 154.

[49] Royal Commission to Inquire into Operation of Acts Relating to Transportation and Penal Servitude. Report, Appendix, Minutes of Evidence [Royal Commission on Transportation and Penal Servitude] (1863) [3190] [3190–I], pp. 13, 23, 40.

[50] Ibid., p. 13.

conduct adopted in Irish and English convict prisons was criticised as was the practice of granting convicts marks for diligence in Irish prison schools.[51] The Commissioners noted differences in the administration of penal servitude legislation in England and Ireland, and commended the 'formidable' rendering of the separate system under Crofton's system in Ireland. In addition to the operation of intermediate prisons, and the supervision of holders of tickets of leave, in terms of the implementation of the separate system during the probationary stage at Mountjoy, they specifically praised the lower, meat-free diet provided during the first four months in separation and limiting work to oakum picking in the first three months.[52] These rigorous elements of the separate system, they argued, increased the 'wholesome effect' on the minds of prisoners.[53] The Commission sought greater severity in sentencing penal servitude convicts, the introduction of the 'progressive' or 'mark system' in English prisons, and tighter implementation of the separate system. Colonel Edmund Henderson, who succeeded Jebb as Chairman of the Directorate of Convict Prisons in 1863, implemented many of these recommendations; the provision of 'extra diets' was prohibited except on medical grounds, hammocks in separate cells were substituted with plank beds, and convicts were to spend the full nine months in separation except in cases of serious injury to mental or physical health.[54]

Lord Carnarvon's 1863 Select Committee was particularly important in shaping policy in local and borough county prisons. Witnesses were quizzed on the high levels of recidivism among prisoners, poorly trained staff and substantial variations in the implementation of regulations. Prison inspectors and other medical and lay experts on penology identified local prisons as particularly problematic, repeatedly criticising them for failing to impose rigorous and uniform systems of discipline, though it was acknowledged that sentences in local prisons were too short for the full application of the separate system. They were also accused of overfeeding prisoners and lax supervision of ticket-of-leave prisoners.[55] When published, the recommendations of the Carnarvon Committee reinforced the social function of prison while its reformative aim was downplayed.[56] The 'moral reformation of character', Carnarvon insisted,

---

[51] Ibid., p. 29.   [52] Ibid., p. 40.   [53] Ibid.
[54] McConville, *The History of English Prison Administration*, p. 406; Correspondence between the Secretary of State for the Home Department and the Directors of Convict Prisons, on the Recommendations of the Royal Commission on the Penal Servitude Acts (1864) [61], pp. 4, 18, 40.
[55] Forsythe, *The Reform of Prisoners*, pp. 146–9.
[56] Report from the Select Committee of the House of Lords on the Present State of Discipline in Gaols and Houses of Correction [Carnarvon Committee] (1863) [499], p. xii.

was 'greatly assisted by a preliminary course of stringent punishment'.[57] While retaining the separate system as the basis for penal discipline in local prisons, Carnarvon sought to configure specific elements of the regime, notably prison labour, diet and the environment of the cell, to heighten the punitive experience.[58]

Carnavon's recommendations set the tone for debate on local prisons across England and Ireland, and specifically shaped the English Prison Act of 1865.[59] In Ireland, Corry Connellan, Inspector General for Prisons, advocated in 1863 for the introduction of many of the committee's recommendations to local prisons. He helped draft a Prisons (Ireland) Bill in 1866, which, if implemented, would have consolidated legislation relating to prisons in Ireland and introduced elements of the 1865 English Prison Act.[60] The Chief Secretary for Ireland, Lord Naas, was an influential proponent of the bill, but, while reaching a second reading in the House of Lords, it fell foul of the extremely busy parliamentary sessions in 1866 and 1867 and did not pass into legislation. Nonetheless, the separate system was scheduled for implementation in local prisons as provision expanded in the 1860s, including the opening in 1863 of a new east wing with over 100 cells for separate confinement at Kilmainham Gaol, Dublin (Figure 3.1).

The remit of the Carnarvon Committee was wide-ranging, and specific aspects of penal discipline, notably what constituted hard labour, prison diet and the conditions and implementation of separate confinement, were forensically examined. The effectiveness of these aspects of prison discipline was debated during subsequent inquiries into English and Irish penal policy over the next three decades, including the 1878 Commission on the Penal Servitude Acts (the Kimberley Commission), and the 1884 Royal Commission on Irish Prisons, which reviewed the implementation of prison legislation in local and convict prisons. Primarily concerned with balancing the punitive and reformative aims of imprisonment, prison officials, penologists and a small number of ex-prisoners debated the deleterious impact of the new disciplinary regimes on prisoners' physical and mental health in their evidence to these inquiries. In addition, as the duties of prison medical officers were

---

[57] Ibid.   [58] Wiener, *Reconstructing the Criminal*, p. 108.
[59] McConville, *English Local Prisons*, pp. 97–148.
[60] RIGPI, 1865 (1866) [3690], pp. xlviii–xlix; Prisons (Ireland) Bill to Consolidate and Amend the Law relating to Prisons in Ireland (1866), iv; Hansard HC Deb, 10 May 1866, vol. 183 cc671–2, Sir Robert Peel. See James Quinn, 'Bourke, Richard Southwell 6th earl of Mayo', *DIB*, https://doi.org/10.3318/dib.000804.v1 [accessed 24 Apr. 2020].

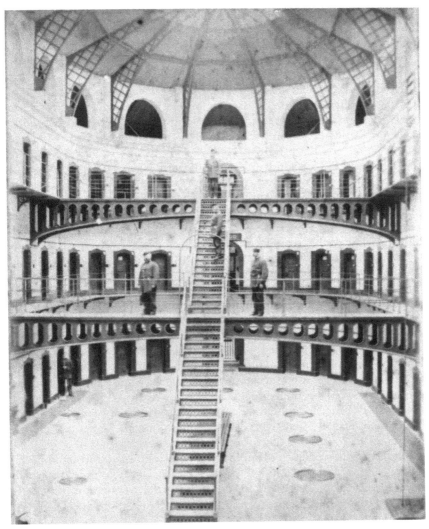

Figure 3.1 Interior of East Wing, Kilmainham Gaol, Dublin by
Thomas Flewett, Deputy Governor, 1860s
Source: Irish Architectural Archive, Dublin

reconfigured and bolstered, some medical officers highlighted the challenges of aligning their roles and responsibilities in safeguarding the
mental health of prisoners with the increasingly penal approach of the
prison environment.

The push for uniform and rigid application of prison discipline across the prison estate in the 1860s and 1870s was partly a response to high-profile reports, including those of physiologist and social reformer, Dr Edward Smith, that highlighted the uneven implementation of prison discipline.[61] In the late 1850s Smith had surveyed the effects of prison discipline on prisoners' health in English county gaols, and his analysis of the dietary requirements of prisoners on hard labour were submitted to the Carnarvon Committee and published in the final report.[62] His work, reported in the *Lancet* in 1858, revealed uneven enforcement of hard labour across the English prison estate, and in some instances he found 'no labour at all'.[63] Smith observed disparities in the types of labour designated as hard labour; in one prison, 'oakum-picking was no labour ... and hard labour in another'.[64] He also claimed women were placed at the crank and treadwheel in some prisons, although George Laval Chesterton, Governor at Cold Bath Fields Prison in Clerkenwell, had complained that women, who 'could not expect the same chivalrous sympathy accorded to their more morally upright sisters', did not work at the treadwheel.[65] Considering the implementation of the separate system in local prisons, Smith reported strict enforcement of all elements in some prisons, including prisoners being compelled to wear masks when moved around the prison, while elsewhere 'hundreds of prisoners sit together in the room picking oakum'.[66] He also drew attention to the varied punishments inflicted on prisoners, noting unequal application of corporeal punishments including whipping by officers using the 'cat'.[67] In his evidence to the Carnarvon Committee, Smith sought absolute uniformity of prison punishments, and claimed prisoners were idle for long periods of each day. He suggested they perform not less than 7½ or 8 hours of work a day when serving hard labour sentences, and a minimum of 10 hours a day for other prisoners.[68]

The imprint of Smith's findings can be identified throughout the report and recommendations of the Carnarvon Committee, which rejected oakum picking, and forms of industrial occupation, originally intended to improve prisoners' minds as well as punish them, as 'light' or

[61] Kenneth J. Carpenter, 'Smith, Edward (1819–1874)', *DNB*, https://doi.org/10.1093/ref: odnb/25794 [accessed 4 Mar. 2020].
[62] Carnarvon Committee (1863), pp. 505–12.
[63] Anon., 'Influence of Prison Discipline on Health', *Lancet*, 72:1820 (17 July 1858), 70–1, at p. 71.
[64] Ibid.
[65] Lucia Zedner, *Women, Crime and Custody in Victorian England* (Oxford: Clarendon Press, 1991), p. 140.
[66] Anon., 'Influence of Prison Discipline on Health', p. 71.   [67] Ibid.
[68] Carnarvon Committee (1863), Evidence of Dr Edward Smith, p. 75.

'immediate' labour, and only accepted punitive work at the treadwheel and crank as 'hard labour' proper (Figure 3.2). Shot drill was permitted when local authorities needed to supplement the treadwheel and crank.[69] In designating these three forms of work as 'hard labour', they explicitly rejected the positive impact of industrial labour on prisoners' minds as 'much less penal, irksome, and fatiguing' in favour of punitive hard labour intended to make prisoners' experiences more unbearable.[70] In Ireland, Connellan advocated Carnarvon's recommendations, lamenting the lack of 'punitive labour' in local prisons, which, he argued had been imperfectly replaced by industrial labour, a change he dismissed as futile. With the publication of the Report of the Carnarvon Committee, he sought its reintroduction to county prisons, and suggested the separate system be extended to prison hospitals to prevent communication among patients.[71]

Several witnesses to the Carnarvon Committee were troubled by some of the proposals. Dr John George Perry, Inspector of Prisons for the Southern and Western Districts and the Medical Inspector of Prisons in England and Wales, emphasised the dangers of the treadwheel to prisoners' health. He sought its abolition 'on account of the inequality of its operation', 'its injurious effect upon the health of many of the prisoners', and 'when unproductive, a waste of labour which might be better bestowed'.[72] Major William Fulford, Governor at Stafford Prison, however, suggested to the committee that he already had the powers to impose a deterrent and severe regime, which in his view should combine hard labour with a low diet and use of the whip:

If I had the means of giving every man who is sentenced to hard labour in Stafford prison the full amount of discipline I am empowered to do by Act of Parliament, for two years, no man alive could bear it: it would kill the strongest man in England.[73]

Other witnesses referred specifically to the 'irritating' impact of the crank and treadwheel on the minds of prisoners, with some prisoners finding unproductive work 'disheartening', 'depressing' and leading them to despair.[74]

Nonetheless, work at the treadwheel was selected as the preferred form of hard labour and prison officials sought its implementation across local prisons. In Ireland, there was variation in the form of hard labour

[69] Ibid., p. vii.   [70] Ibid.
[71] RIGPI, 1863 (1864), Memorandum by Mr Corry Connellan, pp. xlii–lii.
[72] Carnarvon Committee (1863), Evidence of Dr John George Perry, pp. 47, 51.
[73] Ibid., Evidence of Major William Fulford, p. 156.
[74] Ibid., Evidence of Sir Joshua Jebb, p. 116.

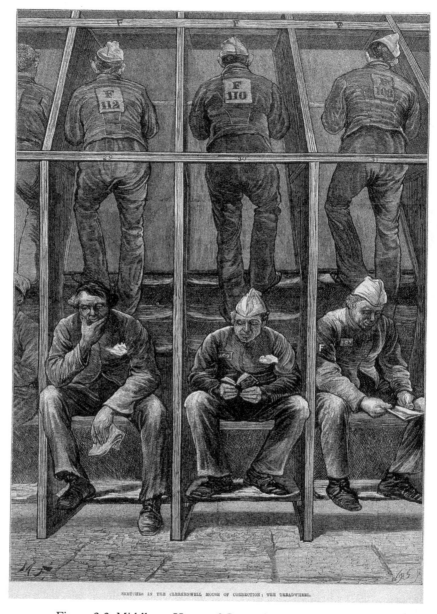

Figure 3.2 Middlesex House of Correction: male prisoners on
treadmill. Wood engraving by W.B. Gardner, 1874, after M. Fitzgerald
Credit: Wellcome Collection. Attribution 4.0 International (CC BY 4.0)

depending on conditions at individual gaols, and the treadwheel was not systematically introduced. However, by 1880, it was implemented at Castlebar, Clonmel, Richmond, and Galway and Cork Male Prisons. At other local prisons, male inmates picked rope junk or oakum, worked at shot drill, which, according to Priestley, was virtually ignored in English local prisons, or broke stones.[75] In prisons with a sizeable female population, such as Belfast, Kilmainham, Cork and Grangegorman, women usually worked at picking rope or oakum.[76] After nationalisation those confined at Mountjoy Male Prison were employed at mat making and picking coir in cells, while convicts in Mountjoy Female Prison made bedding and clothing, and did the laundry for other prisons and institutions.[77] By 1882, however, Frederick Richard Falkiner, Recorder of Dublin, criticised the continued use of the treadwheel and shot drill in some prisons, as well as 'the almost valueless oakum and hair picking, and the mat making' in others.[78] Alongside the deferral of legislative reforms, for him the persistence of such prison labour was evidence of the deterioration of the Irish system, once praised as 'the best solution of the convict problem, and a model for imitation in Europe and America'.[79]

Most parliamentary commissions on prisons were preoccupied with the relationship between prison diet, punishment and discipline, and several witnesses highlighted the potentially negative effects of reduced diet on the minds of prisoners. Jebb stressed the importance of a 'good diet', which Reverend W.L. Clay had dismissed as 'belly bribes' for prisoners serving long sentences at Pentonville Prison in his evidence to Carnarvon's Committee, arguing it counteracted the 'depressing influences of separate confinement'.[80] An advocate of separate confinement, Jebb insisted the separate cell had a 'very corrective effect upon the mind of a prisoner'.[81] As early as 1849, as discussed in Chapter 2, Jebb had, however, become concerned that a severely reduced diet could damage the mental as well as physical health of convicts.[82] Dietary modifications to reduce costs at Wakefield Prison, he claimed, were a false economy

---

[75] Priestley, *Victorian Prison Lives*, p. 166; RGPBI, 1879–80 (1880) [C.2689], pp. 90–109.
[76] RGPBI, 1879–80 (1880), pp. 90–109.   [77] Ibid., pp. 113, 121.
[78] F.R. Falkiner, 'Our Habitual Criminals', *Journal of the Statistical and Social Inquiry Society of Ireland*, 8:60 (Aug. 1882), 317–30, at p. 327.
[79] Ibid.
[80] Carnarvon Committee (1863), Evidence of Reverend W.L. Clay, p. 124; Reverend W.L. Clay, *Our Convict Systems* (Cambridge: Macmillan and Co., 1862), p. 41.
[81] Carnarvon Committee (1863), Evidence of Sir Joshua Jebb, pp. 120, 124.
[82] The National Archives (TNA), HO 45/1451, Lunacy; Poor Law and Paupers; Prisons and Prisoners, Sept. 1846–Jan. 1849, Convict Department at Wakefield, J. Jebb to Home Office, 6 Jan. 1849, Memo by Lieut Colonel Jebb in Reply to Sir George Grey's Queries on Mr Hill's Letter of 18 Dec. 1848.

given that 'imprisonment injudiciously prolonged after unequivocal symptoms of failing health had appeared or an insufficiency of diet', rendered the convicts mentally and physically depressed and unfit for transportation, and was thus a long-term drain on prison resources.[83] Two years earlier, William Milner, Medical Officer at Wakefield Prison, had become concerned about the 'unmanageable' delusions among prisoners in separate confinement, and in response had increased dietary allowances and periods of exercise, modifications that appeared to have benefited the prisoners.[84]

The importance of a 'sufficient' diet was stressed by Inspector Perry, who commented on the restorative and medicinal use of diet by prison surgeons not only to 'treat disease but to prevent it'. He sought extra dietary allowances to restore the constitutions of enfeebled and physically debilitated prisoners, especially vagrants.[85] Nonetheless, there were those who advocated for sparser dietary scales, including Fulford at Stafford, on the grounds that prisoners on shorter sentences were not required to perform hard labour.[86] Concerns about prisoners becoming too enfeebled and physically incapacitated to work on release, the threat of epidemic disease outbreaks in prisons, and maintaining prisoners' capacity to perform labour, prompted the Carnarvon Committee to defer any proposals for a national, uniform dietary scale for local prisons, and concluded that prison diet was not to be used as an instrument of punishment.[87]

The quality and quantity of prison diet in Ireland was also scrutinised in the 1860s. As in England, diet in local prisons was sparser than in convict prisons; nonetheless, these dietary scales had been criticised for their generosity when compared to the diets of the average agricultural labourer, workhouse dietaries and the sparser diets implemented in English local prisons. A lower dietary scale was introduced in 1849, and further reductions implemented in 1854 for prisoners aged fifteen years and under, to align prison and workhouse diets for that age group.[88] Cautioning against further reductions, in 1863 the Irish lawyer and politician Edward Gibson insisted that once a fair, 'sufficiently penal' diet had been agreed, diet should be 'regarded as a medical question'. 'The system of starving crime into surrender', Gibson argued, if it went

---

[83] Ibid. (emphasis in original).
[84] Wakefield Record Office, QS 10/56, Quarter Sessions Order Book, Oct. 1846–Apr. 1850, Wakefield Adjourned Sessions, Surgeon's Report, 9 Dec. 1847, p. 98.
[85] Carnarvon Committee (1863), Evidence of J.G. Perry, pp. 133, 134.
[86] Ibid., Evidence of Major W. Fulford, p. 156.
[87] McConville, *English Local Prisons*, pp. 118–21, 304.
[88] RIGPI, 1849 (1850) [1229], p. ix; RIGPI, 1854 (1854–55) [1956], p. xiv.

below the limit necessary for health, would prompt expensive hospital admissions, with prisoners liable to become burdens on the rates once released. Consequently, the 'superiority' of prison food 'must again be asserted'.[89] The 1863 Commission on Transportation and Penal Servitude recommended that the practice of not providing meat during the first months in separation in Irish prisons be extended to English convict prisons, and, while they did not advocate for the reduction of diet for convicts working in association in public works prisons, they suggested some experimentation 'to ascertain whether any reduction can safely be made'.[90]

From 1863 the disciplinary regime applied to penal servitude convicts in separation became more punitive, and by 1878 the Kimberley Commission concluded that the sentence was 'generally an object of dread to the criminal population'.[91] Dietary privileges, including those allowed at Mountjoy Convict Prison, were abolished and the reduced diet for convicts during the first three months of their sentences was enforced.[92] These changes prompted concern from penologists, including Crofton, who defended the relatively generous dietary scales for convicts against criticism from the Board of Superintendence of Dublin City Prisons on the grounds that convicts were required to preform hard labour.[93] In 1863, Reverend Charles Bernard Gibson, Chaplain at Spike Island, also warned against reducing convict diets further, but he reasoned that depriving convicts of employment during their first months in 'solitary cells' was more damaging as it deprived 'the mind of its proper food'.[94] Responding to these concerns, a medical committee, comprising the eminent physician Dr William Stokes, Dr John Hill, the Poor Law Medical Inspector, and Dr William M. Burke, Medical Superintendent at the General Register Office, were appointed to inquire into dietary scales in Irish county and borough gaols.[95] On their

[89] Edward Gibson, 'Penal Servitude and Tickets of Leave', *Journal of the Statistical and Social Inquiry Society of Ireland*, 3:23 (Apr. 1863), 332–43, at pp. 334, 335; Patrick Maume, 'Gibson, Edward 1st Baron Ashbourne', *DIB*, https://doi.org/10.3318/dib .003457.v2 [accessed 16 Mar. 2020].

[90] Royal Commission on Transportation and Penal Servitude (1863), pp. 41, 42.

[91] Kimberley Commission (1878–79), p. xxvi.   [92] Ibid., pp. xvi, xxiii.

[93] Walter Crofton, 'Irish Convict System', *The Irish Times*, 17 Jan. 1863.

[94] Charles Bernard Gibson, *Life among Convicts* (London: Hurst and Blackett, 1863), p. 56.

[95] Helen Andrews, 'Stokes, William', *DIB*, https://doi.org/10.3318/dib.008336.v1 [accessed 16 Mar. 2020]; see Hill's obituary in *BMJ*, 1:529 (18 Feb. 1871), 184; Dr William Malachy Burke (1819–79) was physician at Dr Steeven's Hospital, Dublin, and Physician in Ordinary to the Lord Lieutenant of Ireland, 1866–68 and 1874–76. He was Medical Superintendent in the General Register Office from 1864 to 1876. See C.A. Cameron, *History of the Royal College of Surgeons in Ireland* (Dublin: Fanin and Company, 1916), p. 557.

recommendation, in 1868 prison governors were ordered to improve the quality of the food.[96] In their final published report, the commissioners highlighted the tensions inherent in the role of the prison surgeons. It was, they noted, inconsistent 'with the character and the objects of medical science, that the Surgeon should be compelled to watch for the time when the punishment can be no longer endured, and so virtually to become, in his own capacity, an assistant to the execution of a sentence'.[97]

The nationalisation of both prison systems under the 1877 Prison Acts reopened the debate on prison diet. The Acts enabled prison boards to further enforce the punitive and disciplinary regimes in both convict and local prisons. Rationalisation, frugality and disciplinary rigour preoccupied Du Cane and Charles Bourke, and Du Cane established a scientific committee on prison diet, which reported in February 1878.[98] Comprising Henry Briscoe, Inspector of English Prisons, Dr Robert Gover, Medical Officer at Millbank Prison, and C. Hitchman Braddon, Medical Officer at Salford Hundred County Prison, it was charged with considering whether changes to prison discipline brought in under the 1877 Act necessitated new dietary scales, especially in cases when the period prisoners spent at hard labour was reduced. The committee members framed imprisonment as a 'physiological rest' when the 'struggle for survival is suspended', with prisoners guaranteed food and other necessities. Considering the psychology of prisoners, they contended that 'Tranquility of mind and freedom from anxiety are leading characteristics of his [the prisoner's] life. From the moment that the prison gates close behind him, the tendency, in most cases, is to lessened waste of tissue; he lives, in fact, less rapidly than before.'[99] Labour exacted on inmates in local prisons, they argued, was not 'excessive', while 'wholesome' work, whether mental or physical, was not normally lethal. 'Worry', however, was more dangerous, as it was a 'rust, which eats into the blade and destroys it', although prisoners, 'as a rule' were free from it.[100] The committee's published report repeatedly referenced the 'mental peace' and tranquillity of life in prison, which was characterised as a protected and insulated existence, with prisoners free from the

[96] Report of the Committee on Dietaries in County and Borough Gaols, Ireland (1867–68) [3981], p. 33.
[97] Ibid., p. 29.
[98] Smith, 'The Irish General Prisons Board, 1877–1885', p. 134; McConville, *English Local Prisons*, pp. 220, 304.
[99] Report of the Committee Appointed to Inquire into the Dietaries of the Prisons in England and Wales subject to the Prison Acts 1865 and 1877 (1878) [C.95], p. 5.
[100] Ibid.

emotional strife that can 'exhaust the vital energies' in everyday life. The prisoner 'rarely experiences domestic grief or disappointment; and, as a general rule, he has no pride capable of receiving a wound'.[101] While briefly acknowledging that 'the restraints of discipline' and the loss of liberty could be irksome and a 'severe trial', and 'that what appears to us to be peace and order may to the inmates be often indistinguishable from gloom and monotony', the overall tone of the report minimised the difficulties of prison life.[102] Deviating from the 1868 recommendations of the medical committee on Irish dietary scales, Du Cane's committee did not highlight any potential tension in the role of the prison medical officers and instead reiterated the importance of the judgement of the prison doctor in deciding whether prisoners should be allocated extra allowances of food.[103] The committee recommended that prison medical officers retain discretionary power to approve extras, and, while noting that diet should not be diminished where health was damaged, they cautioned against prison doctors allocating too liberal a diet.[104]

A modified version of English prison diet, scheduled for Irish prisons under the 1877 Prison Act, was delayed owing to disagreement among the Irish medical profession on its suitability. However, a second medical commission, established by the Irish General Prisons Board in 1880, concluded the new scales were 'sufficiently liberal'. As with the English commission, they agreed prison doctors should be permitted to make minor alterations for 'diseased' prisoners, but disapproved 'of any interference with the dietary scales as laid down for healthy prisoners'.[105] They also introduced amendments to the convict prison diets at Spike Island and Mountjoy Male and Female Prisons.[106] The 1884 Royal Commission on Irish Prisons claimed that changes to prison diet contributed to increased expenditure.[107] Nonetheless, the Commission recommended enhanced dietary allowances for specific classes of prisoners owing to the inferior bodily condition of Irish prisoners, whose previous habits, poor quality of foodstuff and their 'generally low physical condition of health render them more susceptible to the effects of prison discipline'.[108] Despite earlier attempts by the General Prisons Board to halt such practices, the Commission noted that medical officers frequently prescribed improved diets as a prophylactic against illness among

---

[101] Ibid., p. 6.   [102] Ibid.   [103] Ibid., p. 29.
[104] McConville, *English Local Prisons*, p. 306.
[105] RGPBI, 1880–81 (1881) [C.3067], p .2.   [106] Ibid., p. 15.
[107] Royal Commission on Prisons in Ireland, Second Report (1884) [C.4145], pp. 15, 31.
[108] Royal Commission on Prisons in Ireland, Vol. 1. Reports, Digest of Evidence, Appendices; Minutes of Evidence, 1884 (1884–85) [C.4233] [C.4233–I], p. 34.

'juvenile offenders, nursing mothers, and aged prisoners ... although as a matter of fact such prisoners are in excellent health'.[109]

While debates on prison diet and the implementation of hard labour dominated discussions of penal discipline in the late nineteenth century, other aspects of prison discipline, which affected prisoners' mental and physical health, were critically reviewed, including hammock-style bedding, which had been used in separate cells since the implementation of the separate system. Following Carnarvon's recommendations, hammocks, believed to be too comfortable, a 'self-indulgence', were replaced with plank beds usually without any mattress, for inmates serving the first stage of sentence.[110] Inspector Perry, however, warned against their widespread use, as they caused repeated sleepless nights and impaired mental and physical health.[111] In 1884 the leading Irish nationalist parliamentarian Charles Stewart Parnell, who viewed prison diet and the treadwheel as too severe a punishment, noting the 'semi-starved' aspect of the prisoners at Kilmainham Gaol, described the plank bed as a 'punishment attended with physical torture'.[112] Society, Parnell argued, was not entitled 'to enfeeble the bodies of prisoners in order to reform their minds, or with a view of maintaining discipline amongst them'.[113] Dr Hercules McDonnell, echoing Parnell in his objection to the plank beds, insisted 'punishment should not include cruelty, nor should it impair health'. He argued against their use 'in long term sentences ... from a moral point of view. It engenders a mental state of resistence [sic] to authority, and renders the prisoner less amenable to discipline or the better influences which ought primarily to be cultivated.'[114]

MacDonnell was one of many detractors of the revised disciplinary regimes of the 1860s and 1870s and the relentless drive to impose a uniform punitive system. Witnesses at Carnarvon and subsequent committees cited the potential damage the harsher disciplinary regimes could inflict on prisoners' spirits, and ultimately their minds, and their implementation elicited further debate on the link between the separate system of confinement and incidences of mental disorder and distress in prisons.

---

[109] Ibid., pp. 26, 27, 178. See Ciara Breathnach, 'Medical Officers, Bodies, Gender and Weight Fluctuation in Irish Convict Prisons, 1877–95', *Medical History*, 58:1 (2014), 67–86.

[110] Carnarvon Committee (1863), p. 121.

[111] Ibid., pp. 21–22 and Evidence of Inspector Perry, pp. 120, 149.

[112] Royal Commission on Prisons in Ireland, 1884 (1884–85), pp. 339, 343.

[113] Ibid., p. 339.

[114] Hercules MacDonnell, 'Notes on Some Continental Prisons', *Journal of the Statistical and Social Inquiry Society of Ireland*, 9:64 (July 1886), 81–95, at p. 88.

In their critiques, prison medical officers, chaplains and other prison officials explicitly connected mental disorder among prisoners and convicts to the new punitive prison regimes, and modified versions of the separate system were introduced to some local prisons in England and Ireland. Proponents of the new penal regimes, meanwhile, persistently argued that many prisoners entered prison predisposed to mental weakness and were constitutionally unable to withstand its rigour or benefit from it, rather than blaming the regime for prompting mental breakdown and insanity.

In 1863 a number of key prison administrators, including Inspector Perry, Herbert Voules, the Inspector for the Northern District, and Edward Shepherd, Governor at West Riding Prison, Wakefield, objected to various measures proposed for local prisons, citing the potential for damage to the minds of prisoners. Perry, for example, contended that prisoners found unproductive labour such as the treadwheel and the crank demoralising, degrading and irritating, having a 'prejudicial effect on the temper of the men' and 'resulting in 'insubordination produced by irritation and despair'.[115] Jebb, who acknowledged the 'depressing influence' of unproductive labour, also downplayed it, insisting that 'some prisoners will resist anything that is disagreeable to them'.[116] Such commentary highlighted an enduring ambiguity: on the one hand, prison administrators commented on the harm inflicted on prisoners by prison discipline and environments, and, on the other hand, demonstrated a persistent faith in the overall efficacy of prison discipline and in the separate system. Voules agreed that 'unproductive employment', such as the treadwheel, led to the degradation and irritation of the minds of prisoners and that separation was a 'severe punishment' to prisoners.[117] Yet he insisted that the separate system was 'the only safe foundation of prison discipline ... it forces a man to reflect; it makes him feel that employment is a boon ... and it separates him from [the] contaminating influence of other prisoners'.[118] In 1863, Jebb suggested the 'depressing influences' of separation were partly a consequence of the reduced amount of exercise required of convicts while working at a trade, but that 'any deleterious effect' on prisoners would be mitigated with sufficient fresh air and exercise.[119] Dr Clarke at Pentonville, however, noted that prolonged periods in separation produced a 'debilitating effect upon

[115] Carnarvon Committee (1863), Evidence of J.G. Perry, pp. 51, 116, 117; Clay, *Our Convict Systems*, p. 41.
[116] Carnarvon Committee (1863), Evidence of Sir Joshua Jebb, p. 116.
[117] Ibid., p. 187, Evidence of Herbert Voules, pp. 192–3, 203.   [118] Ibid., p. 186.
[119] Ibid., Evidence of Sir Joshua Jebb, p. 126.

men', and in 1870 observed that the moral influence of solitary confinement was, 'if not hurtful to the mind, at least negative for good'.[120] However, defending the separate system, Dr William Guy, Medical Superintendent of Millbank Prison, observed:

> Our system of separate confinement does not appear to affect the mind injuriously. I do not mean to say that a prisoner who comes into prison upon the verge of unsoundness of mind, might not develop into full unsoundness in that time, partly because of the separation; but I am of opinion, also that a prisoner should expect that this may happen to him, and that the possibility of unsoundness must be taken into account as one of the results of his being in prison at all.[121]

Irish prison staff showed similar disquiet and ambivalence. In 1862 Dr Maurice Corr, Medical Officer at Philipstown Prison, which housed a large number of invalids, noted the 'great irritability and total destitution of self control' among prisoners whose 'mental disease' was 'generated and fostered in prison', while Michael Cody, Roman Catholic chaplain at Mountjoy Male Prison, objected to subjecting prisoners to separate discipline for eight months.[122] Disagreeing with the Directors of Convict Prisons in 1869, at a time when the prison population at Mountjoy had declined by two-thirds, Cody argued 'that to subject the prisoners to the separate discipline for eight months is calculated to injuriously affect them mentally as well as physically' as the regime had 'the effect of gradually causing depression of spirits, nervousness, eccentricity, and causing, what is most to be deplored, loss of that controlling power by which man governs his imagination, course of thought, and inferior appetite'.[123]

Despite these concerns, and the disastrous experiences at Pentonville in the 1840s, in the late nineteenth century support for separate confinement remained entrenched among senior prison officials. Medical Inspector Dr Gover, commenting favorably on conditions in Millbank Prison in 1870, noted that among the 27 convicts certified as insane, 25 were sick on admission and two had histories of mental illness. Defending the disciplinary regime, he observed that 'No case came under my observation, of which it could be said that the mental disease had been brought on by the discipline of the prison.'[124] In 1874

---

[120] Cited in David Nicolson 'Parliamentary Blue Books: Reports of Directors of Convict Prisons, in England, Ireland and Scotland, for the Year 1870', *Journal of Mental Science*, 18:82 (July 1872), 256–62, at p. 260.
[121] Carnarvon Committee (1863), Evidence of Dr William Guy, p. 370.
[122] RDCPI, 1861 (1862) [2983], p. 47; RDCPI, 1869 (1870) [C.108], p. 18.
[123] RDCPI, 1869 (1870), p. 18.
[124] RDCP, 1870 (1871) [C.449], Millbank Prison, p. 77.

Millbank's chaplain described separate confinement, 'as the only chance' of bringing prisoners under 'moral or religious influence', insisting the prison's regime had no injurious mental or physical consequences. While acknowledging that strict implementation of separation for the whole sentence of penal servitude was harmful, he advocated in favour of minimum association among prisoners as 'the most successful in its reformatory and deterring effects on the criminal'.[125]

Despite Hercules McDonnell's criticisms, there was greater acknowledgement during the 1884 Royal Commission on Irish Prisons of the dangers the separate system posed to prisoners' minds. Captain John Barlow, Director of Irish Prisons, under questioning from Dr George Sigerson, conceded that 'The cellular discipline of Mountjoy would I suppose tend to develop insanity.'[126] Sigerson claimed 'the number of male convicts becoming insane at Mountjoy would exceed three times' the number found in prisons that were not operating the separate system.[127] The final report criticised prison medical officers for failing to rigorously examine prisoners on reception to identify incipient diseases, especially symptoms of mental illness, and recommended reception wards be provided in prisons to allow for the close observation of prisoners on admission. With early identification such prisoners could be quickly removed to hospitals, or carefully observed, and so 'prevent the infliction of punishment for breaches of discipline committed by prisoners suffering from nervous irritability, who really are more properly subjects for medical treatment than for punishment'.[128]

'A Servant of the Board'? Medical Officers and Prison Practices and Regimens

While the degree of uniformity originally sought by senior prison officials, including Du Cane, was never realised, cumulatively the legislative and policy changes of the 1860s and 1870s had a striking impact on prison life and prisoners. McConville has suggested that conditions in English local prisons were especially harsh with little support for the reformative objective of imprisonment. For inmates the prison environment became more taxing, rigorous, and in some instances brutal, especially in prisons that were overcrowded, insanitary and the physical

---

[125] RDCP, 1874 (1875) [C.1346], Millbank Prison, p. 210.
[126] Royal Commission on Prisons in Ireland, 1884 (1884–85), p. 277.   [127] Ibid.
[128] Royal Commission on Prisons in Ireland, Second Report (1884), p. 22.

infrastructure dilapidated.[129] Conditions in Irish local prisons were like-
wise severe, and, in terms of sanitation, often dangerous, though, as
Beverly Smith has argued, it is unclear whether these conditions reflected
a coherent penal policy or the General Prisons Board's bad management.[130] Officers in some local prisons struggled to maintain discipline
and order, and their efforts to implement prison regimes could be fierce
and relentless, especially when managing irritable, destructive and violent prisoners, many of whom were described as mentally ill-equipped
and unable to withstand prison discipline. There were also instances of
neglect, cruelty and poor management by badly trained staff.

As noted above, the 1865 English Prison Act tightened regulations to
ensure regular medical visitations to local prisons, while in the early
1860s individual boards of superintendence of county gaols in Ireland
published bye-laws and detailed schedules of doctors' duties and responsibilities. Overall in both settings, these expanded regulations required
prison medical officers to attend prisons regularly, to examine every
prisoner each week, and to visit daily sick prisoners on extra diet and
those confined in punishment cells, recording treatments in journals and
report books. They were also required to attend prison staff and their
families, to supervise and train hospital warders, inspect the entire prison
building on a regular basis, report structural faults in prison ventilation
and drainage, and to assess the quality of bedding, clothing and food, and
when necessary, implement public health measures to prevent the spread
of infectious diseases.[131] They were also to investigate prisoner deaths.
Finally, the regulations enforced doctors' active involvement in the
administration of prison discipline, requiring them to adjudicate on
prisoners' fitness for hard labour and punishments. The regulations
specifically outlined prison medical officers' duties in terms of safeguarding the minds of prisoners, and watching for signs of mental deterioration
or other adverse health effects related to the disciplinary regime. Doctors
were to report cases to the prison governor with directions for treatment,
which usually included extra food and exercise. They were also permitted
to consult medical advisors from outside the prison. These duties and
regulations not only placed prison doctors under considerable pressure,
they also involved them in the disciplinary aims of penal regimes, regard-
less of whether or not they endorsed these.

[129] See McConville, *English Local Prisons*, for a comprehensive discussion of the brutalising
impact of the change of policy.
[130] Smith, 'The Irish General Prisons Board'.
[131] For detail on Irish regulations, see the Royal Commission on Prisons in Ireland, 1884
(1884–85), Appendix XXII, pp. 168, 172, 175, and for English regulations, see 28&29
Vict., c.126 (1865) and 40&41 Vict., c.21 (1877).

Many prison doctors in England and Ireland, like prison governors, transferred from military careers into the prison service and would have been used to a working environment that stressed discipline and order, though increasingly by the second half of the century they devoted their entire careers to prison medicine. They pressed regularly for improved conditions and salaries, framing these requests as being beneficial to the prisoners they cared for. In Ireland, the Association of Gaol Surgeons, with Dr Hercules MacDonnell as Honorary Secretary, was formed to lobby for the interests of the profession as the duties of prison medical officers were expanded under the 1877 Act without, they argued, appropriate remuneration.[132] In 1882, these duties, as originally laid out in the legislation, were partly amended, but the Association continued to pursue a campaign against the General Prisons Board, lasting several years. Acrimonious and bitter, it highlighted the hostility prison doctors felt towards the Board, which was accused of 'insidious encroachment', 'illiberality' and 'attempted bullying'.[133] To improve relationships, the 1884 Royal Commission on Irish Prisons recommended the appointment of a Medical Inspector to the General Prisons Board, and a year later Dr Frederick McCabe, Local Government Inspector, commenced in post. Though complimentary about McCabe, the *Medical Press and Circular* claimed that he and the prison 'medical department' had been 'subordinated' by making the post holder 'a servant of the Board', compromising McCabe's capacity to act and comment independently.[134]

In much of their early correspondence with local prison governors, the General Prisons Board vigorously enforced new prison rules, demanding that prison officers, including surgeons, adhered to the new orders, prompting the resentment of prison medical officers.[135] Medical officers were frequently admonished for interfering with or ignoring the decisions of the Board, and exceeding their powers. In May 1880, following the death of prisoner J. Connors after an attempted suicide, the Board rebuked the Governor at Waterford Prison for exhibiting 'a great want

[132] They separated from the Association of Infirmary Surgeons and Medical Officers of Gaols: Royal Commission on Prisons in Ireland, 1884 (1884–85), Appendix XXII, p. 169. A similar body does not appear to have been formed in England.
[133] Anon., 'Prison Surgeons', *Medical Press and Circular* (14 Mar. 1883), 233–4; see also Anon. (22 Nov. 1882), 451; Anon. (12 Sept. 1883), 223–4; Anon. (31 Oct. 1883), 381.
[134] Anon., 'The Medical Department of the Irish Prisons Board', *Medical Press and Circular* (4 Mar. 1885), 200.
[135] Anon., 'Retrospect of 1884 – The Irish Prison Service', *Medical Press and Circular* (31 Dec. 1884), 578. For examples of the Board's censorial approach see NAI, General Prisons Board (GPB)/Minute Books (MB)/Vol. 1, Nov. 1877–May 1881, at 25 June 1879, 3 July 1879, 3 Aug. 1879.

of judgment ... in not requiring the prisoner to be visited frequently during the night after he had been placed in muffs & that it was considered he attempted suicide'.[136] The Board subsequently drafted a circular requiring that prisoners under mechanical restraint be visited at night and medical officers called on to regularly attend prisoners who attempted suicide.[137]

The work of medical officers was complicated further by varied prison populations and conditions for inmates. While it is unlikely that the many prisoners serving short sentences spent prolonged periods in separation, its implementation remained the aim of prison officials.[138] As some English prisons were closed or amalgamated, others saw a rise in numbers and overcrowding in the late nineteenth century. Liverpool Borough Prison had a particularly large number of female committals, many 'professedly prostitutes'.[139] On 20 September 1869, 1,097 male and female convicts were confined in 1,001 cells certified for separate confinement at Liverpool and two-thirds of the 12,785 admissions that year were recommittals.[140] The persistent problems of overcrowding and reoffending among female prisoners had first emerged in the 1850s.[141] By 1877, the prison's Roman Catholic minister, Reverend James Nugent, an ardent temperance reformer, observed that among the 4,571 females under his charge in that year, only 648 had never before been in prison.[142] Some 1,310 were committed after being found drunk or accused of riotous conduct, and 1,555 for disorderly behaviour on the

---

[136] NAI, GPB/MB/Vol. 1, Nov. 1877–May 1881, 13 May 1880, p. 282.

[137] Ibid., 21 May 1880, p. 282.

[138] For example, see Catherine Cox and Hilary Marland, '"Unfit for Reform or Punishment": Mental Disorder and Discipline in Liverpool Borough Prison in the Late Nineteenth Century', Social History, 44:2 (2019), 173–201.

[139] LRO, 347 MAG 1/2/2, Proceedings of the Meetings of the Liverpool Justices of the Peace, Minutes 1870–78, Quarterly Session of Justices of the Borough of Liverpool for Regulating the Boro' Gaol, 27 Apr. 1871, Report of the Prison Minister, p. 43.

[140] LRO, 365.32 BOR, Reports of the Governor, Chaplain, Prison Minister and Surgeon, of the Liverpool Borough Prison, Presented to the Court of Gaol Sessions, Holden on the 28th Day of October, 1869, Report of the Chaplain, p. 21.

[141] Cox and Marland, 'Unfit for Reform or Punishment', n. 87; LRO, 347 JUS 4/1/2, Minutes of Justices Sessions Gaol and House of Correction, Oct. 1864–Jan. 1870, Minutes of Justice, 29 Dec. 1869, p. 232; LRO, 365.32 BOR, Reports of the Governor, Chaplain, Prison Minister and Surgeon, of the Liverpool Borough Prison, 28th Day of October, 1869, Report of the Chaplain, p. 14; Report of the Inspectors of Prisons of Great Britain, Northern District (1876) [C.1500], p. 6 and (1877) [C.1724], p. 8.

[142] LRO, H352 COU, Borough of Liverpool. Proceedings of the Council, 1876–77, p. 556, Report of the Prison Minister, p. 18. Nugent was the first Catholic Chaplain appointed to Liverpool Borough Gaol under the 1863 Prison Ministers Act. D. Ben Rees, 'Nugent, James (1822–1905)', DNB, https://doi.org/10.1093/ref:odnb/54013 [accessed 1 Apr. 2020].

streets. Nugent, in his final report for the prison before his retirement, observed:

Drink is making terrible havoc upon the female population of this town; not only demoralizing the young, and leading them step by step into crime and the lowest depths of vice, but destroying the sacred character of family life, and changing wives and mothers into brutal savages.[143]

Flagging up the close association between excessive drinking and mental breakdown, Nugent observed that 'Not a week passes without some one being brought to the prison whom drink has maddened and robbed of all female decency, whose language and actions are so horrible that they seem no longer rational beings, but fiends.'[144] In 1898, Dr W.C. Sullivan and Dr Stewart Scholar, the latter Deputy Medical Officer at Liverpool Prison, reported on the link between alcoholism and suicidal impulses as revealed in 142 cases of persons charged with attempted suicide and remanded in Liverpool Prison. They argued that women's 'generative organs', were 'peculiarly susceptible to the alcoholic poison', which produced 'emotional alterations of the personality' that could prompt suicidal tendencies.[145]

In Ireland, the local prison population declined in the decades immediately after the Great Famine. In his evidence to the 1878 Commission on the Penal Servitude Acts, Reverend Lyons, Roman Catholic Chaplain at Spike Island, when pressed on whether he believed prison discipline acted as deterrent, was ambivalent and instead argued that during the Great Famine 'The kind of people who were convicted were peasantry who had no notion of ever committing a crime.'[146] Nonetheless, there was anxiety about high rates of reoffending. The Inspectors General of Prisons in Ireland, concerned at the expansion of the local prison population, noted a 5.5 per cent increase in committals between 1862 and 1863, when they totalled 33,940, highlighting a rise in short sentences and a troubling growth in recommittals especially among women.[147] Frederick Falkiner observed in 1882 that among prisoners in custody for the January quarter of his court sittings, 76 per cent of the male prisoners had previous convictions; the average was five each while three

143 LRO, H352 COU, Borough of Liverpool. Proceedings of the Council, 1876–77, p. 556, *Report of the Prison Minister*, p. 18.
144 Ibid.
145 W.C. Sullivan and Stewart Scholar, 'Alcoholism and Suicidal Impulses', *Journal of Mental Science*, 44:185 (Apr. 1898), 259–71, at pp. 268–9, 271.
146 Kimberley Commission (1878–79), Evidence of Reverend Lyons, pp. 1072–3, at p. 1073; see P. Sargent, *Wild Arabs and Savages: A History of Juvenile Justice in Ireland* (Manchester: Manchester University Press, 2014).
147 RIGPI, 1863 (1864) [3377], pp. x–xii.

had been imprisoned more than twenty times.[148] Among women the average number of previous convictions was seventeen.[149] Falkiner further noted that 'with these unfortunates, men and women, the coming and going in this world is from the streets to the prison, from the prison to the streets, and back again with the certainty of recurrent tides – more contaminating and more contaminated with every flux and reflux'.[150]

By the final decades of the nineteenth century, there was a 'remarkable decrease' in the size of the English and Irish prison populations.[151] Yet, while the overall figures supported claims that there was 'a decline in the spirit of lawlessness', the high rates of recommittals, especially for minor offences such as those related to alcohol, remained a cause of disquiet among prison officials.[152] At some prisons, not least Liverpool, the sheer size of the prison, combined with frequent overcrowding, the large numbers of prisoners on short sentences, and the high rates of recommittals, especially among women, prompted harsh responses from overburdened prison staff, including its medical officers working to rigorously implement new prison regulations.[153] In 1866, the Visiting Justices imposed work on the treadwheel or crank as first-class hard labour of the 'most penal kind' for able-bodied male adults, employing extra officers to enforce this. Other prisoners, including women, were set to oakum picking.[154] By 1868, prisoners were placed on the treadwheel for five hours during the first month of their sentence, and Liverpool's Governor subsequently increased this to six hours a day, and then seven hours.[155] The treadwheel accommodated forty-five prisoners who were compelled to ascend 9,240 feet daily, and by 1876 a daily average of 148 male prisoners worked on it.[156]

For prisoners, especially those serving their first sentences, hard labour was felt keenly, and authors of prison memoirs and some prison officials highlighted its mental as well as physical toll. In 1850, William Hepworth Dixon evoked the mental anxiety associated with hard labour, 'the dull,

---

[148] Falkiner, 'Our Habitual Criminals', p. 317.   [149] Ibid., p. 318.   [150] Ibid.
[151] Report of the Commissioners of Prisons, 1890 [C.6191], p. 2.
[152] Cited in Wiener, *Reconstructing the Criminal*, p. 217.
[153] Cox and Marland, '"Unfit for Reform or Punishment"'; LRO, 347 JUS/4/1/2, Minutes of Justices Sessions Gaol and House of Correction, Oct. 1864–Jan. 1870, 25 July 1867, *Report of the Chaplain*, p. 16, *Report of the Governor*, p. 123.
[154] LRO, 365.32 BOR, *Report of Visiting Justices of the Borough Gaol*, n.d., 1868–69, p. 5; 347 JUS/4/2/2, *By-Laws of the Liverpool Borough Prison for the Regulation of All Such Matters as Lie within the Discretion of the Visiting Justices* (1865–74), p. 3.
[155] LRO, 347 JUS/4/1/2, Minutes of Justices Sessions Gaol and House of Correction, Oct. 1864–Jan. 1870, 30 July 1868, *Report of the Governor*, pp. 157, 177; ibid., 29 Oct. 1868, *Report of the Governor, Chaplain, Prison Minister and Surgeon for 1868*, pp. 5, 154.
[156] Report of the Inspectors of Prisons of Great Britain, Northern District (1871) [C.372], p. 42 and (1876), p. 57.

soughing voice of the wheel, like the agony of drowning men – the dark shadows toiling and treading in a journey which knows no progress – force on the mind involuntary sensations of horror and disgust'.[157] Uninitiated prisoners dreaded the treadwheel and were said to find it 'very irksome and severe'; in his evidence to the 1878 Kimberley Commission, Captain Henry Kenneth Wilson, Governor of Maidstone Gaol, described it as a 'very unfair punishment'.[158] The Manchester Merchant, confined to Kirkdale Gaol in the late nineteenth century, 'pitied the treadwheel men as they went out to their labour'; after a spell on it, it was not unknown for 'big, strong fellows' to be 'led away crying'.[159] 'One Who Has Tried It', who served time in a local prison in England in the 1890s, referred to being in a 'bath of perspiration' and feeling 'quite crushed' when he returned to his cell after his first experience on it.[160] Governor Wilson, however, 'noted that experienced prisoners preferred the wheel to picking oakum', which was a dirty, slow job.[161] The rope was covered in tar and the strands were difficult to prise apart. Usually set as 'task' work, inexperienced prisoners fell behind, resulting in punishments, reduced diet or loss of marks, prompting intense feelings of mental anxiety.[162] Experienced prisoners shared 'tricks' to mitigate hard labour; one prisoner advised 'One Who Has Tried It' on how to ride the treadwheel, 'to sway the body from right to left' and allow the 'rising wheel to assist the upward movement', and explained he should use a nail, smuggled into the cell, for oakum picking.[163]

Prisoners' capacity to withstand hard labour was also related to their physical condition when committed, and in the late nineteenth century, prison staff and penologists commented on a marked deterioration in prisoners' physical and mental states, with many ill-equipped to withstand the regime. The Liverpool Visiting Justices estimated that 10 to 15 per cent of prisoners were 'unfit for hard labour of first class on account

---

[157] Cited in Priestley, *Victorian Prison Lives*, p. 125.
[158] Kimberley Commission (1878–79), Evidence of Captain Henry Kenneth Wilson, p. 387.
[159] *Kirkdale Gaol: Twelve Months Imprisonment of a Manchester Merchant* (Manchester: Heywood & Son, 1880), p. 49; John Hay, *A Gross Miscarriage of Justice: Seven Years Penal Servitude or the Value of a Royal Pardon* (London: The Literary Revision Society, 1894), p. 32. Cited in Priestley, *Victorian Prison Lives*, p. 128.
[160] One Who Has Tried It, 'What Prison Life Is Really Like', *The Windsor Magazine* (2 July 1895), 197–201, at p. 200.
[161] Kimberley Commission (1878–79), Evidence of Captain Henry Kenneth Wilson, p. 387.
[162] Priestley, *Victorian Prison Lives*, pp. 121–2.
[163] One Who Has Tried It, 'What Prison Life Is Really Like', p. 200.

of bodily health'.[164] Considering the zeal at Liverpool for the new prison regime and for maximising the use of the treadwheel, this may have been a conservative assessment. Dr Francis Archer, Surgeon at Liverpool, who was responsible for assessing all prisoners, noted in 1869 that one-fifth of prisoners – 399 out of 2,023 – sentenced to hard labour on the treadwheel were unfit and excused from hard labour on medical grounds.[165] Acknowledging that hard labour at Liverpool was of a 'more severe character', Archer and Governor Jackson did not introduce the new dietary scales proposed by the Carnarvon Committee.[166]

At Wakefield Prison, the 'physical tests' introduced by the Visiting Justices to assess the condition of prisoners demonstrated they 'were now in feebler condition, bodily and mental, than had been the case some years back'.[167] In 1871, the prison surgeon reported prisoners' health as 'good', noting only 'one suicide, three pardons on medical grounds, and three cases of insanity', who had been found insane after admission and removed to a lunatic asylum.[168] Three years later, there were two suicides, and twelve removals to the lunatic asylum, an increase from 'an average of three for the previous seven years'.[169] At Liverpool, the prison surgeon reported '11 deaths from natural causes, and one case of suicide by hanging, and three pardons on medical grounds' in 1876.[170] The General Prisons Board also commented on the impoverished state of Irish prisoners in the 1870s, noting their poor physical and mental conditions and linking them to bad harvests and the agrarian distress of 1879 and 1880.[171] In 1886 Dr Hercules MacDonnell noted that

our criminals suffer from periods of semi-starvation, prolonged fits of intoxication, bad housing, clothing, and many other hygienic defects, it can be readily understood why prison *regime* does not cause any appreciable deterioration. Cleanliness, regularity, and a sufficiency of food account for this.[172]

Similar comments were made about 'the deterioration of female criminals' in the late nineteenth century, with Miss Pumfrey, Lady

[164] LRO, 365.32 BOR, *Report of Visiting Justices of the Borough Gaol*, n.d., 1868–69, p. 7.
[165] LRO, 365.32 BOR, *Reports of the Governor, Chaplain, Prison Minister and Surgeon, of the Liverpool Borough Prison, 1869, Report of the Surgeon*, p. 26.
[166] LRO, 347 MAG 1/3/1A, Proceedings of the Meetings of the Liverpool Justices of the Peace, Minute Book, 19 Feb. 1856–25 Sept. 1866, Meeting of Visiting Justices, 28 June 1865, p. 147.
[167] Turner, *The Annals of Wakefield House of Correction*, p. 246.
[168] Report of the Inspectors of Prisons of Great Britain, Northern District (1871), p. 44.
[169] Turner, *The Annals of Wakefield House of Correction*, p. 246.
[170] Report of the Inspectors of Prisons of Great Britain, Northern District (1876), p. 59.
[171] RGPBI, 1879–80 (1880), p. 9.
[172] MacDonnell, 'Notes on Some Continental Prisons', p. 89 (emphasis in original).

Superintendent at Winchester convict refuge, acknowledging in 1878 that most of her charges were habitual criminals 'the residuum ... of the criminal population'.[173] In Liverpool particular concern was expressed at the persistently high numbers of female admissions, well over half, 12,518 of the 21,602 admissions in 1884.[174] Efforts to rehabilitate 'unhardened', young female prisoners centred on releasing them into female refuges run by religious orders. At Liverpool Nugent, inspired by his campaign to protect young women against 'vicious lives', removed Roman Catholic women to a Magdalen Asylum run by the Good Shepherd religious order and to similar institutions in Canada.[175] Towards the end of their sentences, women were transferred to the convict refuges at Winchester and Goldenbridge, Dublin, run by Protestant and Roman Catholic religious orders.[176] While the refuges in England only held prisoners, a 'principal point' of the Goldenbridge institution was that convict women mixed with women who had never been sentenced, a system Du Cane doubted to be beneficial for the 'free' women.[177]

Refuges were intended to imitate the workings of the intermediate prisons for men, with the women prepared for release through work.[178] In England female convicts were transferred to refuges nine months prior to discharge while in Ireland they were transferred for a sixteen-month period. The Sisters of Mercy, the order that managed Dublin's Goldenbridge refuge, refused the admission of infirm convicts from Mountjoy on the grounds that physical illness added to the difficulties in reforming women, while the burden of accommodating sick, infirm prisoners added to expenses.[179] Such women, apparently small in number, were released on licence, which Barlow implied was preferable to languishing in a refuge too infirm to work.[180] Even with the establishment of female refuges, opportunities for reform and rehabilitation were limited, especially as most women served short prison terms.[181]

Given the enfeebled condition of male and female prisoners, medical officers questioned the utility and impact of repeated punishments for misdemeanours and bad behaviour in terms of prisoners' mental health.

[173] Kimberley Commission (1878–79), Evidence of Eliza Pumfrey, p. 607.
[174] LRO, 347 MAG 1/3/3, Proceedings of the Meetings of the Visiting Committee, Apr 1878–June 1897, 30 Jan. 1885, *Annual Report for 1884*, p. 46; 347 MAG 1/3/4, Proceedings at the Meetings of the Visiting Committee, Visiting Committee Minutes, July 1897–Oct. 1904, 4 Jan. 1898, p. 20.
[175] LRO, H352 COU, Borough of Liverpool. Proceedings of the Council, 1876–77, Prison Minister's Report, 25 Oct. 1877, p. 18.
[176] Kimberley Commission (1878–79), Evidence of E.F. Du Cane, p. 38.   [177] Ibid.
[178] Ibid., Evidence of Captain J. Barlow, p. 791.   [179] Ibid.   [180] Ibid.
[181] Ibid., pp. 38, 791.

They queried whether repeated punishments were an effective means of forcing prisoners to amend behaviour, or of convincing them to accept imprisonment as an appropriate sanction for their crimes. Medical officers adjudicated on prisoners' fitness to undergo punishments, including the implementation of bread and water diets, confinement in dark cells and inflicting corporeal punishment while also guarding against unnecessary cruelty. Prison visiting justices, governors, surgeons and chaplains were required to be alert to the 'mind or body of prisoners[s] injuriously affected by discipline or treatment', while at Liverpool the governor was to 'see that all insane prisoners are removed from prison as speedily as the law allows'.[182] As the 1867 medical commission on diet in Irish prisons noted, however, the speed with which prison doctors and others intervened to protect the mental and physical health of prisoners was determined by rules that permitted them to do so only when injury or impairment had been inflicted.[183]

In 1866, Dr Robert McDonnell at Mountjoy Male Prison, who would later describe himself as leaning 'too much towards the side of humanity', argued that prolonged punishments could have a 'maddening effect', the prisoner is 'irritated by it; and if there is any tendency to mental disease, this irritation becomes highly injurious'.[184] Chaplain Cody, commenting on the decline in the number of punishments in 1869, noted: 'to punish a man for petty infractions of rules, arising from human infirmity, inadvertence, strong provocation, or other extenuating cause, has an evil effect on the minds of the majority of the convicts. When the prisoner was treated like a man, and he conducted himself like a man; he was docile and manageable.'[185] Often prisoners who attempted suicide had been repeatedly punished for disruptive behaviour, including earlier suicide attempts. Patrick Byrne, a twenty-one-year-old prisoner who commenced his sentence of six months' hard labour for larceny at Clonmel Prison on 2 June 1887, committed suicide one month later by hanging himself with a bed strap tied to one of the bars of his cell window. He had been placed on a punishment diet on five different occasions in June for talking to other prisoners. The coroner's inquest found that he had been temporarily insane at the time of the attempt although the medical officer did not refer to any abberant behaviour in his report.[186] These difficult

---

[182] LRO, 347 JUS/4/2/1, *Rules and Regulations for the Government of the Liverpool Borough Gaol and House of Correction at Walton-on-the-Hill, near Liverpool* (1855).
[183] Report of the Committee on Dietaries in County and Borough Gaols, Ireland (1867–68), p. 28.
[184] RDCPI, 1866 (1867) [3805], p. 19.   [185] RDCP, 1869 (1870) [C.204], p. 17.
[186] NAI, GPB/Incoming Correspondence (CORR)/1887/Item no. 9419: Correspondence relating to suicide of prisoner Patrick Byrne, Clonmel, Aug. 1887.

and disruptive prisoners refused to comply with prison discipline, and were repeatedly punished, sometimes over several years. While a minority of cases were transferred to asylums, for the most part they were suspected to be cases of malingering and carefully observed by the medical officers.[187]

The difficulties faced by prison medical officers in managing disruptive and dangerous behaviour among prisoners, often related to mental illness, were highlighted in an inquest report into the death of a convict at Spike Island in 1870. The convict had died of ascites, and, according to the report of the *Medical Press and Circular*, the jury had expressed, 'in the strongest terms, their "total disapproval of the frequent punishment he suffered in cells, on bread and water for several days in succession, during his imprisonment in Spike Island"'.[188] The unnamed convict had been transferred by McDonnell from Mountjoy Prison as unfit for cellular discipline, but not as an 'invalid' although he had been suspected of suffering from epilepsy. McDonnell had kept him in the prison infirmary for several months as the 'only means of keeping him from the system which might have been injurious to him'.[189] Defending the actions of Dr Jeremiah Kelly at Spike, the *Medical Press and Circular* noted that Kelly had not received the 'convict as a sick man, nor had he any reason to know that he was unfitted for the usual bread-and-water discipline of Spike Island'.[190] The article also reflected on the difficult position of Kelly and McDonnell in relation to the prison authorities when advocating for or protecting the health of their charges. Citing the example of McDonnell, described as 'an inconveniently compassionate medical officer', who, they argued, had been removed from his position at Mountjoy for the 'fearless discharge of his duty' in defending untried Fenian prisoners from excessive punishment, the article speculated that the same fate might befall Kelly had he countermanded orders to punish the convict. The jury's censure of Kelly, 'for undue severity of punishment', provided, they argued, the opportunity for prison authorities 'to shift their responsibility to Dr Kelly and expurgate themselves by throwing him overboard'.[191] The article sought enhanced protection for prison medical officers who, in discharging their duties and responsibilities in relation to prisoners, were liable to be 'McDonnellized' or made to 'suffer for official sins'.[192]

---

[187] See NAI, GPO/PN/4 and GPO/PN/5: Philipstown Character Books, 1847–62 for examples. See ch. 4 for asylum transfers and ch. 5 for a discussion of feigning.

[188] Anon., 'Death of a Convict at Spike Island', *Medical Press and Circular* (9 Mar. 1870), 193–7, at p. 196.

[189] Ibid.   [190] Ibid.   [191] Ibid.   [192] Ibid.

The new rules introduced after nationalisation heightened the anxieties of Irish prison medical officers who argued that the regulations further compromised their capacity to protect the 'health of prisoners under their charge'.[193] In a submission to the 1884 Royal Commission on Irish Prisons, the Association of Gaol Surgeons highlighted the tension between surgeons' responsibilities to their prisoner patients and ensuring the disciplinary function of prison sentences was not 'unduly mitigated'.[194] They also emphasised the potential damage to professional reputations should they miss cases of malingering.[195] The Association's Honorary Secretary, Dr Hercules MacDonnell, expanded on these points in his address to the Statistical and Social Inquiry Society of Ireland in May 1885, which was also forwarded to the General Prisons Board and published in the *Daily Express*.[196] MacDonnell stressed that while 'neither the diet nor surroundings should be such as to make imprisonment agreeable … punishment should not include cruelty, nor should it impair health'.[197] In his review of prison regimes in Belgium, Germany and Italy, published in 1886, he reiterated the point that 'Punishment must be deterrent. Loss of personal liberty and deprivation of all usual enjoyments act under this head. Under no circumstances should this partake of the character of vengeance.'[198]

As shown in Chapter 2, allegations of cruelty, abuse of power by prison officials and severe punishments, involving excessive infliction of crank work, repeated floggings and dangerous restriction of diet, resulting in several suicides, were unmasked at Birmingham and Leicester Gaols in the 1850s. While casting a long shadow over the nineteenth-century prison, the scandals did not undermine support for the separate system or the authority of prison officers, and while prison officials such as Inspector Herbert P. Voules suggested the investigation would deter prison officials from over-severe measures, in case they faced 'another Birmingham inquiry', there were other instances involving severe implementation of disciplinary regimes.[199] At Liverpool, punishments become more commonplace, and the annual report for 1869 listed 'stoppage of diet' for 818 male and 35 female prisoners, alongside confinement in solitary or dark cells for 579 males and 1,131 females and whipping for

[193] Royal Commission on Prisons in Ireland, 1884 (1884–85), Appendix XXII, p. 168.
[194] Ibid., pp. 168–9.   [195] Ibid., p. 168.
[196] NAI, GPB/MB/Vol. 3, Nov. 1883–Dec. 1886, 19 May 1885, p. 237.
[197] Hercules MacDonnell, 'A Review of Some of the Subjects in the Report of the Royal Commission on Prisons in Ireland', *Journal of the Statistical and Social Inquiry Society of Ireland*, 8:63 (July 1885), 617–23, at p. 619.
[198] MacDonnell, 'Notes on some Continental Prisons', p. 88.
[199] Forsythe, *The Reform of Prisoners*, p. 116.

six male prisoners.[200] The Wakefield justices noted that there had been no cases of corporal punishment for prison offences for seven years despite the steady rise in committals, especially cases of drunkenness. However, in 1876 there were 453 punishments by bread and water in dark cells, and 1,305 by bread and water in light cells.[201] In the annual report for 1876 they noted 'three punishments by whipping, 2,386 by solitary or dark cell, and 553 by stoppage of diet' were carried out that year. Though only two were reported to be insane on committal, eight prisoners were removed to lunatic asylums and there were 47 deaths in the prison.[202]

After nationalisation, punishments could entail confinement in punishment cells, dietary punishment, birching, deprivation of marks and demotion of prisoners who, through good behaviour, had progressed through the various stages or classes. Medical Officer Dr Quinton supported the implementation of dietary punishments for 'unruly prisoners', acknowledging that he knew 'nothing approaching a scientific excuse for its use, except the principle upon which a horse has its oats reduced in order to tame his spirit'.[203] In Ireland, the numbers punished for offences between 1878–79 and 1879–80 rose from 10,475 to 13,304, a significant increase according to the General Prisons Board. The Board speculated that it was caused by 'the exercise of a closer supervision, and the enforcement of a stricter discipline, and an increased amount of industry, as the officers have become more familiar with the operation of the new rules and system'.[204] Under the new regulations ill-conducted or idle prisoners could be placed on a bread and water diet for three days only followed by an interval of a 'stirabout' diet and then returned to the bread and water diet. Officially, the period on punishment diets was not to exceed fifteen days and such prisoners were not required to perform labour.[205]

Incorrigible and disobedient prisoners, who refused to work on the treadwheel, were flogged or birched. In 1887 Surgeon Hammond at Liverpool ordered prisoner Joseph Leeane be given twelve strokes of the birch rod for refusing to work at the wheel. Leeane argued his sentence was unjust and insisted hard labour was not 'proper punishment' for his crime of begging.[206] Hammond frequently rejected

---

[200] Report of the Inspectors of Prisons of Great Britain, Northern District (1871), pp. 41, 44.

[201] Turner, *The Annals of Wakefield House of Correction*, pp. 246, 247; Report of the Inspectors of Prisons of Great Britain, Northern District (1876), p. 209.

[202] Report of the Inspectors of Prisons of Great Britain, Northern District (1876), p. 210.

[203] Cited in Sim, *Medical Power in Prisons*, p. 42.   [204] RGPBI, 1879–80 (1880), pp. 7–8.

[205] Ibid., p. 27.

[206] LRO, 347 MAG 1/3/3, Proceedings of the Meetings of the Visiting Committee, Apr. 1878–June 1897, 1 Dec. 1887, p. 68.

prisoners' requests for mitigation on grounds of poor health, declaring prisoners fit to work on the wheel and being quick to punish prisoners he suspected of feigning insanity.[207] As discussed in Chapter 5, prisoners went to great lengths to secure mitigated conditions, including feigned suicide attempts. On 26 May 1893, a sixteen-year-old prisoner, James Allender, undergoing a sentence of nine months' hard labour, was threatened with further birching if he made a second attempt at suicide. On the first attempt he tried to hang himself with a rope made from oakum, and when found assaulted the warder, insisting he would 'break a pane of glass and then cut my throat'. On inquiring into the incident, Allender admitted to the Governor he 'never intended to do anything to myself as sure as there is a God in Heaven'. His punishment was twelve strokes with a birch rod, and Dr Beamish, the prison medical officer, commented that Allender was 'not strong but was fit to be birched'.[208]

By the late nineteenth century, there was growing distaste for corporal punishment and the infliction of pain, on moral as well as rational grounds, and by the time of the Gladstone Committee of 1895, the view that 'every form of punishment is objectionable' was more widely endorsed.[209] By then, the use of the 'entirely dark cell' had been discontinued in Ireland and there was evidence of a decline in corporal punishments in local prisons after 1893.[210] While the Report of the Gladstone Committee opposed corporeal punishment, especially in the case of habitual criminals, individual prisons resisted these changes. In the case of Liverpool, a deputation of the Visiting Committee petitioned the Home Secretary, in July 1898, for permission 'to retain the power to order such corporal punishment as hitherto allowed'.[211]

II MEDICAL EXPERTISE AND KNOWLEDGE PRODUCTION

Medical Management of Mental Disorder in Convict and Local Prisons

Prison doctors, working in environments shaped by deterrence, adopted various treatment and management strategies when dealing with

---

[207] Cox and Marland, 'Unfit for Reform or Punishment'.
[208] LRO, 347 MAG 1/3/3, Proceedings of the Meetings of the Visiting Committee, Apr. 1878–June 1897, Special Inquiry Held at H.M. Prison on 30 May 1893, p. 257.
[209] Under-Secretary of State, Sir G. Lushington, cited in Gladstone Committee (1895), p. 15; Wiener, *Reconstructing the Criminal*, pp. 334–5.
[210] Gladstone Committee (1895), p. 16.
[211] LRO, 347 MAG 1/3/4, Proceedings at the Meetings of the Visiting Committee, Visiting Committee Minutes, July 1897–Oct. 1904, 20 July 1898, pp. 45–6.

prisoners experiencing symptoms of delusion, mania and depression of spirits. These varied across the prison estates and depended on conditions within individual prisons and individual doctors' practices. Prisoners were typically retained in prison while their mental states were monitored and assessed, moved in and out of prison hospitals, kept under cellular observation, or placed in cells with fellow prisoners who watched over them. These measures were not always successful; at Chatham prison, one convict committed suicide in the prison hospital, 'under the eyes of ... fellow prisoners'.[212] He had shown symptoms of melancholia for several days and had been admitted to the prison hospital for observation.[213] At Mountjoy, Dr James W. Young, McDonnell's successor, assisted by the chief prison warder, closely watched those on probation for signs of mental distress. When 'a tendency to insanity in a prisoner' was observed, the warder reported the prisoner to Young, who, with the governor's approval, authorised more 'open air exercise'. Commenting on Young's system of observation at the Kimberley Commission in 1878, convict E.F., who had been held at Mountjoy and Spike Island Prisons, claimed 'dozens of men ... who had been decidedly affected in the head, have by this simple arrangement been able to complete their sentence, learn a trade, and must have become good members of society'.[214] By the 1880s, the Prison Medical Inspector for Ireland was required to testify that prison medical officers implemented systems for observing prisoners and identifying those unfit for the regime.[215]

Overburdened prison medical officers struggled to manage convicts and prisoners whose mental and physical decline was accompanied with eccentric, erratic and violent outbursts, particularly in England where prisoner numbers and the number of such cases were higher. Despite the impact on their workloads, the medical officers devoted time and effort to treating individual cases to halt further deterioration. Convict William Williamson, also known as John O'Hare, a forty-nine-year-old American, serving a five-year sentence for larceny at Mountjoy, was in poor physical condition on his admission in October 1882. Described as 'spare' in frame, he was transferred to Maryborough Invalid Prison in September 1885. His medical sheet, which travelled with him as he was moved around the prison estate, records an extensive list of weekly prescriptions intended to bolster his physical and mental health. By March 1887, Williamson was repeatedly fed with a stomach pump, as he was no longer

---

[212] RDCP, 1887–88 (1888) [C.5551], p. xxxviii.   [213] Ibid.
[214] Kimberley Commission (1878–79), Evidence of Convict E.F., p. 838.
[215] RDCP, 1888–89 (1889) [C.5880], p. vii.

eating, and he was transferred to Dundrum Asylum in April 1887.[216] Another convict, thirty-four-year-old James Slattery, serving a five-year sentence at Mountjoy, was described on committal in December 1881 as stout and strong. Following his removal to Spike Island, his health declined, he became 'febrile' and was diagnosed with bronchitis. He was then transferred to Maryborough Invalid Prison, as a 'spare' and 'weak' prisoner in October 1884; by then his weight had fallen from 160 to 141 pounds. Discharged from Maryborough in November 1885, he was back at Mountjoy in January 1887, and a month later was reported to be abstaining from food. After being fed with a stomach pump throughout February, he was discharged to Dundrum Asylum in April 1887.[217]

This level of attention was not unique to the convict system or the smaller Irish prison estate. In July 1901 the Visiting Committee at Liverpool Prison heard a complaint from prisoner John Pearson about medical treatment for his bad chest. Pearson claimed he had not been 'sounded' and had received only 'occasional doses of medicine', though the Deputy Medical Officer, Dr Frank A. Gill, insisted he had visited Pearson forty-three times over three months.[218] At that time, the prison was dealing with many disruptive prisoners; male and female prisoners broke up their cells, were violent, refused to work, and assaulted officers.[219] Even so, prison staff explored several options to secure the safe removal of another prisoner, Albert Halliwell, who was reported to be an epileptic, including a medical discharge. Halliwell had not experienced any epileptic fits while in the prison, and the medical officer argued he could not certify him insane and remove him to an asylum. In an effort to resolve the question of Halliwell's care, Liverpool officials contacted the Prison Commission enquiring whether it would bear the cost of 7 shilling 6 pence a week to pay for his care at an epileptic colony near Liverpool. The colony was full and instead it was suggested that Halliwell be pardoned on medical grounds and transferred to a 'suitable home'. By June 1905, however, it was reported that a suitable destination for Halliwell could not be found and it is unclear whether he was discharged on medical grounds without accommodation.[220]

[216] NAI, GPB/Penal Files (PEN)/3/41, William Williamson, otherwise John O'Hare.
[217] NAI, GPB/PEN/3/61, James Slattery.
[218] LRO, 347 MAG 1/3/4, Proceedings at the Meetings of the Visiting Committee, Visiting Committee Minutes, July 1897–Oct. 1904, 8 July 1901, pp. 204–5.
[219] Ibid., 27 Jan. 1899, pp. 79–82.
[220] LRO, 347 MAG 1/3/5, Proceedings at the Meetings of the Visiting Committee of Liverpool Prison, Nov. 1904–Sept. 1912, 7 Apr. 1905, p. 24, 5 May 1905, p. 25, 2 June 1905, p. 29.

Prison medical officers also conducted detailed investigations into attempted suicides. These provoked great concern among prison officers as they indicated a failure of the prison to safeguard its inmates. Mountjoy Prison saw frequent suicide attempts, though prisoners were often suspected of feigning.[221] The Governor of Galway Prison reported two separate suicide attempts in December 1884 and January 1885. One of these, John Burke, protesting against the prison diet, tied his trouser braces together, and fastened one end to the handle of the bell in his cell and the other tightly round his neck. Burke, who was on the first scale of the third-class diet, had complained of hunger to Medical Officer Dr R.J. Kinkead, who on weighing him concluded that he had gained five pounds while confined. Kinkead insisted that Burke's suicide attempt was not genuine but carefully staged to ensure he would be seen, and was an attempt to secure 'increased diet, or to be placed in association'.[222] While it is unclear what happened to Burke, his suicide attempt prompted the medical officer to recommend that bell handles be removed from prison cells and replaced with electric bells. Kinkead also suggested the hooks and chains that supported hammocks be replaced with 'solid supports from the wall'.[223] The ubiquity of suicide attempts led the Chairman of the General Prisons Board to order safety netting for local prisons in 1885, particularly for institutions where 'gallery railings are not sufficiently high to prevent prisoners committing suicide'.[224]

As Halliwell's case suggests, a small number of prisoners, in a poor condition and with little hope of improvement, were eventually discharged on medical grounds. Chapter 2 has investigated the caution surrounding medical discharges at Pentonville in the 1840s, and by the late nineteenth century, pardoning and releasing prisoners on medical grounds was still unusual. In 1891, for example, only one convict was released from Irish convict prisons on the grounds of physical illness, while six were transferred to the Dundrum Criminal Lunatic Asylum.[225] These cases received only a perfunctory reference in official records. In 1884 the prison inspectors deftly noted two male and nine female prisoners were pardoned on medical grounds at Liverpool Prison, while in 1885 twelve prisoners were discharged on medical grounds, though no

[221] NAI, GPB/MB/Vol. 3, Nov. 1883–Dec. 1886, 14 Jan. 1884, p. 26.
[222] NAI, GPB/CORR/1885/Item no. 571, Documents Relating to Suicide Attempt/ Prevention.
[223] Ibid.
[224] NAI, GPB/CORR/1886/Item no.7076, Documents Referring to Alterations to Fabric of Prisons to Prevent Suicides, Feb. 1885–June 1886.
[225] RGPBI, 1890–91 (1891) [C.6451], pp. 23, 136.

details were given.[226] When details were noted, life-threatening physical ailments such as respiratory or heart diseases were recorded and women were also discharged in the final months of pregnancy.[227] In 1886 Dr Gover estimated that the rate of medical releases among convicts was only 1.9 per 1000.[228] Objecting to such releases, he claimed prisoners survived for longer periods when retained in prison hospitals, as most were discharged without resources or into the care of relatives with limited means.[229] In Ireland, authorisation for medical releases was at the discretion of the 'Judge of the Court by whom such Prisoner was committed', and in June 1880 the General Prisons Board felt compelled to remind Kilmainham Prison's Medical Officer of the regulation, suggesting that releases had taken place illegally.[230]

While prison medical officers devoted significant time to assessing and managing prisoners' physical health, the ubiquity of mental breakdown among prisoners added significantly to their workload. It involved differentiating between a range of complex symptoms, keeping prisoners under medical observation in prison hospitals, or in individual cells with other inmates for weeks, sometimes months. Campbell reproduced some of the conditions of a lunatic asylum at Woking, including a hospital diet, sometimes supplemented by extra items, close attendance of inmates, and provided insane prisoners with books and crafts to occupy them. He noted that such occupation occasionally resulted in cures and prisoners were returned to convict prisons.[231] For some prison doctors, however, holding potentially insane prisoners in prison was undesirable. Dr Hercules MacDonnell, for example, expressed concern about the lengthy detention of the insane in prisons lacking provision for care and specialised medical treatment.[232]

In England, convicts showing symptoms of insanity were removed to Millbank, which was utilised as a form of collection and assessment centre for the close observation of such prisoners, and, as discussed in Chapter 5, to check for signs of feigning. Criticising the length of time convicts were kept at Millbank – up to three to four months during which time the convicts had no employment – the 1878 Kimberley Commission insisted that the detention period be shortened and convicts required to work, especially as 'one third' of those sent there were 'found not to be

[226] LRO, 347 MAG 1/3/3, Proceedings of the Meetings of the Visiting Committee, Liverpool Borough Gaol, Apr. 1878–June 1897, 30 Jan. 1885, p. 46, 8 Feb. 1886, p. 54.
[227] RGPBI, 1890–91 (1891), pp. 18, 57–8.
[228] RDCP, 1886–87 (1887) [C.5205] [C.5205–I], p. xxxiii.   [229] Ibid.
[230] NAI, GPB/MB/Vol. 1, Nov. 1877–May 1881, 14 June 1880, p. 293.
[231] Campbell, Thirty Years, pp. 86–103.
[232] MacDonnell, 'The Royal Commission on Prisons in Ireland', p. 621.

really insane'.[233] Following a period of medical assessment at Millbank, these convicts were then removed to different institutions; for example, among 54 convicts under medical observation at Millbank in 1861, nine were removed to Bethlem Hospital as insane, fifteen to invalid prisons, nine kept in association on medical grounds, five removed to able-bodied prisons, and a further nine remained under medical observation. One Irish convict, returned to Millbank from Bermuda owing to his mental condition, was subsequently sent on to Spike Island.[234]

The removal of prisoners showing signs of mental disorder to public works prisons and invalid prisons burdened prison medical officers with the difficult task of distinguishing those inmates who were unfit for or unable to withstand the full rigour of prison discipline from the 'truly' insane. Unlike prisoners certified insane, those diagnosed as weak-minded or invalids were retained in prison, although the full rigours of the separate system of confinement and hard labour were ameliorated. Significant numbers accumulated; Dr William Guy, reported that some 200 convicts 'unsound in mind ... and yet not deemed quite fit for the lunatic asylum' were confined at Millbank in 1869.[235] Divisions or wings of individual prisons served as repositories for mentally ill prisoners at various points during the late nineteenth century, including Woking Invalid Prison, which opened in 1859, and where, in 1874, a separate wing was designated for male lunatic convicts to alleviate pressure on Broadmoor. Prior to that only a small number of prisoners with mental diseases were transferred there; Campbell noted only fifteen cases during 1863.[236] Woking and Parkhurst contained specific divisions devoted to accommodating weak-minded and 'imbecile' convicts. Parkhurst, a prison for juveniles from 1838 to 1863, catered for prisoners invalided as weak-minded or imbecile from 1869; by 1882 there were around 140 prisoners confined at Parkhurst.[237] Woking Invalid Prison remained the main repository for invalid convicts in the late nineteenth century. According to Campbell, by the 1870s there were almost 200 mentally ill prisoners, the majority weak-minded, in the prison.[238] Owing to concerns about the legality of retaining the insane

[233] Kimberley Commission (1878–79), p. xlii.   [234] RDCP, 1861 (1862) [3011], p. 444.
[235] William A. Guy, 'On Insanity and Crime; and on the Plea of Insanity in Criminal Cases', *Journal of the Statistical Society of London*, 32:2 (June 1869), 159–91, at p. 186.
[236] RDCP, 1863 (1864) [3388], Woking Invalid Prison, p. 263.
[237] Davie, *Tracing the Criminal*, p. 70; see John A. Stack, 'Deterrence and Reformation in Early Victorian Social Policy: The Case of Parkhurst Prison, 1838–1864', *Historical Reflections/Réflections Historiques*, 6:2 (1979), 387–404 for the early history of Parkhurst.
[238] RDCP, 1871 (1872) [C.649], Woking Invalid Prison, p. 415.

in prisons, the wing catering for male lunatic convicts at Woking was closed in 1888.[239]

In Ireland, after 1855 weak-minded convicts were deposited in Philipstown Prison, and, following its closure, by December 1863 they, along with the aged and other invalid prisoners, had been removed to Spike Island, which held 901 convicts in that year.[240] In 1861, when Philipstown was scheduled for closure, there were ten certified lunatics awaiting accommodation at Dundrum among the 145 convicts, and 'large numbers of invalid and other prisoners labouring under deficient intellectual powers with great irritability and total destitution of self-control'.[241] Dr Maurice Corr, Medical Superintendent at Spike Island, noted that in some cases the illness had 'commenced with curable weakness of intellect, and terminated in dangerous incurable insanity', insisting that the growth of 'mental disease' had been 'generated and fostered in prison'.[242] Weak-minded convicts were usually separated from other convicts at public works prisons such as Spike Island and Dartmoor, a practice endorsed in the Report of the Kimberley Commission in 1878 following the presentation of evidence that the eccentric behaviour of the weak-minded prisoners aggravated the other inmates.[243]

In 1872, as invalid prisoners accumulated in Spike Island, prison inspectors and officials sought alternative, separate accommodation for them. Their proposals included the construction of a purpose-built building at Spike Island, erecting two iron huts in Mountjoy Male Prison garden, and redesignating Smithfield Prison in Dublin as a dedicated invalid prison similar to Woking.[244] Though these proposals were not implemented, Inspector Barlow and Crofton persisted in advocating for a separate institution for weak-minded convicts, and by 1878 the local prison at Maryborough was repurposed as a prison for invalid, weak-minded and imbecile male convicts. In 1884 the Royal Commission on Irish Prisons specified that in 'every case where there are unmistakeable signs of disease, mental or bodily, such as would warrant transfer to an invalid prison, the convicts should be at once moved to Maryboro', so that the disease may be checked in its earlier stages'.[245] From July 1885,

---

[239] Report of the Commission to Inquire into the Subject of Criminal Lunacy (1882) [C.3418], Report, p. 17.

[240] RDCPI, 1863 (1864), pp. 25, 29, 34.   [241] RDCPI, 1861 (1862), pp. 40, 47.

[242] Ibid.

[243] Kimberley Commission (1878–79), Evidence of Captain J. Barlow, p. 775.

[244] NAI, Chief Secretary's Office Registered Papers (CSORP)/1874/Item no. 4814, Weakminded Prisoners, Letter from Captain Barlow to Inspector Bourke, 18 May 1872.

[245] Royal Commission on Prisons in Ireland, 1884 (1884–85), p. 41.

Maryborough was constituted solely as an invalid prison for male convicts, having ceased to operate as a local prison, although by 1887 the prison also housed convicts removed from the recently closed Lusk Intermediate Prison.[246] Among the 57 convicts held at Maryborough on 31 March 1886, thirty were serving penal servitude sentences and another ten were serving life sentences, suggesting that most had been in separation for a portion of their sentence.[247] Campbell also noted the 'great number' of invalid prisoners at Woking who had been subjected to 'long-continued solitary confinement'. Describing the 'ulterior effects' of the separate system to be 'in many cases, most injurious', he recalled that convicts who had been subjected to the regime frequently 'gave evidence of impairment both bodily and mental, marked by great depression, a semi-idiotic expression and the dilation of the pupils'.[248]

Weak-minded or imbecile convicts comprised the largest group of 'mental cases' at Woking; in 1861, among its 786 convicts, Woking received 130 such cases from Millbank and a further 116 from Dartmoor.[249] While 'pretty manageable', Campbell reported that they also displayed eccentric habits, were liable to fits of excitement and to break out.[250] Convicts invalided owing to physical conditions also suffered from 'impairment of mental facilities', and at the temporary Invalid Convict Depot at Lewes, established in 1857, the medical officer noted in 1860 that 'the mental faculties of most of the paralysed men were a good deal impaired'.[251] Convict M.E. at Lewes, for example, was suffering from 'paralysis and debility' when received in 1859. The medical officer described his habits on admission as 'dirty', and he walked with difficulty. As his mental condition deteriorated, he became noisy, violent and excitable, experienced delusions, such as 'fancying himself the proprietor of large estates', and he was eventually removed to a lunatic asylum.[252] Aged and infirm convicts were 'frequently very peculiar and eccentric', while those reported to have dementia were said to become violent, intractable and disruptive, prompting their removal to asylums.[253] In 1863 Campbell transferred nine such cases to the private lunatic asylum, Fisherton House.[254] Among those invalided for physical ailments, he contended that their persistent insubordination, violence and other conduct was inconsistent with sound minds.[255] While at

[246] RGPBI, 1885–86 (1886) [C.4817], p. 42.   [247] Ibid., p. 13.
[248] Campbell, *Thirty Years*, p. 34.   [249] RDCP, 1861, Woking Invalid Prison, p. 318.
[250] RDCP, 1863, Woking Invalid Prison, p. 263.
[251] RDCP, 1859 (1860) [2713], Lewes Invalid Convict Establishment, p. 360.
[252] Ibid., p. 320. See ch. 4 for a discussion of general paralysis of the insane in prisons.
[253] RDCP, 1863, Woking Invalid Prison, p. 263.   [254] Ibid.
[255] RDCP, 1873 (1874) [C.1089], Woking Invalid Prison, p. 439.

Woking convicts with 'disorders of the intellect' required constant medical supervision, including those whose mental and physical health improved under the regime. Some invalided convicts were noted to be quiet and amenable for long periods, yet liable to 'break out when least expected'.[256] Campbell regarded the physical and mental diseases of invalided convicts to be linked to their criminality, a product of 'depraved habits, intemperance, and hereditary predisposition' and their long careers in vice and crime, alongside their bad tempers and disgusting propensities, rendered them more unmanageable than ordinary lunatics.[257]

The burden on medical officers employed at the large public works prisons, such as Spike Island and Dartmoor, and at invalid prisons, was especially heavy, owing to the sheer numbers and categories of prisoners held there. John Campbell, when Medical Officer at Dartmoor Prison in the 1850s, claimed healthy men were a minority.[258] Dr R.E. Power, who had been Assistant Surgeon at Portsmouth Prison for five years, and then Medical Officer at Dartmoor, where he supervised an assistant surgeon, dealt with nearly 1,000 convicts, as well as '500 women and children' and 200 officers.[259] Conditions at the public works prisons were exacting and severe, with healthy prisoners working in association outdoors for long hours at heavy labour, excavating earth, quarrying and undertaking other arduous tasks. Invalid prisoners, including the weak-minded, were usually employed at 'sedentary' tasks.[260] Defending conditions at Dartmoor, with its damp, foggy and stormy climate, Campbell insisted that the invalid class, 'greatly enfeebled by long standing diseases' and possessed of constitutions undermined by 'intemperance and other depraved habits', benefited from the 'elevated position' of the moor.[261] He described the regulation that required medical officers to classify prisoners according to fitness for different kinds of work, as a tax on medical men's knowledge and expertise because of the 'diversity of ... physical and mental condition' and the large number of prisoners.[262] He also sought increased allowances of food for men at public works labour, to 'compensate for the wear and tear of the body'.[263] Austin Bidwell, sentenced to penal servitude for life in 1873, and transferred to Chatham prison after a year in separation at Pentonville, described his amazement when he first witnessed a convict work party: 'their famished,

[256] Ibid., p. 418.   [257] Ibid., pp. 436, 439.
[258] Campbell, *Thirty Years*, p. 33; RDCP, 1867 (1867–68) [4083], Dartmoor Prison, p. 235.
[259] Kimberley Commission (1878–79), Evidence of R.E. Power, p. 757.
[260] Campbell, *Thirty Years*, p. 33.   [261] Ibid., p. 34.   [262] Ibid., p. 135.
[263] Ibid., p. 136.

wolfish looks – thin, gaunt and almost disguised out of all human resemblance by their ill-fitting, mud-covered garments and mud-splashed faces and hands ... the weary, almost ghastly spectre march I had witnessed constantly haunted me'.[264]

Labour at these prisons was often enforced through punishment and prisoners were frequently suspected of malingering. The evidence of convict E.F. to the Kimberley Commission highlighted the brutal treatment of convicts at Spike Island and the deleterious impact on convicts' minds. E.F., convicted in 1875 and released early on medical grounds in 1878, claimed punishments were 'the order of the day at Spike Island' and prisoners were threatened, starved and flogged. He described the prison staff at Spike as 'inferior' to those at Mountjoy, and in their interactions with prisoners, 'more irritating and annoying, and growling at [prisoners] unnecessarily'.[265] He dismissed Medical Officer Dr Patrick Kelly as a 'dispensing doctor' who inflicted 'inhumane cruelty' by placing 'poor maniacs in perpetual cells until reason had become undermined from hunger, flogging and deprivation of the air of heaven'.[266]

Labelling, Taxonomies and Knowledge Production

Drawing on their work assessing, diagnosing and managing numerous cases of mental disorder, medical officers increasingly laid claim to extensive and unique expertise in understanding mental illness in the context of the prison. Some, including Gover, Campbell and notably Nicolson, published on the topic, producing a sizeable body of literature. They critiqued the expertise of asylum doctors, including their evidence in court, and argued that their experience enabled them to distinguish between true and feigned insanity. As prison psychiatry emerged as a discrete field of activity and prison doctors asserted their expertise, they developed a separate taxonomy to describe the range of mental conditions they encountered in prisons. Their concern was primarily diagnosing and labelling the conditions they observed, and less with treatment, although some prisoners were reported to have recovered while in the prison hospital and the timely removal of convicts out of separation could limit the damage inflicted on the minds of prisoners. In 1867 McDonnell described two prisoners, who he noted to be '"dangerous," and of

---

[264] Austin Bidwell, *From Wall Street to Newgate via the Primrose Way* (Hartford, CT: Bidwell Publishing Co., 1895), p. 39.
[265] Kimberley Commission (1878–79), Evidence of Convict E.F., p. 824.
[266] Ibid., p. 838.

frenzied passion and irritability', who had been 'reclaimed' by removing them to the prison hospital, where they received 'judicious moral and physical treatment'.[267]

The emergence of a discrete language and set of categories to describe the minds of prisoners can be traced to the years following the introduction of separate confinement. Thereafter prisoners, whose violent and erratic behaviour prompted speculation among staff about their mental state, were recorded and described by prison surgeons in specific terms. Prisoners were noted to be 'sullen', 'irritable', 'obstinate', 'passionate', 'impatient' and 'dull', as well as delusional.[268] At Pentonville 'irritability' was used to denote a more general prevailing mood among the convicts and within the prison, as well as the absence of self-control in individual cases. In his report for 1849 Dr Owen Rees described, in reference to the general condition of the prisoners, 'that there is an "irritability" observable which I have never before observed in men confined'.[269] In 1855 Governor Grace at Philipstown also noted the 'troublesome state' of the prison, which he linked to the irritable, violent and uncontrollable passion of prisoners, including juveniles.[270] Conditions of the mind were closely observed and recorded; at Pentonville prisoners demonstrated 'sullen obstinacy', a combination of 'cunning and weakness', 'knavery and almost imbecility of mind', while those removed from Mountjoy to public works prisons on medical grounds had 'great nervousness', 'irritability', and were 'exciteable' and 'eccentric'.[271] John Daughton, an eighteen-year-old convict who had spent nine months in separate confinement in Mountjoy Prison, and then transferred to Philipstown in February 1858, was described by the medical officer as 'sullen', 'morose' and 'very eccentric', while Andrew McQuirk, imprisoned in January 1861, was reported to be 'excitable, 'mischievous' and 'irritable'.[272] Medical officers commented on the condition and health of the minds of prisoners who persistently broke rules, yet seemed indifferent to repeated punishments. In considering suicide attempts,

---

[267] Anon., 'The Psychology of Punishments', *BMJ*, 1:330 (27 Apr. 1867), 484–5, at p. 484.

[268] Report of the Commissioners for the Government of the Pentonville Prison (1847) [818], pp. 41–2, 51; NAI, GPO/PN/4–5, Philipstown Character Books, 1847–62.

[269] TNA, PCOM 2/96, Pentonville Prison, Middlesex: Visitors Order Book 1849–50, 20 Feb. 1850.

[270] NAI, GPO/CORR/1855/ Philipstown/Item no.18, Letter from Governor Grace to the Directors of Convict Prisons, 11 Jan. 1855.

[271] Report of the Commissioners of the Pentonville Prison (1847), pp. 41–2; NAI, GPO/ PN/4–5, Philipstown Character Books, 1847–62.

[272] NAI, GPO/PN/4–5, Philipstown Character Books, 1847–62, John Daughton, Andrew McQuirk.

McDonnell related the case of prisoner J. Murphy, who had become excited, refusing to declare his religious denomination. He was sent to the punishment cell on a bread and water diet, and McDonnell 'soon satisfied myself that the prisoner was not insane, but simply irritated to an extreme degree by a punishment that did not appear just to him'.[273]

The labels used to describe women reflected the gendered conceptualisation of mental disorder and criminality. Women's 'irritability' involved 'a restiveness and a longing for some change or variety of circumstance' that could only be gratified through misconduct.[274] David Nicolson commented that the 'unreasonable acts of destruction' committed by women in prison 'doubtless arise strange and pleasurable feelings of a triumphant nature' as the prisoner was 'temporarily in command of the situation'.[275] The violent outbursts of female prisoners, referred to as 'breaking out' in English prisons, perplexed and disturbed prison medical officers. In Ireland prison doctors noted similar behaviours among women, although use of the phrase 'breaking out' was not widespread. In 1873 Nicolson commented that 'Female convicts are not only liable to give way to destructive emotions when disappointed or irritated; but they afford, in what has been termed their "breakings-out", an illustration of a state of mind whose aspect is even more distinctly morbid' than among male convicts.[276] This violence was distinguished in the opinion of prison doctors from that observed among female patients in lunatic asylums, consisting 'of a frantic outburst, in which destructiveness is the main feature, a special partiality being displayed for the shivering of window panes and the tearing of blankets and sheets into fragments'.[277]

In his evidence to the 1878 Kimberley Commission, Dr Henry Westwood Hoffman detailed his management and treatment of women considered to be 'bordering on insanity' at Fulham Female Refuge, where women worked in association following transfer from Millbank and Woking (Figure 3.3). Drawing on the example of convict Hughes, who, he argued, was not of sound mind yet at other times was 'perfectly rational', Hoffman explained that despite her difficult behaviour she was not a fit case for punishment or suitable for transfer to Millbank. Hughes was 'quarrelsome, irritable, jealous, and not amenable to discipline', and, while she did not suffer from delusions, he argued that when she 'breaks out, she is not responsible'.[278] She had been sent to two lunatic asylums

---

[273] Anon., 'The Psychology of Punishments', p. 484.
[274] David Nicolson, 'The Morbid Psychology of Criminals', *Journal of Mental Science*, 19:87 (Oct. 1873), 398–409, at p. 402.
[275] Ibid., p. 401.   [276] Ibid.   [277] Ibid.
[278] Kimberley Commission (1878–79), Evidence of Dr Henry Westwood Hoffman, p. 844.

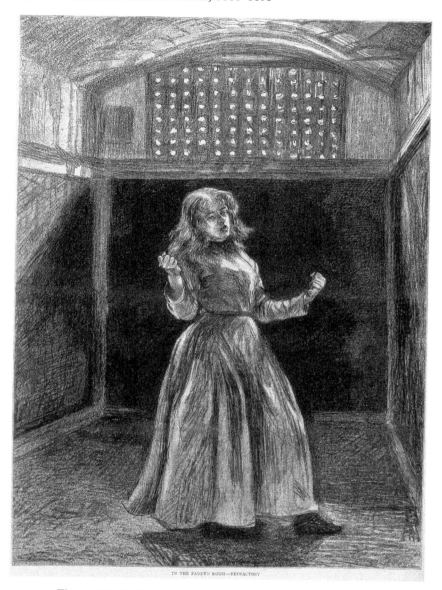

IN THE PADDED ROOM—REFRACTORY

Figure 3.3 Woking Convict Invalid Prison: a woman prisoner in solitary confinement. Process print after P. Renouard, 1889
Credit: Wellcome Collection. Attribution 4.0 International (CC BY 4.0)

for treatment, one of which was Broadmoor, but when her behaviour 'passes off' she was released. While he could not decide whether Hughes was insane he did not suspect her of feigning insanity.[279] Despite his heavy workload, Hoffman was reluctant to request a second opinion from Millbank's medical officers, insisting his *locum tenens* provide it.[280] As discussed in Chapter 5, prison doctors alleged that women planned these destructive outbursts, which were prompted not by 'provocation, angry excitement or disappointment', but by a desire for change.[281] That these destructive impulses were more often provoked by trivial causes among women, Nicolson argued, was 'attributable to functional causes which present themselves in connection either with the normal menstrual flow or with its derangement' and women's need for companionship with some prisoners deliberately 'getting into trouble in order that she may be near to her "pal", and bear her company in punishment'.[282] While their behaviour was regarded as outrageous, manipulative and distinctly unfeminine, it could also be interpreted as an expression of women's agency and resistance to the prison environment and routine.[283]

In developing a distinct set of categories to explain such mental conditions and psychiatric states, medical officers linked criminality and criminal behaviours with prisoners' apparent inability to adapt to, or benefit from, the discipline of the prison. They also drew on specific characteristics and dispositions, as well as environmental factors, commonly evoked in general rhetoric on criminal behaviour in the late nineteenth century. Consequently, prison psychiatric categories were connected to familiar tropes that characterised criminals as inherently violent, quick tempered, duplicitous, sly, lacking in self discipline and control, and childlike. In 1870 Gover argued that among female prisoners with symptoms of mental distress 'hereditary defects' were 'doubtless ... aggravated by the influence of bad example and vicious training', and mental illness caused by a loss of self-control and excess passion.[284] When assessing the case of convict Richard Murphy, alias Thomas Doyle, who had 'feigned' suicide in his cell, McDonnell at Mountjoy concluded that Murphy belonged to

that class of cases which are unquestionably of a nature most difficult for a medical man to deal with ... cunning, deceitful, passionate, and impatient of

---

[279] Ibid., p. 845.   [280] Ibid.   [281] Ibid.

[282] Nicolson, 'The Morbid Psychology of Criminals', p. 402.

[283] See Rachel Bennett, '"Bad for the Health of the Body, Worse for the Health of the Mind": Female Responses to Imprisonment in England, 1853–1869', *Social History of Medicine*, 34:2 (2021), 532–52.

[284] Cited in Nicolson 'Parliamentary Blue Books', pp. 258, 259.

control yet in my judgement having naturally bad disposition complicated by a certain admixture of disease which tends to make the mind more fretful, irritable, and uncontrollable ... such disease should be treated as firmly yet as gently as the circumstances ... will admit.[285]

Murphy's 'cunning' and deceitfulness were simultaneously characteristics of his criminality and of his mental condition. While disciplined and punished for their 'criminal' traits, the behaviour of these inmates also prompted medical officers to debate the impact of frequent punishment on the minds of prisoners, and to explore the relationship between punishment and prisoners' mental capacity to improve and comply with prison rules. At Mountjoy, McDonnell warned against punishing prisoners in cellular confinement suffering from forms of 'mental disturbance' that fell short of 'insanity', arguing such treatment resulted in them becoming 'irritable, peevish, sullen, morose and gloomy, liable to burst into passion on the most trifling provocation, fancy everyone to be an enemy and quite unable to control their bursts of frenzy'.[286]

Highlighting the cases of two convicts, J. Croughwell and Patrick Maher, McDonnell insisted repeated punishments had not only failed to improve their behaviour, but had also led them into the 'most miserable condition'. Such convicts, McDonnell argued, fancied that they were 'without a kindly feeling from anyone; wronged and misunderstood by all the world; friendless and in despair. This is doubtless the condition which leads onto suicide.'[287] Convict Croughwell, fifteen years old when he was convicted of robbery in October 1851, was originally sentenced to ten years, and then given an additional four years' penal servitude for assaulting a prison officer. His conduct was reportedly very bad, and he acquired a spectacularly long punishment sheet.[288] Between November 1857 and May 1859, he attempted suicide three times, and, while repentant and well behaved in hospital, McDonnell felt he was not fit for the disciplinary regime at Mountjoy and recommended he be removed to an associated prison.[289]

In the case of Patrick Maher, who attempted suicide in June 1863 and was violent towards the warders, McDonnell first placed him in a padded cell and then transferred him to the prison hospital. McDonnell concluded Maher's life was not in danger, and that he was sane and fit for punishment. When dealing with such cases, however, McDonnell argued

[285] NAI, GPO/CORR/1860/ Mountjoy (Male) Prison/Item no. 6.
[286] RDCPI, 1866 (1867) [3805], p. 19.   [287] Ibid., pp. 18–19, at p. 19.
[288] NAI, GPO/PN/4–5, Philipstown Character Books, 1847–62.
[289] NAI, GPO/CORR/1859/Mountjoy (Male) Prison/Items nos. 91, 124, Letter from Robert McDonnell, Prison Medical Officer to Governor of Mountjoy Male Prison, 25 May 1859.

that the wrong type of punishments prompted or exacerbated morbid feelings, leading to further suicide attempts. 'The slow class of punishment', such as the curtailment of diet or close cellular confinement, made 'a prisoner like Maher moody and sullen'.[290] Punishments 'of short duration', including corporal punishment, were more suitable as it was less likely to contribute to mental disorder.[291] 'Viewing punishment in its medical aspect (psychological)', McDonnell argued that prisoners should believe the punishments inflicted on them were fair, commensurate with the misdemeanour and deserved. In the absence of 'a clear conception of his guilt', prison staff risked prompting mental distress among prisoners: 'the punishment becomes an extreme source of mental irritation.... In the one case, he bears his punishment and is the better of it, in the other, he is irritated by it; and if there is any tendency to mental disease, this irritation becomes highly injurious.'[292]

Campbell also warned against dietary punishments, especially when repeated frequently, and applied to weak-minded prisoners. Not only did these punishments fail to deter; they impaired prisoners' minds and bodies, especially among those with a hereditary tendency to diseases such as scrofula, which laid the foundations for maladies of a fatal nature.[293] Contrasting the criminal or convict class with that of the habitual offender and semi-imbecile, Campbell argued that 'encouragement and punishment seem alike ineffectual in restraining ... [the] bad dispositions' of the latter.[294] Nonetheless, medical officers argued there were some benefits in punishing such prisoners, and again these were understood in the context of their criminal natures. In 1873, David Nicolson justified punishments on the grounds that 'fear in its moral aspect' did not restrain prisoners; rather 'the selfish fear or dread of physical chastisement and pain, more or less immediate, with which he will be visited' was effective when managing volatile prisoners prone to emotional outbreaks.[295]

Prison officers also questioned the efficacy of punishing female prisoners and their mental capacity to withstand punishments, while simultaneously expressing shock at their extreme and unfeminine behaviour. Reflecting on his time as Assistant Chaplain at Millbank Prison in the 1860s, Reverend James Francis noted the women there 'were in a most excited, irrepressible condition; I never saw anything like it'.[296] He

[290] NAI, GPO/CORR/1863/Mountjoy (Male) Prison/Item no.129, Letter from Robert McDonnell, Prison Medical Officer to Governor of Mountjoy Male Prison, 2 June 1863.
[291] Ibid.   [292] RDCPI, 1866 (1867), p. 19.   [293] Campbell, *Thirty Years*, p. 120.
[294] Ibid.   [295] Nicolson, 'The Morbid Psychology of Criminals', p. 399.
[296] Kimberley Commission (1878–79), Evidence of Reverend James Francis, p. 881.

claimed the dark punishment cells were 'continually full with raving, screaming women' who were noisy and disruptive when excited, kicking on doors and disrobing sick prisoners held nearby.[297] Crofton contended that 'irritable' women, subjected to repeated punishments while in strict prison discipline, fared better when removed out of separate system and transferred to refuges.[298] Special measures were introduced to manage female convicts who were perceived to be especially unsuited for separate confinement. In 1869 Dr Young rejected the new dietary scales introduced in 1868, instead placing women at Mountjoy on a diet with greater quantities of milk and bread. He observed that 'after long periods of confinement, [the diet] was loathed by the prisoners' owing to the lack of variety, and 'great quantities of the bread rejected. This led to insubordinate conduct, malingering, and punishment.'[299] From 1878 women at Mountjoy were kept in strict separation for four months, though specific measures were introduced to mitigate aspects of the separate regime, especially for women who were susceptible to extreme and volatile outbursts when punished.[300] Second-class female convicts were permitted to work and sit in their cells with the doors opened on alternate days, allowing them to observe prison activities. Women were also granted more generous remissions for good conduct than men.[301] Captain Barlow, Director of Convict Prisons, for example, was reluctant to cut women's hair, a practice permitted for hygienic or disciplinary purposes, as he found it had a very negative effect; the women found it 'very cruel' and for some he feared it would make them 'half mad'.[302]

In England there was similar disquiet among prison doctors and staff dealing with female convicts and ambiguity concerning women's capacity to endure the disciplinary regime. Hoffman at Fulham Female Refuge objected to placing women on bread and water punishments, arguing only 'strong' women could withstand it for more than two days and that women fared better in terms of behaviour and temperament on their usual diet while punishment diets 'hardened' women.[303] Superintendent Pumfrey at the Winchester Refuge complained that some women arrived in very enfeebled physical health as well as in 'bad' character, once again blending their medical condition with their alleged criminal dispositions. Describing one woman transferred to the refuge, Pumfrey noted how she 'never knew her mother and was

[297] Ibid.   [298] Ibid., Evidence of Sir Walter Crofton, p.1040.
[299] RDCP, 1869 (1870), p. 34.
[300] Kimberley Commission (1878–79), Evidence of Captain J. Barlow, p. 789.
[301] Ibid.   [302] Ibid., p. 793.
[303] Ibid., Evidence of Dr Henry Westwood Hoffman, p. 846.

regularly dragged out of the slums'. She had behaved 'very badly' while in Woking Prison and arrived at Winchester in very poor health, which Pumfrey attributed to her being placed on punishment diet of bread and water, confined to the dark cells and with her ankles fastened together in 'hobbles'.[304]

By embedding contemporary ideas on the intrinsic deviant inheritance of criminals, and their poor morals and character, with psychiatric categorisations of mental illness and insanity in the prison context, medical officers, however, largely defended prison regimes, arguing they did not cause mental collapse among prisoners whose criminality was evidence of an inferior mental condition. They argued the expertise in identifying the traits and symptoms of this 'admixture' of criminality and insanity resided with them, with their extensive experience of observing both the insane and the criminal. As Wiener has contended, from the late 1860s English doctors in regular contact with criminals developed a scientific conception of the criminal, though their heavily inflected physicalist 'scientific reinterpretation of criminality' dissipated in the early 1870s.[305] Yet those working in prisons continued to speculate on the specific forms of mental disorders they encountered. Major Arthur Griffiths, Deputy Governor at Millbank Prison from 1870 to 1872, described the particular challenges of this work, contending that prisoners were liable to special and exclusive phases of insanity that included strange and intense delusions, religious mania, claims of persecution, exaggerated destructive tendencies, curious attempts at suicide and persistent feigning.[306]

Dr David Nicolson, his experience built up at several convict prisons and subsequently Broadmoor, published his theories of the criminal mind in the 1870s. Wiener noted that Nicolson moved away from the 'oversweeping claims of the physicalists', which were present in the articles he published between 1873 and 1875, to a position from which he argued only a minority of criminals possessed distinctive physical characteristics.[307] In his understanding of delusions, Nicolson differentiated between 'ordinary' delusions experienced by all human beings and the 'special delusions' experienced by many prisoners. These arose in the

---

[304] Ibid., Evidence of Eliza Pumfrey, p. 601.
[305] Wiener, *Reconstructing the Criminal*, p. 233.
[306] Arthur Griffiths, *Memorials of Millbank, and Chapters in Prison History* (London: Henry S. King & Co., 1875), pp. 177–8. Major Arthur Griffiths (1838–1908) was Inspector of Prisons and deputy governor of several prisons: Bill Forsythe, 'Griffiths, Arthur George Frederick (1838–1908)', *DNB*, https://doi.org/10.1093/ref:odnb/33581 [accessed 3 Jan. 2018.]
[307] Wiener, *Reconstructing the Criminal*, p. 234.

particular circumstances of prison life, and Nicolson connected them with the irritable condition of the criminal mind.[308] Delusions of the 'irritative type' were most often found among prisoners, who claimed they were unjustly punished or treated, or believed their food had been poisoned. Such delusions, he argued, were more common in men than women, and expressed through vigorous resistance to authority, and demonstrations of resentment, threats, food refusal and 'personal violence'.[309] Arising from 'irritation and feelings of resentment', these delusional prisoners were especially dangerous and careful precautions were advocated.[310] Prisoners' minds were unable to withstand the 'irksome experiences' of prison life and disciplinary regimes, especially separate confinement, the pressure of 'labour' was distasteful, and eventually the 'chronic grumble' assumes 'mastery'.[311] Nicolson insisted that through closely observing the workings of 'diseased' minds, prison medical officers and those experienced in prison psychiatry were able to study, test and sort 'phenomena' in the context of their uniform and standard prison experience, and develop new psychiatric knowledge beneficial to practice outside the prison.[312]

Much of the debate on psychiatric conditions in prisons in the late nineteenth century occurred in the context of concerns about high rates of recidivism and habitual criminals. By the 1880s, official statistics suggested that the inexorable climb in criminality had at least slowed, if not halted, yet the reasons for persistence of criminal behaviour among some groups continued to preoccupy penologists and prison doctors. Though estimates vary, some reports suggest that between 1888 and 1892 recommittal rates to English local prisons rose to 48 per cent.[313] In Ireland among the 29,916 confined between 1879 and 1880, only 18,183 had never been in prison, 818 had been committed over twenty times, and 1,041 confined between twelve and twenty times.[314] Frederick Falkiner noted the physical and mental weakness of this class of prisoner, observing that they were unable and unlikely to benefit from reformative regimes. He sought harsher and longer sentences, insisting that 'habitues in street crime cannot maintain reform in the streets'.[315] Barlow, who had responsibility for the Registry of Habitual Criminals under the 1871 Prevention of Crimes Act, which followed the 1869 Habitual Criminals Act, described criminals in Irish prisons as 'the dregs

[308] David Nicolson, 'The Morbid Psychology of Criminals', *Journal of Mental Science*, 20:89 (Apr. 1874), 20–37, at pp. 20–1.
[309] Ibid., pp. 23, 24.   [310] Ibid., pp. 30, 31.   [311] Ibid., p. 23.   [312] Ibid., p. 28.
[313] McConville, *English Local Prisons*, p. 576.   [314] RGPBI, 1879–80 (1880), p. 11.
[315] Falkiner, 'Our Habitual Criminals', p. 320.

of the towns, a different class of men altogether'.[316] In 1878, William Fagan, Director of Convict Prisons for England, with responsibility for Millbank, Wormwood Scrubs, Brixton and Portsmouth prisons, and George Clifton, Governor of Portland Prison, referred to prisoners as being 'the waste of all the large towns and of London particularly'. Their prisons were populated with the 'thieves and the worst description of men from the large cities, broken down in constitution from vice and debauchery'.[317] Dr Henry Francis Askham, Medical Officer at Portland, who had previously served at Dartmoor and at Woking Female Prison, also observed in 1878 that 'As a class they are greatly deteriorating.'[318]

The implementation of the Habitual Criminals Acts, which imposed harsher penalties and sentencing for repeat offenders, who were usually confined in local prisons, rendered this cohort of offender more visible to prison authorities, and prompted further commentary on the mental and physical 'quality' of prisoners. At Woking, Campbell asserted, many of those first received as lunatic criminals were of an 'insubordinate type' and had pursued 'a life-long career of crime and deception, spending most of their time in prisons, asylums and workhouses'. He absorbed stereotypical criminal traits into his emerging psychiatric categories. 'Even in the more favourable or hopeful cases', Campbell argued, 'it must be remembered that we had to deal with lunatics that were also criminals, and it was sometimes difficult to discriminate between these two elements of character.'[319] In urban prisons, a large proportion of habitual offenders were committed on drunk and disorderly charges, leading Dr Moore, Belfast Gaol's Medical Officer, to advocate for 'habitual drunkards' to be committed to prison for an indefinite period, only to be released when cured.[320] Dr Rogers, Medical Superintendent at Rainhill Lunatic Asylum, exemplifying the position adopted by some asylum psychiatrists on habitual drunkards, argued they fell into the category of criminals with limited responsibility. He opposed committing such 'poor persons to prison', insisting they required treatment and that it was 'unjust' to punish them.[321] Echoing Moore's demands in the 1890s, the Visiting Committee at Liverpool Prison, contending with a

---

[316] Kimberley Commission (1878–79), Evidence of Captain J. Barlow, p. 797.
[317] Ibid., Evidence of William Fagan and George Clifton, at pp. 177, 718.
[318] Ibid., Evidence of Dr Henry Francis Askham, p. 739.
[319] Campbell, *Thirty Years*, pp. 85–6.
[320] Anon., 'The British Medical Association: Psychological Section', *Medical Press and Circular* (15 Aug. 1877), p. 138.
[321] 'The British Medical Association', *BMJ*, 2:870 (1 Sept. 1877), 308. For detailed discussion on the changing position of the habitual drunkard, see Wiener, *Reconstructing the Criminal*, pp. 294–300; Zedner, *Women, Crime and Custody*, ch. 6.

large number of repeat offenders, many of whom were convicted for drunk and disorderly offences, however, wrote to the Home Office pleading for a system of reformatory detention, as 'Criminals – like lunatics – should be detained till they are cured.'[322]

Regarded as irredeemable and hopeless cases, the 'habitual' criminals' alleged dislike of hard labour was interpreted as an indication of mental weakness, as well as being further evidence of innate criminal propensities. Director Fagan claimed that the 'rough working criminal' preferred separate confinement over public works prisons. Labour in separation, Fagan insisted, was of a 'milder industrial labour, with perhaps a touch of the wheel or something of that sort'.[323] The prisoner in separation was not driven the same way as on public works labour, and preferred the 'idleness' of separation.[324] Campbell argued the habitual or 'casual' criminal was 'so thoroughly debased and hardened as to resist any system of treatment'.[325] Repeat offenders, he claimed, laboured under physical defects, with an inherited propensity to criminality and vagrancy from childhood. So 'degenerate in body and in mind' they were unable to earn a livelihood and determined to 'persist in their evil courses', rendering prison discipline and reformation futile.[326] Inspector Gover explicitly linked their resistance to prison discipline to the condition of their minds, observing in 1870 that 'The moral obtuseness of habitual criminals graduates insensibly into insanity, and a similar remark would apply to those prisoners who habitually commit breaches of discipline.'[327]

In the late nineteenth century prison medical officers increasingly categorised prisoners and convicts who refused to work, resisted or were unable to conform to prison discipline, and seemed impervious to repeated punishments, as 'weak-minded'. From the 1860s, as Davie argues, the term weak-minded was not a 'clearly defined medical condition'. Rather it was used as a 'pragmatic means to identify inmates considered incapable of bearing the punishment regime', although, as Saunders demonstrates, there was agreement among psychiatrists that the weak-minded were 'not capable of being certified as insane'.[328] Amid

[322] TNA, HO 45/9695/A9757, Prisons and Prisoners (3) Prisoners – Visiting Committee and Boards of Visitors: Liverpool Prison. Annual Reports of Visiting Committee, Letter to the Home Secretary, 18 Feb. 1892.
[323] Kimberley Commission (1878–79), Evidence of William Fagan, p. 716.   [324] Ibid.
[325] Campbell, *Thirty Years*, p. 130.   [326] Ibid., p. 131.
[327] Cited in Nicolson 'Parliamentary Blue Books', p. 257.
[328] Neil Davie, 'The Role of Medico-Legal Expertise in the Emergence of Criminology in Britain (1870–1918)', *Criminocorpus, revue hypermédia* [Online], *Archives d'anthropologie criminelle* and related subjects, 3 [11 Oct. 2010], http://criminocorpus.revues.org/316; Janet Saunders, 'Institutionalised Offenders: A Study of the Victorian Institution and

heightened anxieties about recidivism, high-profile prison doctors, such as Guy at Millbank, linked criminal weak-mindedness to repeat offenders.[329] Medical officers repeatedly stressed that weak-minded habitual offenders had an inordinate dislike of 'honest industry' and of public works. They should be separated from casual and first offenders, and prevented from returning to their homes on release. Instead, it was recommended that they be secluded in a separately designated 'refuge' or, in the case of habitual offenders in Ireland, forced to emigrate.[330]

While not perceived as being as dangerous as other categories of convicts, weak-minded convicts and prisoners were observed to be prone to irresponsible and eccentric behaviour, and

peculiarly subject to sudden and ungovernable outbursts of temper and passion, to commit strange and eccentric acts of violence, to irritate their fellow prisoners and are easily excited by them, and are not amenable to the ordinary influences of self-interest or fear of punishment.[331]

At Spike Island Prison, Medical Officer Jeremiah Kelly recommended 'eccentric' and 'slightly weak-minded' convicts, unfit for separation and labour, to be permitted to work in association, while the 'weak-minded' worked in association at picking oakum.[332] Kelly referred to these convicts as 'irresponsible', 'troublesome' and 'unmanageable'; they committed acts of insubordination and restraint was 'absolutely' required.[333] In his evidence to the 1878 Kimberley Commission, Dr Henry Roome, at Parkhurst Prison, noted the weak-minded formed a large proportion of the habitual criminal class and were a constant annoyance and 'perplexity'.[334] Inspector Barlow reported that the weak-minded were a 'constant cause of misconduct', committed small offences and acts of insubordination.[335] Campbell also noted the 'eccentricities' of Woking's weak-minded convicts, although he argued the 'great majority' of these prisoners were harmless and some were 'even industrious'.[336] Observations by Campbell and others on the annoyance the weak-minded caused fellow inmates gave support to those advocating for separate prisons or prison wings for weak-minded convicts.[337]

Its Inmates, with Special Reference to Late Nineteenth Century Warwickshire' (unpublished University of Warwick PhD thesis, 1983), p. 258.

[329] Saunders, 'Institutionalised Offenders', p. 258.

[330] Campbell, *Thirty Years*, p. 132; Falkiner, 'Our Habitual Criminals', p. 329.

[331] Kimberley Commission (1878–79), p. xliii.   [332] RDCPI, 1863 (1864) [3367], p. 34.

[333] Ibid.

[334] Kimberley Commission (1878–79), p. xliii and evidence of Dr Henry Roome, p. 644.

[335] Ibid., Evidence of Captain J. Barlow, p. 775.   [336] Campbell, *Thirty Years*, p. 76.

[337] Wiener, *Reconstructing the Criminal*, pp. 233–5; Davie, *Tracing the Criminal*, pp. 202–3.

In day-to-day practice and management, decisions relating to weak-minded convicts and prisoners and their disposal were muddled and haphazard. While Barlow argued such convicts were not to be punished as they were not responsible for their actions, at the same time he noted that 'doctors cannot certify them as mad, but they are certainly irresponsible'.[338] Some weak-minded prisoners were well treated, such as Kate Moroney, an inmate of Limerick Female Prison in 1895. Previously committed on several occasions to a lunatic asylum, as a 'weak-minded' patient, in prison she was confined to bed on beef tea and two glasses of whisky.[339] There are more examples, however, of severe treatment. Patrick Gordon, a thirty-year-old convict sentenced to seven years' penal servitude in November 1881 for breaking and entering, was noted to be 'obscene' and 'eccentric' on his committal to Mountjoy. Gordon had been convicted on ten previous occasions since June 1875. According to the medical report drawn up by Drs Young and Minchin when Gordon was transferred to Dundrum Lunatic Asylum in 1882, soon after his committal they had observed 'evident symptoms of weak-mindedness', laughing on unsuitable occasions and 'quite idiotic in his deportment'. Despite claims that such prisoners were not punished, Gordon had been frequently placed in close confinement on a reduced diet for various offences related to unruly behaviour, including destroying prison clothing.[340] As his behaviour deteriorated, the punishments became more severe and in May 1882 he was held in close confinement on a punishment diet for seven days. Concluding that because of his state of mind it was 'impossible to subject him to the discipline of a prison', he was removed to Dundrum Asylum in July.[341] Oscar Wilde recorded the cruelty of punishing the weak-minded and the reactions of fellow prisoners while confined at Reading Gaol from 1895 to 1897. In one of the letters he published in the *Daily Chronicle* following his release, Wilde described one prisoner, a soldier, as 'silly', 'noisy' and 'half-witted'; he was frequently punished, placed in solitary confinement and flogged. Following one such flogging, recommended by the doctor who suspected the soldier of feigning, Wilde observed the man at exercise:

His weak, ugly, wretched face [was] bloated by tears and hysteria almost beyond recognition.... He was a living grotesque. The other prisoners all watched him, and not one of them smiled. Everybody knew what had happened to him, and that he was being driven insane – was insane already.[342]

[338] Kimberley Commission (1878–79), Evidence of Captain J. Barlow, p. 775.
[339] NAI, GPB/CORR/1895/Item no. 1810, Case of Prisoner Kate Moroney, Limerick Female Prison.
[340] NAI, GPB/PEN/3/13, Patrick Gordon.   [341] Ibid.
[342] 'To the Editor of the Daily Chronicle', *Daily Chronicle*, 28 May 1897.

The unpredictable volatility of weak-minded prisoners, who were otherwise docile and quiet, was repeatedly commented on, as in 1894 when twenty-three-year-old Jemima Overend, convicted for vagrancy and held in Belfast Female Prison for three months with hard labour, was reported to be 'disorderly'. She 'attempted to damage her utensils, and threatened to break her window & cell furniture'.[343] With a history of abusive language and of damaging her cell, she had been confined to the punishment cell on bread and water diet several times. In February 1894 the acting medical officer, Dr E.C. Bigger, had her restrained in muffs, describing her as 'one of those eccentric and weak-minded individuals who sometimes becomes violent without any provocation, and settles down again, and goes on quietly for some time'.[344] Nonetheless, Bigger certified her as fit for restraint, confinement and the punishment diet. In 1886 Governor A.C. Bulkeley at Maryborough described invalid convicts as 'notoriously troublesome' who 'usually commit breaches of prison discipline'.[345] In spite of the link made between invalid and weak-minded convicts and habitual criminality, among the 57 convicts held in Maryborough on 31 March 1886, 25 had never been in prison before, and only six had been confined more than six times.[346]

Determining whether weak-minded inmates were eligible for removal to 'specialist' facilities depended on the type of sentence they were serving as well as their medical diagnosis. Convicts serving penal servitude sentences were removed to Woking and Marybourgh Invalid Prisons, where they received less severe treatment. Prisoners not serving sentences of penal servitude, who were ineligible for transfer to invalid convict prisons, languished in local prisons or were transferred to other quasi-penal institutions. One such case was prisoner Michael Quinn, who came to the notice of the Irish General Prisons Board in 1884. Quinn, arrested while concealed in a farmer's outhouse, was in poor physical condition, covered in vermin, and unable to give an account of himself. Tried for vagrancy at Athboy Petty Sessions, he was committed to Kilmainham Prison where the medical officer determined he was 'undoubtedly weak-minded' and listed him as an 'imbecile' on the prison record. While confined, Quinn was 'not be required to do much work' and was 'allowed a bed'. On encountering Quinn at Kilmainham, Inspector Bourke determined he was not 'a fit subject for confinement in a prison', and, presumably because he was not charged with a serious

---

[343] NAI, GPB/CORR/1894/Item no. 2235, Case of Prisoner Jemima Overend, Belfast Female Prison, under restraint Feb. 1894.
[344] Ibid.   [345] RGPBI, 1885–86 (1886), pp. 147, 150, 152.   [346] Ibid., p. 149.

offence, released Quinn from custody to the South Dublin Union workhouse.[347]

As the case of prisoner Quinn highlights, medical officers utilised both 'imbecile' and 'weak-minded' to describe this category of prisoner. Saunders notes the term 'imbecile' was 'convenient shorthand for prison officials when describing prisoners who refused to conform to the model of stoical acceptance demanded of them by the penal regime'.[348] According to psychiatric categorisation, in the last quarter of the nineteenth century, 'idiots were at the lowest end of the ability range, followed by imbeciles and finally the "weakminded" at the end of the range nearest normality'.[349] Prisoners described as 'imbecile' accumulated in convict and local prisons, alongside the mentally ill and the weak-minded, prompting medical officers to speculate on the nature of their mental states, how to manage them, and whether prison discipline had the potential to improve their minds. In 1874, there were eighteen convicts described as 'imbecile' and requiring 'special treatment' working in the oakum room at Spike Island, and a further '12 to 20 others on the Public Works and in the Garden Party who are considered more or less imbecile or weak-minded but not to such an extent as to unfit them altogether from the works'.[350] Gover estimated there were 140 imbecile convicts in 1880 at Parkhurst and a further 40 at Woking.[351] Florence Maybrick, who was sentenced to fifteen years' penal servitude, served at Liverpool, Woking and Aylesbury prisons, observed female prisoners in Woking who 'hover on the borderland of insanity for months, possibly for years'.[352] Advocating separate institutions for weak-minded convicts, and noting that weak-minded, epileptic and consumptive prisoners were not isolated at Woking, Maybrick's comments reflect the challenges this group of prisoners presented:

They are recognized as weak-minded, and consequently they make capital out of their condition, and by the working of their distorted minds, and petty tempers, and unreasonable jealousy, add immeasurably not only to the ghastliness of the 'house of sorrow,' but are a sad clog on the efforts to self-betterment of their level-minded sisters in misery.[353]

---

[347] NAI, GPB/CORR/1884/Item no. 15050, Nov. 1884.

[348] Saunders, 'Institutionalised Offenders', p. 257.

[349] Ibid. Also see Janet Saunders, 'Quarantining the Weak-Minded: Psychiatric Definitions of Degeneracy and the Late-Victorian Asylum', in W.F. Bynum, Roy Porter and Michael Shepherd (eds), *Anatomy of Madness: Essays in the History of Psychiatry*, vol. 3 (London: Routledge, 1988), pp. 273–96.

[350] NAI, CSORP/1874/Item no. 4814, 7 Apr. 1874.

[351] Commission on Criminal Lunacy (1882), Evidence of R.M. Gover, p. 56.

[352] Florence Elizabeth Maybrick, *Mrs. Maybrick's Own Story: My Fifteen Lost Years* (New York and London: Funk & Wagnalls, 1905), p. 82.

[353] Ibid., pp. 82–3.

By the end of the century, prisoner W.B.N. described Parkhurst Prison as 'half a hospital and half a lunatic asylum', owing to the invalids and weak-minded prisoners who were brought from other convict prisons when their condition was considered serious. In 1900 a new hospital wing at Parkhurst was designated for criminal lunatics when Broadmoor became too full.[354] W.B.N. described the 'great many who are more or less touched in the top story, or who succeed in making it believed that they are so'. They were the 'weak-minded' or 'balmies', of feeble intellect or partially demented. By the end of the nineteenth century, it was estimated there were about ninety at Parkhurst, and many, W.B.N. added, were difficult to manage and very offensive to staff and prisoners.[355]

Defining an imbecile as someone labouring under an 'original congenital defect' and 'incapable of recovery', in evidence to the 1882 Commission on Criminal Lunacy, Gover claimed that such prisoners, when released into 'ordinary life', were frequently reconvicted to local prisons, where, serving short sentences, the condition of their minds was not diagnosed.[356] In these cases imbecility was 'not so marked as to constitute insanity', and these prisoners were not certified as criminal lunatics.[357] Only imbeciles who were also habitual criminals and serving penal servitude sentences were removed to Parkhurst where, Gover claimed, they would be 'better treated'.[358] Those held in local prisons were detained, but, he insisted, not punished, as medical officers, recognising that these prisoners suffered mental or physical defects, moderated the prison discipline, although he also acknowledged 'it may take some little time to ascertain whether a man is an imbecile'.[359] Gover opposed the removal of criminal imbeciles to local workhouses, claiming they were 'the most treacherous and dangerous set of men you can imagine', 'savage and thoroughly intractable', while others were 'very easily influenced, and tractable'.[360] Gover sought their removal from workhouses, as well as prisons, arguing that while the minds of some imbeciles could be improved when placed in the correct environment in a special institution, in the case of criminal imbeciles, there was no hope of recovery.[361] When confined in convict prisons these inmates were subjected to a modified form of discipline, yet, Gover insisted, they were not completely unfit for the disciplinary regime.[362]

---

[354] W.B.N., *Penal Servitude* (London: William Heinemann, 1903), pp. 148–9.
[355] Ibid., p. 150.
[356] Commission on Criminal Lunacy (1882), Evidence of R.M. Gover, p. 56; Saunders, 'Institutionalised Offenders', p. 257.
[357] Commission on Criminal Lunacy (1882), Evidence of R.M. Gover, p. 56.   [358] Ibid.
[359] Ibid.   [360] Ibid., pp. 57, 59.   [361] Ibid., pp. 57, 59. 63.   [362] Ibid., p. 63.

In evidence to the 1882 Commission on Lunacy, Broadmoor's Medical Superintendent, Dr Orange, also argued that in Broadmoor the uncertain 'moods and tempers' of imbeciles resulted in dangerous and unpredictable behaviour.[363] Orange claimed the mental conditions of 'weak-minded' and 'imbecile', while recognisable to medical men, were not as clearly defined as lunacy although there were some similarities such as deficient powers of self-control.[364] As imbeciles who were also habitual criminals already 'constantly in the habit of committing a crime', these deficiencies were grounds for detaining them.[365] While agreeing with prison medical officers that punishing these convicts would not influence their behaviour, Orange proposed they be trained and managed along lines 'adopted to influence children', to alter and improve their behaviour.[366]

As Orange's comments imply, psychiatrists and prison medical staff disagreed on the distinction between lunatics and imbeciles in the prison context. During the 1882 Commission on Criminal Lunacy, Guy and Dr Arthur Mitchell, Deputy Commissioner of Lunacy for Scotland, clashed over the operation of the Lunacy Acts as they related to imbeciles and over Guy's advocacy of a separate institutional provision, a National Imbecile Asylum.[367] Guy and Mitchell submitted separate memoranda on the subject to the Commission, both emphasising their expertise in understanding the minds and nature of imbeciles, Guy in the context of the convict prison and Mitchell in his role on the Lunacy Board for Scotland visiting adult imbeciles 'at large' and in asylums and prisons over '12 or 14 years'.[368] In his submission Guy elucidated on his interpretation of criminal imbecility as defined under the Criminal Lunatics Acts, arguing that the legislature drew a clear distinction between 'persons suffering from unsoundness of mind, other than those styled indifferently idiots or imbeciles', and those 'who suffer from imbecility of mind'. He noted that 'The one class are [sic] made inmates of the asylum with a view to the protection of life and property, the other as unfit for penal discipline.'[369] Guy argued that criminal imbeciles constitute most

---

[363] Ibid., Evidence of W. Orange, p. 48; for Orange, see J.V. Shepherd, 'Broadmoor's Victorian Superintendents': https://voicesfrombroadmoor.wordpress.com/2015/06/22/broadmoors-victorian-superintendents/; David Nicolson, 'Obituary. William Orange', *BMJ*, 1:2924 (13 Jan. 1917), 67–9.

[364] Commission on Criminal Lunacy (1882), Evidence of W. Orange, p. 53.   [365] Ibid.
[366] Ibid.
[367] Ibid., Memorandum by W.A. Guy, 'The Insane and the Asylum', pp. 161–4; Arthur Mitchell, 'Notes on Dr. Guy's Memorandum entitled the "Insane" and the "Imbecile"', pp. 164–7.
[368] Ibid., Mitchell, 'Notes on Dr. Guy's Memorandum', p. 166.
[369] Ibid., Guy, 'The Insane and the Asylum', p. 162.

of the 'beggars, thieves, mendicant thieves, tramps and vagrants' who 'infest our thoroughfares and fill the minds of the weaker, more helpless members of society with constant apprehension'. Echoing Gover's evidence to the Commission, and combining definitions of the criminal nature of imbecility with psychiatric diagnosis, Guy described imbeciles as 'dangerous to life and property', incurable and not amendable to improvement through education.[370] On this basis, Guy argued all imbeciles, not only those who committed crimes or were found unfit for penal discipline, should be placed in safe custody. Criminal behaviour, including dangerous or serious crimes such as rape, he contended, were embedded in the criminal imbecile's nature, the majority of whom were habitual criminals. As their criminal natures did not cease with the termination of the penal sentence, he justified the retention of criminal imbeciles in institutions under the remit of the convict prison system.[371]

Emphasising his expertise as a psychiatrist, Mitchell opposed Guy's proposal for a separate imbecile asylum, and objected to retaining imbeciles in institutions after the expiration of sentences on the grounds that such a measure would deny their legal rights. Once prisoners ceased to be criminals and, by Guy's logic, they could not be defined as lunatics under the Criminal Lunatics Acts, medical men, Mitchell insisted, had no legal grounds to detain them. In his critique of Guy's categorisation of imbecility as inherently criminal, Mitchell countered that Guy's experience of prison medicine, and of imbeciles in prison, had resulted in him studying the 'very worst of them', which were 'a mere handful of the whole body'.[372] Imbeciles, Mitchell argued, were not 'malicious destroyers of property' but could be easily 'led to abstain from doing wrong', as many had been 'trained to vicious practices by vicious sane persons'. Rejecting Guy's 'dark view of imbeciles', he also argued that environmental factors such as poverty and neglect were the main drivers of their criminal behaviours.[373] In a commentary on a census of imbecile and weak-minded prisoners held in convict prisons on 14 December 1879, and published in the 1882 Commission report, Mitchell drew attention to the varied uses and definitions of the terms 'weak-minded' and 'imbecile' convicts employed by prison governors, medical officers and chaplains in their assessments of individual cases.[374] He picked up on previous histories of poverty and neglect and the 'guilelessness' of

---

[370] Ibid.   [371] Ibid., pp. 161–4.
[372] Ibid., Mitchell, 'Notes on Dr. Guy's Memorandum', p. 166.
[373] Ibid. See also Saunders, 'Quarantining the Weak-Minded', pp. 286–8, for the clash between Guy and Mitchell.
[374] Commission on Criminal Lunacy (1882), 'Return of Lunatics, Weak-Minded and Imbecile Prisoners in Convict Prisons during December 1879', p. 147.

criminal imbeciles, a point Griffith had also noted in his assessment of imbeciles who he described as 'tools' of 'others more intelligent and more designing'.[375]

In developing these psychiatric categories, medical officers, including Guy and Mitchell, related particular forms of mental disorder to specific crimes, again focusing on habitual criminals. In 1869, Guy, in an analysis of the English convict prison population, concluded that 'men who suffer from diseases of the mind and nervous system are especially addicted to sexual offences, to arson and to acts of violence other than burglary; also in a less marked degree to cattle stealing'. He attributed 'sexual offences, the fire-raisings and the burglaries' to weak-minded male convicts, crimes of violence to the epileptic.[376] Commenting on a case of acute mania at Woking in 1869, Campbell also noted that the young male prisoner had 'some peculiarity of manner ... together with a conviction for arson, which is a crime suggestive of mental weakness'. The prisoner, who had been seized in a sudden manner while in the oakum room and had an aversion to food, was very violent and had been in a 'febrile excitement'.[377] Gover noted that criminal imbeciles were 'wayward and impulsive', 'grown-up' children addicted to wandering, acts of mischief and of cruelty such as arson.[378]

This individualised and practical orientation of prison medicine distinguished the work of Campbell, Guy, Nicolson and MacDonnell from their continental counterparts. Rejecting theories of the 'born criminal' and generalisations on the nature of the prisoners' minds, developed by the Lombrosian school and based on surveys of prison populations, prison medical officers emphasised the importance of treating and assessing individual prisoner patients in their quest to understand mental disorder among prisoners and manage such cases in challenging prison environments. Largely unsympathetic to theories that criminals were predetermined or programmed to commit crime, those who had some sympathy with these arguments in the early 1870s, such as Nicolson, rebuffed scientific claims that hereditary defects, including insanity and criminality, were identifiable by anatomical or physiological stigmata. Instead they stressed the 'value and influence of domestic and social environment, and of education and training, in moulding and forming

[375] Ibid.   [376] Guy, 'On Insanity and Crime', p. 171.
[377] RDCP, 1869 (1870), Woking Invalid Prison, p. 314.
[378] Commission on Criminal Lunacy (1882), Evidence of R.M. Gover, pp. 59, 60.

the character'.[379] In 1899 MacDonnell, also dismissing Lombrosian theories, noted that 'environment and example are two large factors' in the production of crime.[380] As discussed above, prison medical officers devoted considerable time to managing and treating individual cases, prescribing drugs and enhanced food allowances, and, in some cases, force-feeding prisoners. They stressed their unique experience and access to such cases, which Guy noted provided him with 'the special information which nearly seven years of office as medical superintendent of a convict prison, with a daily attendance subject to few interruptions, could not fail to have afforded me'.[381]

This emphasis on individual case studies was repeatedly enforced, with Nicolson arguing in 1895 that 'Each case must be taken on its own merits, and above all, and first of all, the man must be allowed to speak for himself, and to give his own "reason for the hope that is in him"'.[382] He dismissed the 'criminological method' as 'useless' and 'misleading' in daily practice and, citing statistics on juvenile reformatories, disagreed with claims that the majority of criminals could not be reformed and emphasised the significance of environmental factors such as poverty as motivating factors.[383] Ever wary of attacks on their professional status, there were also concerns that the generalised methodology of these theories reduced the function of the prison doctor to a technician who sorted prisoners according to several degenerate categories and institutions rather than providing individual diagnoses.[384] Arguing that prisoners were 'not passive victims of hereditary', Guy claimed the majority retained responsibility and the capacity to 'prefer thieving, with all its concomitant risk, to more reputable, if more laborious, modes of maintaining themselves'.[385] In his extensive publications, he sought a prestigious and expert role for prison doctors, who were uniquely positioned to understand the minds of prisoners, one that went beyond stamping '"criminals" as lunatics or quasi-lunatics, or to place them on a special morbid platform of mental existence'.[386]

Pentonville's Medical Officer, Dr John Baker, adopted a similar position in the 1890s. He characterised Lombroso's theories as 'extravagant

[379] David Nicolson, 'Presidential Address at Fifty-Fourth Annual Meeting of the Medico-Psychological Association', *Journal of Mental Science*, 41:175 (Oct. 1895), 567–91, at p. 581.
[380] Hercules MacDonnell, 'Prisons and Prisoners. Suggestions as to Treatment and Classification of Criminals', *Journal of the Statistical and Social Inquiry Society of Ireland*, 10:79 (Apr. 1899), 441–52, at p. 443.
[381] Guy, 'On Insanity and Crime', pp. 159–60.
[382] Nicolson, 'Presidential Address', p. 580.   [383] Ibid., pp. 577–80.
[384] Ibid., p. 580.   [385] Ibid.   [386] Ibid.

views held by a section of continental criminologists' and concluded that attempts to identify 'physical and psychical' stigmata among English felons do not 'warrant the assumption that there exists a special criminal type or a distinct criminal neurosis'.[387] From his close work in prison, he linked forms of mental disorders with specific crime noting, for example, 'the violence of epileptic insanity, the proneness of general paralytics to acts of petty larceny, the dangerous nature of delusional insanity, and the aimless crimes of dements'.[388] Baker suggested that the arsonist had a 'defective mental capacity' or was 'weakminded' and that there was 'a general relation of acts of incendiarism to the various forms of insanity'.[389] Baker went on to claim that prisons removed 'dangerous and insane criminals' from society and 'annually eliminated [them] from the ranks of the community', thus underlining the important role played by prison medical officers.[390]

Conclusion

By the end of the nineteenth century, vocal critics inside and outside of prisons highlighted the high incidences of mental illness among prisoners, and the excessively harsh aspects of prison discipline, including the separate system of confinement as it then operated in prisons in England and Ireland, which they argued could be harmful to the minds of prisoners. In 1894, Reverend William Morrison, chaplain at Wandsworth Prison between 1887 and 1898, claimed insanity rates in English local prisons had reached 113 per 10,000 between 1875 and 1877, increasing to 226 per 10,000 in 1890–92.[391] These high figures may in part have reflected a greater willingness by medical officers to diagnose prisoners as insane towards the end of century. Witnesses to the 1895 Gladstone Committee criticised the treatment of insane prisoners, while members of the Howard Association claimed that prisons produced an 'undue amount of insanity' among inmates, and these criticisms, among others, prompted the dismantling of the Du Cane system in England and, as examined in Chapter 6, the eventual decline of the separate system.

---

[387] John Baker, 'Insanity in English Local Prisons, 1894–95', *Journal of Mental Science*, 42:177 (Apr. 1896), 294–302, at p. 294.

[388] Ibid., p. 301.

[389] John Baker, 'Cases of Incendiarism with Commentary', *Journal of Mental Science*, 35:149 (Apr. 1889), 45–54, at pp. 46, 54.

[390] Baker, 'Insanity in English Local Prisons', p. 295.

[391] William Douglas Morrison, 'Are Our Prisons a Failure?', *The Fortnightly Review*, 55:328 (Apr. 1894), 459–69, at p. 468.

Such claims did not go uncontested, and, in response to allegations that the separate system produced mental disorders, prison commissioners, administrators and staff repeatedly defended the regime, insisting that prisoners were likely to be insane on admission, had a hereditary predisposition to insanity, were weak-minded or were feigning insanity.[392] In his report for the year 1897, Dr Herbert Smalley, the Medical Inspector of English Prisons, denied that 'prison is a manufactory for the production of lunacy', while Dr A.R. Douglas, an ally of Smalley's, argued that the high incidences of mental disorder among prisoners was a consequence of the 'material which is subjected to the penal environment'.[393] Although the first-time offender might initially experience feelings of depression, nonetheless, he argued, 'this individual is of sufficient mental calibre to have enabled him to take up to the time of his arrest a fairly successful part in the battle of life, it is absurd to suppose that this depression should deepen in intensity and become acute Mental pain'.[394] In the case of recidivists, however, prison was a 'normal condition' and while some 'take their imprisonment as a matter of course', others 'make it their business to give as much trouble as they can'.[395] In a robust defence of prison medical officers, the *Journal of Mental Science* argued that prisoners, owing to inherent mental weaknesses, had already demonstrated their inability to adapt to non-penal environments and 'oscillated' between asylums and prisons.[396] 'Depression must constantly follow imprisonment' owing to 'minds so ill-developed and ill-balanced, and often already depressed by anxiety arising from fear of detection in wrong-doing' and 'the sudden withdrawal of habitual excitation (mental or physical)'. While in prison 'depression is often exaggerated by their low physical powers and by onanism'.[397] The social role of the prison was emphasised as the 'beneficial results of the healthful [prison] regime and withdrawal from excesses' outweighed any negative results.[398]

Prison officials and medical officers made similar comments on the 'quality' of prisoners in Ireland. In 1905 a report of the medical committee appointed to inquire into removals of prisoners to Dundrum Asylum, noted that 'by parentage, education and association', prisoners' 'minds

[392] Kimberley Commission (1878–79), Evidence of M. Murphy, p. 943.
[393] Report of the Commissioners of Prisons and the Directors of Convict Prisons, 1896–97 (1897) [C.8590], p. 37; A.R. Douglas, 'Penal Servitude and Insanity', *Journal of Mental Science*, 44:185 (Apr. 1898), 271–7, at p. 271.
[394] Douglas, 'Penal Servitude and Insanity', p. 272.   [395] Ibid.
[396] Anon., 'Insanity in Prison', *Journal of Mental Science*, 43:80 (Jan. 1897), 115–16, at p. 116.
[397] Ibid.   [398] Ibid.

are impregnated and identified with ideas and habits of a vicious and criminal nature which show themselves during sane not less than during insane periods'. The medical committee, which included David Nicolson and Dr George Plunkett O'Farrell, Inspector of Lunatic Asylums in Ireland, also argued that the management of such cases in prisons required an 'extension of the area of sanity so as to include prisoners for whom ordinary penal discipline has to be relaxed and enables prisoners of this exceptional type to be detained in prison'.[399] While acknowledging that such prisoners were unable to withstand the full rigour of prison discipline, the medical committee regarded them as primarily as criminals who were also lunatics, a distinct label and category examined in Chapter 4. Meanwhile, over the last quarter of the nineteenth century, the professional confidence of prison medical officers had steadily grown, and rooted in decades of close observation of individual cases of mental illness in the prison, many published widely on the topic, advocated for their professional interests and contributed to official debates on penal policy. Though still negotiating a pathway through the complex demands of providing medical care on the one hand and complying with the requirements of prison discipline on the other, prison medical officers were confidently asserting a role as 'the recognised and responsible protector of the prisoner from any harsh treatment that may tend to his physical and mental detriment'.[400] They also increasingly laid claim to the advancement of professional psychiatric practices and the production of new knowledge that could be applied outside as well as inside the prison.

[399] NAI, CSORP/1905/12904, *Report on the Committee of Inquiry into Certain Doubtful Cases of Insanity amongst Convicts and Person Detained*, 1905, p. 10.
[400] Quinton, *Crime and Criminals 1876–1910*, p. vi.

4   Criminal or Lunatic, Prisoner or Patient?
Confining Insanity in the Late Nineteenth Century

> Whether the fifty insane convicts in Pentonville are of prison manufacture, or have found their way thither through judicial bungling, it is certain that their incarceration in such a place is highly improper.... Their presence in prison must seriously embarrass the officers, and interfere with its regular administration; and the denial to them of medical treatment at the time when it might be of service in rescuing them from lifelong insanity, is a cruel wrong.[1]

By the late nineteenth century, it was widely acknowledged that many insane criminals were languishing in prisons in England and Ireland. However, this statement, appearing in the *British Medical Journal* (*BMJ*) in June 1880, was unusually forthright about this state of affairs, with its comment on judicial bungling and claim that the prison could 'manufacture' insanity. The article was triggered by the suicide of one of the Pentonville 'lunatics', and, describing the special measures that had been put in place to deal with the fifty insane prisoners in Pentonville, its governor explained that twenty cells were under observation, and that many prisoners had been deprived of their tin knives for fear that they would harm themselves. The article went on to state that it was very likely that the discipline of the prison was to some degree responsible for the prisoners' insanity and suicidal propensities, but also that some prisoners had suffered a miscarriage of justice, being insane at the time of their trial, and ought never to have been Pentonville in the first place.[2]

While highlighted as a pressing issue by the *BMJ*, the annual report of the Directors of Convict Prisons for 1880, far from being 'embarrassed', referred to the suicide in a curt, matter-of-fact manner, without further comment. Prisoner G.77 had committed suicide by hanging himself in his cell. He had been subject to epileptic attacks, sometimes preceded by 'periods of excitement', but he had never exhibited any suicidal tendency

---

[1] Editorial, 'Lunatics in Prisons', *British Medical Journal* (*BMJ*), 2:1035 (30 Oct. 1880), 710–11, at p. 711.
[2] Ibid., pp. 710–11.

and his mental condition had been certified as 'sound' on his reception into the prison.[3] It was also reported that over the course of the year nine prisoners had been moved to other prisons as 'insane', together with an additional sixteen patients with 'mental afflictions other than insanity'.[4]

The suicide of prisoner G.77 illuminates the mounting disquiet concerning the mental wellbeing of prisoners and the 'disposal' of those suspected of suffering from mental illness, which by the second half of the nineteenth century increasingly preoccupied English and Irish prison administrators and medical officers, psychiatrists working outside of the criminal justice system and the medical press. Questions were raised about how prisons dealt with inmates who developed symptoms of mental disorder following their trial and removal to prison, many of whom appeared to be mentally disordered on their committal. While prison administrators and medical officers were concerned to pinpoint cases of feigned insanity, the subject of the following chapter, and to downplay the deleterious impact of prison regimes on the mental health of prisoners, by the late nineteenth century they too were expressing dismay and frustration at the accumulation of large numbers of lunatics in prisons ill-equipped to deal with them.

The scale of the problem was illustrated in 1889 when the Commissioners of Prisons for England and Wales reported that 349 insane persons had been held in prison that year, of whom 210 had been moved on to asylums. According to Dr R.M. Gover, Medical Inspector of Prisons, as many as 290 were found to be insane on reception.[5] Gover complained that 'local prisons ... are at present used to some extent as hospitals for the treatment of mental and bodily disease'. As they were not intended or adapted for that purpose, he continued, 'this practice should as far as possible cease'.[6] In Ireland the story was similar, though the numbers involved were smaller, and by the 1880s it appears that most insane prisoners were being moved on to asylums. The 1884 Report of the Royal Commission on Prisons in Ireland highlighted, as one of the 'most serious points' brought to their notice, the large number of prisoners certified insane in the Irish convict prisons of Mountjoy and Spike Island, remarking, 'The existence of such an excess ought certainly to have attracted the notice of the authorities to a greater

---

[3] Report of the Directors of Convict Prisons (RDCP), 1880–81 (1881) [C.3073], Pentonville Prison: Extracts from the Medical Officer's Report, pp. 317, 321.

[4] Ibid., Table IV, 'Cases of Insanity and of Mental Affections other than Insanity', p. 321.

[5] Anon., 'Report of the Commissioners of Prisons', Lancet, 134:3455 (16 Nov. 1889), 1012; R.M. Gover and Pugin Thorton, 'Report of the Commissioners of Prisons, To the Editors of the Lancet', Lancet, 134:3456 (23 Nov. 1889), 1085–6, at p. 1085.

[6] Anon., 'Report of the Commissioners of Prisons', Lancet (16 Nov. 1889), p. 1012.

extent than it appears to have done.'[7] Dr Hercules MacDonnell, Medical Officer at Dundalk Prison, criticised the Royal Commission, however, for its 'curt dismissal' of the concerns of witnesses relating to the lengthy detention of lunatics in prisons, noting

It is impossible to conceive any course more likely to prove hurtful to persons who have become insane, than that of subjecting them to the discipline and regime necessary in prison life. These cases require the most skilled personal attention, which it is quite impossible for them to obtain in gaols ... and when it is borne in mind that in the majority of prisons there is no adequate provision for the proper nursing of even sick prisoners, it can be readily seen that lunatics must fare very badly.[8]

In 1888, 85 insane prisoners were moved from local gaols to asylums in Ireland and in 1892, 71.[9] The General Prisons Board complained regularly in their reports about this objectionable state of affairs, a complaint upheld by the *Lancet*: 'It is not alone the inhumanity of subjecting lunatics to the unsuitable discipline of an ordinary prison which calls for remark, but also the waste of power involved in providing by means of makeshift arrangements for their safety.'[10] While the *Lancet* castigated the Irish prison authorities for their negligence on this score, it is clear that both English and Irish prisons were under enormous pressure to deal with large numbers of insane prisoners in environments unsuited for their confinement.

An impressive literature has explored trial proceedings involving the insanity plea, the role of doctors as 'expert witnesses' and the processes of deciding whether defendants were 'mad' or 'bad', acting under an insane impulse and thus not to be held responsible for their actions or guilty of a criminal act.[11] As Roger Smith has demonstrated, it became more common over the course of the nineteenth century for medical men to

---

[7] Royal Commission on Prisons in Ireland, Vol. 1. Reports, Digest of Evidence, Appendices; Minutes of Evidence, 1884 (1884–85) [C.4233] [C.4233–I], p. 40.

[8] Hercules MacDonnell, 'A Review of Some of the Subjects in the Report of the Royal Commission on Prisons in Ireland', *Journal of the Statistical and Social Inquiry Society of Ireland*, 8:63 (July 1885), 617–23, at p. 621.

[9] Anon., 'The Prison Reports', *Lancet*, 132:3395 (22 Sept. 1888), 589; Anon., 'General Prisons Board Report', *Lancet*, 140:3617 (24 Dec. 1892), 1472.

[10] Anon., 'The Prison Reports'.

[11] Roger Smith, *Trial by Medicine: Insanity and Responsibility in Victorian Trials* (Edinburgh: Edinburgh University Press, 1981); Roger Smith, 'The Boundary between Insanity and Criminal Responsibility in Nineteenth-Century England', in Andrew Scull (ed.), *Madhouses, Mad-Doctors, and Madmen: A Social History of Psychiatry in the Victorian Era* (London: Athlone, 1981), pp. 363–84; Joel Peter Eigen, *Witnessing Insanity: Madness and Mad-Doctors in the English Court* (New Haven, CT and London: Yale University Press, 1995); Joel Peter Eigen, *Mad-Doctors in the Dock: Defending the Diagnosis, 1760–1913* (Baltimore, MD: Johns Hopkins University Press, 2016); Tony

put forward a plea of insanity, though such pleas were not necessarily successful.[12] Notwithstanding, many defendants were found to be insane prior to or during their trials, and, based on the verdict of 'not guilty by means of their insanity', and in Ireland 'guilty but insane', moved to lunatic asylums or, after 1850 in Ireland and 1863 in England, to state criminal lunatic asylums at Dundrum and Broadmoor.[13]

This scholarship has, however, focused only in a limited way on the detection of mental illness among prisoners after their conviction and imprisonment, the transfers of prisoners to asylums, and the debates surrounding the appropriate placement and care of insane offenders, many of whom ended up traversing back and forth between asylums and prisons.[14] Yet, as Janet Saunders has pointed out with regard to England, in addition to decisions reached during trials, the issue of the disposal of mentally disordered offenders became increasingly important after mid-century. Alongside the removal of prisoners labelled as 'insane convicts', county and borough asylums became 'the major receivers of offenders found insane in local prisons', typically accused of mundane

---

Ward, 'Law, Common Sense and the Authority of Science: Expert Witnesses and Criminal Insanity in England, ca. 1840–1940', *Social and Legal Studies*, 6:3 (1997), 343–62; Katherine Watson, *Medicine and Justice: Medico-Legal Practice in England and Wales, 1700–1914* (Abingdon: Routledge, 2019); Martin J. Wiener, 'Murderers and "Reasonable Men": The "Criminology" of the Victorian Judiciary', in Peter Becker and Richard F. Wetzell (eds), *Criminals and Their Scientists: The History of Criminology in International Perspective* (Cambridge: Cambridge University Press, 2006), pp. 43–60; Pauline M. Prior, *Madness and Murder: Gender, Crime and Mental Disorder in Nineteenth-Century Ireland* (Dublin: Irish Academic Press, 2008); Pauline M. Prior, 'Mad, Not Bad: Crime, Mental Disorder and Gender in Nineteenth-Century Ireland', *History of Psychiatry*, 8:32 (1997), 501–16; Pauline M. Prior, 'Prisoner or Patient? The Official Debate on the Criminal Lunatic in Nineteenth-Century Ireland', *History of Psychiatry*, 15:2 (2004), 177–92.

[12] Smith, 'The Boundary between Insanity and Criminal Responsibility', p. 364.

[13] For Broadmoor, see Jade Shepherd, '"I Am Very Glad and Cheered When I Hear the Flute": The Treatment of Criminal Lunatics in Late Victorian Broadmoor', *Medical History*, 60:4 (2016), 473–91; Harvey Gordon, *Broadmoor* (London: Psychology News Press, 2012); Mark Stevens, *Broadmoor Revealed: Victorian Crime and the Lunatic Asylum* (Barnsley: Pen & Sword, 2013). For Dundrum, see Prior, *Madness and Murder*; Brendan Kelly, 'Poverty, Crime and Mental Illness: Female Forensic Psychiatric Committal in Ireland, 1910–1948', *Social History of Medicine*, 21:2 (2008), 311–28; Brendan Kelly, *Custody, Care & Criminality: Forensic Psychiatry and Law in 19th Century Ireland* (Dublin: History Press, 2014).

[14] Janet Saunders, 'Institutionalised Offenders: A Study of the Victorian Institution and Its Inmates, with Special Reference to Late Nineteenth Century Warwickshire' (unpublished University of Warwick PhD thesis, 1983), especially ch. 7, which focuses on criminal lunatics and practices of referral by magistrates. See also Janet Saunders, 'Magistrates and Madmen: Segregating the Criminally Insane in Late-Nineteenth-Century Warwickshire', in Victor Bailey (ed.), *Policing and Punishment in Nineteenth Century Britain* (London: Croom Helm, 1981), pp. 217–41.

crimes and sentenced to short prison terms.[15] While prison doctors expressed extreme concern about the number of cases of insanity in prisons, asylum superintendents were up in arms about the clusters of insane criminals accumulating in their institutions, 'the pests of all asylums'.[16] They were described as difficult to manage and disruptive for the other patients, at a point when many asylums were under great pressure to admit increasing numbers of pauper lunatics and facing severe shortages of accommodation. Yet at the same time, asylum superintendents were often highly critical of prison medical officers for their failure to detect and move genuinely insane prisoners to asylums where they could receive appropriate care.

Chapters 2 and 3 have demonstrated how concerns about damage limitation shaped policy and practical responses to the treatment of the mentally disordered in English and Irish prisons. Highlighting mental illness and removing prisoners out of the prison system into asylums ran the risk of being interpreted as the failure of prison regimes to improve the minds of prisoners or linked to accusations that the discipline itself had triggered mental breakdown. This was a problem for both the showcase convict prisons and local prisons attempting to implement the separate system as effectively as possible. As Chapter 5 explains, concern about prisoners' efforts to feign mental illness led to extreme caution in transferring prisoners to asylums, and many prisoners whose insanity was doubted would remain in prison until their sentences terminated. Nonetheless, many prisoners were moved out of prisons, to Broadmoor and Dundrum, or to county, district and private asylums, and it is the mechanisms through which decisions were reached to prompt removals, and the experiences of prisoners who were declared insane following their incarceration that is the main focus of this chapter. For a number of prison surgeons, the business of assessing prisoners began in the courtroom or during the remand process, while for others the mundane processes of diagnosing mental illness and authorising transfers to asylums, and oftentimes back to prison became part of their day-to-day workload.

This chapter is divided into two sections. Section I investigates the series of legislative changes and institutional provisions that were put in place in England and Ireland from early in the nineteenth century to manage the allocation of patients to prisons and asylums, as well as

[15] Saunders, 'Magistrates and Madmen', pp. 220, 223.
[16] [W. Charles Hood], 'Criminal Lunatics. A Letter to the Chairman of the Commissioners in Lunacy', *Journal of Mental Science*, 6:34 (July 1860), 513–19, at p. 513.

focusing on the courtroom as the site where prisoners declared insane around the time of their trials would, in theory, be sifted out of the prison system. Yet, as explored in section II, many prisoners suffering from insanity continued to be committed to prison, while responses to particular prisoners, the limitations of institutional space and resources, and the diverse actions of individual doctors and prison and lunacy administrators demonstrate that legal frameworks were subject to hugely varied interpretations in practice. Such actions were closely related to prison medical officers' growing experience and claims of expertise in psychiatry, expressed in both the courtroom and prison, and their ability to assess and diagnose insanity among criminals, as well as their anxieties about how the accumulation of mentally ill prisoners might conflict with their assertion that they were best equipped to deal with such cases. From time to time, as also examined through exploration of a select number of such cases in section II, the regular business of assessment and transfer exploded into high-profile disputes surrounding removals, triggered by insane prisoners arriving in a dreadful state at asylums, with severe injuries or close to death. These cases illuminate the depth of intraprofessional antagonism and completing claims of knowledge and expertise that could arise around the issue of dealing with mentally disordered offenders.

I PROVISION FOR CRIMINAL LUNATICS AND LUNATIC CRIMINALS

Accumulating in Prisons and Asylums: Legislative Change and Institutional Provision

The question of where to house the criminally insane taxed prison and asylum administrators from the early nineteenth century. As asylum facilities began to be set up in England and Ireland, accommodating the criminally insane within them presented enormous challenges in terms of the availability of space, governance and their impact on the welfare of the other patients. In England the 1800 Criminal Lunatics Act first made provision for the custody of criminal lunatics, those found unfit to plead or acquitted of an offence on the grounds of insanity at 'His Majesty's Pleasure', which could mean indefinitely.[17] In effect, however, with no provision for the costs of their maintenance, most criminal lunatics continued to be confined in workhouses or more commonly

---

[17] Prompted by the trial of James Hadfield, who in 1800 attempted to assassinate George III. See Nigel Walker, *Crime and Insanity in England, Volume One: The Historical Perspective* (Edinburgh: Edinburgh University Press, 1968), pp. 74–83.

gaols, often in terrible conditions, where 'the poor criminal lunatics became objects of sport to their unfeeling fellow-prisoners, by whom they were taunted, ridiculed and tormented'.[18] In 1808 the County Asylum (Wynn's) Act authorised counties to set up asylums on a permissive basis with provision for pauper patients and criminal lunatics. It was also recommended that a separate asylum for criminal lunatics be set up at Bethlem to serve the whole country, supported at the state's expense, and in 1816 two wings opened at Bethlem to accommodate sixty criminal patients.[19] A few years later it was found necessary to double the accommodation at Bethlem, and in 1849 a separate ward was erected at Fisherton House private asylum for the excess of criminal lunatics.

In 1816 further provision was made to transfer convicted criminals who became insane during their sentences, with a warrant from the Home Secretary, and in 1840 this was extended to unsentenced prisoners and prisoners awaiting execution. Those transferred under these acts were to be certified insane by two magistrates and two medical men, and would only be returned to prison with the approval of the Secretary of State.[20] These provisions initially applied only to those prisoners who were tried by a jury for more serious crimes, but after 1840 petty offenders showing signs of insanity might be sent to a county asylum.[21] Even with the absorption of criminal lunatics into the slowly expanding county asylum system (with twenty-four established in England and Wales by 1850), and the expansion of its facilities, Bethlem was overwhelmed by this class of patient, so much so that the *Lancet* was prompted in 1855 to describe the asylum as a mere receptacle of insane criminals rather than a curative institution 'into which the waifs of criminal law are swept, out of sight and out of mind'.[22] In 1857 the Commissioners in Lunacy referred to the indiscriminate mixing of patients without regard for their previous

---

[18] W. Charles Hood, *Suggestions for the Future Provision of Criminal Lunatics* (London: John Churchill, 1854), p. 107.

[19] David Nicolson, 'A Chapter in the History of Criminal Lunacy in England', *Journal of Mental Science*, 23:102 (July 1877), 165–85, at pp. 169–70; Jonathan Andrews, Asa Briggs, Roy Porter, Penny Tucker and Keir Waddington, *The History of Bethlem* (London and New York: Routledge, 1997), pp. 403–5.

[20] Patricia Allderidge, 'Bethlem to Broadmoor', *Proceedings of the Royal Society of Medicine*, 67:9 (Sept. 1974), 897–9; Saunders, 'Institutionalised Offenders', pp. 221–2.

[21] 3&4 Vict., c.54 (1840); Kathleen Jones, *Lunacy, Law, and Conscience 1744–1845* (London: Routledge & Kegan Paul, 1955), p. 219.

[22] 'Notices and Reviews of Books' (John Charles Bucknill, *Unsoundness of Mind in Relation to Criminal Acts* (1854)), *Lancet*, 65:1642 (17 Feb. 1855), 187. See also Andrews et al., *The History of Bethlem*, pp. 502–6. The passing of 1845 County Asylums Act (together with the 1845 Lunacy Act) made it mandatory for counties to establish asylums, and the second half of the century saw sustained growth in their number and size. See Andrew

moral and social condition and the 'skeleton cupboards' of Bethlem in the form of the male criminal lunatic wards, with its 'dens ... more like those which enclose the fiercer carnivora at the Zoological Gardens than anything we have elsewhere seen employed for the detention of afflicted humanity'.[23]

In Ireland, the 1787 Prison Act and Lunatic Asylum Acts of 1817 and 1821 dealt with 'the custody of insane persons charged with offences'. In 1821 provision was made for persons acquitted on grounds of insanity or persons indicted and found insane at the point of their arraignment, allowing for 'safe custody' in prison, prior to transfer to an asylum under a Lord Lieutenant's warrant, and specified that 'the custody of insane persons, charged with offences in Ireland shall be regulated in like manner as in England'.[24] The persistent accumulation of the insane in prisons had been one of the drivers behind the establishment of district asylums, and Ireland set up its national asylum system earlier than England. By 1835 nine asylums had been constructed, but their capacity to absorb the insane prisoners languishing in gaol was limited. Even as asylum superintendents, such as Mr Jackson of Armagh Asylum, referred in 1828 to the 'many hopeless cases admitted from the gaols', criminal lunatics continued to accumulate in prisons.[25] Particular pressure was felt in Dublin, served by Richmond District Asylum and in the areas covered by the district asylums of Armagh and Londonderry, 'where the numbers crowding the County Gaols are truly distressing'.[26] During the 1840s it was proposed that an extra ward be set up at Richmond Asylum dedicated to criminal lunatics, but this was never brought into effect, and by 1849 – swelled by the Great Famine – the number of lunatics confined in gaols had increased to 338.[27]

The situation was complicated in Ireland by the implementation of the Dangerous Lunatic Act in 1838, resulting in a new category, of 'dangerous lunatic', making provision for the certification of individuals 'who displayed a propensity to commit an indicatable crime while denoting a "derangement of mind" and who were perceived to represent a threat to

Scull, *The Most Solitary of Afflictions: Madness and Society in Britain, 1700–1900* (New Haven, CT and London: Yale University Press, 1993), p. 281.
[23] Anon., 'Reports of the Commissioners in Lunacy to the Lord Chancellor', *Quarterly Review*, 101:202 (Apr. 1857), 353–93, at p. 361.
[24] 27 Geo. III, c.39 (1787); 57 Geo. III. c.106 (1817); 1&2 Geo. IV, c.33 (1821).
[25] Report of the Inspectors General of Prisons of Ireland (RIGPI), 1828 (1828) [68], p. 12.
[26] Report from the Select Committee of the House of Lords Appointed to Consider the State of the Lunatic Poor in Ireland (1843) [625], p. x.
[27] Report on the District, Local and Private Lunatic Asylums in Ireland, 1848 (1849) [1054], p. 10; Anon., 'Lunatic Asylums in Ireland', *Dublin Medical Press*, 25:633 (Feb. 1851), 124.

the community'.[28] This group came to account for the majority of the 'lunatics' confined in Irish prisons and asylums, most of whom had not been charged with a criminal offence. The 1843 Report on the State of the Lunatic Poor in Ireland claimed that the number of lunatics in gaols and bridewells had doubled over the previous two years to 214, of whom only forty had been charged.[29] In England, the same legislation also required two Justices of the Peace to commit dangerous lunatics to an asylum or licensed madhouse rather than a gaol. However, its impact was felt far less than in Ireland, and, when applied, tended to result in asylum admissions rather than confinement in prison.[30] In Ireland too danger- ous lunatics, along with those becoming insane in prison, were in principle to be transferred from prisons to district asylums on the recom- mendation of two magistrates, who sought medical advice on such cases from local doctors attached to workhouses, gaols or dispensaries. In 1847 Lunacy Inspectors Dr Francis White and Dr John Nugent issued a circular advising all magistrates to seek medical advice, and after 1848 new certification forms were structured to include more medical information, and gaol governors obliged to ensure that the completed form accompanied persons moved from gaols to asylums.[31] However, until the Dangerous Lunatic legislation was amended in 1867, after which alleged lunatics were to be sent directly to an asylum, the confine- ment of dangerous lunatics put even more pressure on gaols, where they might be held for lengthy periods given the shortage of asylum accom- modation. In 1866 some 685 dangerous lunatics were taken into county and borough gaols, of whom 514 were sent on to asylums. Dublin's Richmond Bridewell housed 95 male lunatics and Grangegorman 98 female lunatics.[32] Up until 1867 such practices 'established an intim- ate link between insanity and criminality', associating the lunatic with the 'degredation of the prison'.[33] Though some had separate lunatic cells or wards, or even padded cells, many public gaols had no effective means of

[28] 1&2 Vict., c.27 (1838); Catherine Cox, *Negotiating Insanity in the Southeast of Ireland, 1820–1900* (Manchester: Manchester University Press, 2012), p. 77. See also Mark Finnane, *Insanity and the Insane in Post-Famine Ireland* (London: Croom Helm, 1981), pp. 88–104 and Damien Brennan, *Irish Insanity* (London and New York: Routledge, 2014), pp. 79–83 for the operation of the Dangerous Lunatic legislation.
[29] Select Committee State of the Lunatic Poor in Ireland (1843), p. ix.
[30] Hansard HL Deb, 18 Mar. 1852, vol. 119 cc1230–44, Earl of Shaftesbury.
[31] Cox, *Negotiating Insanity*, pp. 79–80.
[32] RIGPI, 1866 (1867) [3915], pp. xxv–xxvi. The passing of the 1867 Act resulted in a rapid fall-off in the number of mentally disordered persons defined as 'dangerous lunatics' in prison, from 334 in 1867 to 53 in 1868 and 5 in 1869: Brennan, *Irish Insanity*, p. 83.
[33] Oonagh Walsh, '"The Designs of Providence": Race, Religion and Irish Insanity', in Joseph Melling and Bill Forsythe (eds), *Insanity, Institutions and Society, 1800–1914*

separating the lunatic from the criminal. 'The insane were often', as a result, 'made the sport of the guilty and subjected to indignities and cruel treatment', though White and Nugent also pointed out that association with sane prisoners, alongside the removal of alcohol and other prompts to mental breakdown, might be beneficial.[34]

Both the Lunacy Commissioners in England and Inspectors in Ireland lobbied for the setting up of specialist institutions for criminal lunatics in response to constant complaints about the disadvantages of housing them in the prison system, as well as the grave pressures they placed on asylums.[35] Dr Francis White, who prior to becoming Inspector of Lunatics in 1845 served as Inspector of Prisons with responsibility for overseeing lunatic asylums in Ireland, argued that bringing criminal lunatics together would save expense, increase security and put a stop to the use of district asylums for a purpose that they were never intended to fulfil.[36] In evidence presented to the 1843 Select Committee he provided many examples of failures within both prisons and asylums, including the case of the female lunatics housed in Grangegorman Prison, where there was an absence of proper accommodation, classification, employment and trained keepers: 'They are in a most confined Place, and a great Number of them in Strait Waistcoats and muffed, and Two of them strapped to narrow inconvenient Chairs.' Their presence, White concluded, interfered with prison discipline and in practice they were often cared for by other prisoners.[37] While eager to assert the quality of prison doctors – 'they are all clever Men' – they were unable 'to devote their Time to the treatment of insanity so much as those who are attached to Asylums'.[38] Transfer papers and arrangements were also noted to be defective, and prisoners often arrived at asylums 'in a most

(London and New York: Routledge, 1999), 223–42, at p. 225; Cox, *Negotiating Insanity*, p. 80. See also Oonagh Walsh, 'Lunatic and Criminal Alliances in Nineteenth-Century Ireland', in Peter Bartlett and David Wright (eds), *Outside the Walls of the Asylum: The History of Care in the Community 1750–2000* (London and New Brunswick, NJ: Athlone, 1999), pp. 132–52.

[34] *The Irish Times*, 12 July 1867, p. 2; Cox, *Negotiating Insanity*, p. 81. Despite a tightening up of the law in 1845, the Dangerous Lunatic legislation was also subject to misuse by those attempting to use the procedures to admit family members to asylums, while families also protested about their relatives being retained in prison instead of being transferred to asylums, arguing that asylum treatment might assist in their recovery.

[35] Prior, *Madness and Murder*, pp. 30–1.   [36] Ibid., p. 31.

[37] Select Committee State of the Lunatic Poor in Ireland (1843), Evidence of Francis White, 20 July 1843, p. 15.

[38] Ibid., p. 16.

wretched and deplorable state'. They were also noted to be more prone to escape attempts.[39]

In England too pressure mounted for the creation of a specialist facility, particularly as county asylums were under increased pressure to admit what appeared to be ever-growing numbers of patients, including in some areas of the country many Irish migrants.[40] In 1852 the Commissioners in Lunacy (who after 1850 were also responsible for lunatics confined in gaols) claimed that there were 436 lunatic criminals in asylums: 175 in county asylums, 104 in Bethlem, 108 in provincial private asylums, and 41 in metropolitan private asylums, with the remaining eight being held in hospital.[41] The Report bemoaned the association of criminal lunatics with ordinary patients, to whom they caused pain and disquiet: 'the Language and Habits of criminal Patients being generally offensive, and their Propensities almost invariably bad'.[42] According to the Commissioners, they interfered with the routine and discipline of the asylum, with their efforts to feign insanity and to escape, and their bad habits caused insubordination and dissolution among the other patients. They also required stricter custody and strengthened 'the common delusion that an asylum is a prison'.[43] Such issues were pointed out time after time by the Commissioners, just as they had been in Ireland a decade earlier, as they repeatedly advocated for a state criminal asylum, reaffirming that mentally ill prisoners were 'morally tainted with crime' and 'unfit for association with the ordinary inmates of Asylums'.[44] Including individuals who had murdered fellow-prisoners and assaulted attendants, they terrified the other patients, who came to believe that the asylum was a prison, retarding their recovery.[45]

This campaign was supported by eminent asylum superintendents, such as Dr Charles Hood, who, increasingly frustrated about the overcrowding and conditions at Bethlem, initiated its reform.[46]

---

[39] Report on the District, Local and Private Lunatic Asylums in Ireland, 1846 (1847) [820], Ballinasloe District Lunatic Asylum, p. 28, Limerick District Lunatic Asylum, p. 41. See the final part of this chapter for accounts of the condition of transferred patients and Chapter 5 for escape attempts.

[40] Scull, The Most Solitary of Afflictions, and for the case of asylum expansion in Lancashire, Catherine Cox and Hilary Marland, '"A Burden on the County": Madness, Institutions of Confinement and the Irish Patient in Victorian Lancashire', Social History of Medicine, 28:2 (2015), 263–87.

[41] Report of the Commissioners in Lunacy, 1852 (1852–53) [285], p. 43.

[42] Ibid., p. 33.

[43] Ibid.; Nicolson, 'A Chapter in the History of Criminal Lunacy in England', p. 171.

[44] Report of the Commissioners in Lunacy, 1854 (1855) [339], p. 47.

[45] Hansard HL Deb, 18 Mar. 1852, vol. 119 cc1230–44, Earl of Shaftesbury.

[46] Hood, Suggestions for the Future Provision; W. Charles Hood, Criminal Lunatics: A Letter to the Chairman of the Commissioners in Lunacy (London: John Churchill, 1860). Charles Hood was appointed as Medical Superintendent at Bethlem in 1852 and held the post

Dr John Charles Bucknill, superintendent of the Devon County Asylum at Exminster, agreed that Bethlem was clearly inadequate, but suggested (somewhat at odds with the findings of the Commissioners in Lunacy) that the county asylum could be a useful resource for treating carefully selected criminal lunatics, persons often committing minor offences and lacking true criminal propensities, who could be considered as 'lunatics of criminal disposition'. He also argued that his experience showed him that the other patients could be sympathetic to this class of patient rather than offended by them.[47] One such case was an agricultural labourer, 'generally industrious, but was fond of drink, and then liable to commit [sic] all manner of petty offences'. He was also thought to be 'a little weak in the head'. He was committed to the house of correction for six weeks for indecent exposure and there found to be insane. Taken into Exminster Asylum, his maniacal excitement passed off quickly and he was described as jovial and industrious. After eight months he was discharged recovered by order of the Secretary of State. Three years later the man was again committed to prison 'for want of sureties to keep the peace' and then readmitted to Exminster. At this point Bucknill concluded that 'As he is intensively fond of cider, and as cider causes in him maniacal excitement, the asylum is probably the best place for him.'[48]

Based on his experience at Bethlem, Charles Hood advocated for an improved and specialised state asylum, but also recommended that not all criminal lunatics should be confined together, as this would deter recovery, increase public prejudice and, as a result, create a new 'bastille'. Like Bucknill, Hood suggested, minor offenders should be placed in county asylums.[49] Hood also presented accounts of numerous cases confined in Bethlem, who were no longer insane but who he was unable to discharge. Between 1852 to 1858 120 prisoners charged with murder, attempted murder or personal violence were acquitted and seventy-nine

for ten years. He was responsible for reversing Bethlem's poor reputation and campaigned for the segregation of the criminally insane: https://history.rcplondon.ac.uk/inspiring-physicians/sir-william-charles-hood

[47] John Charles Bucknill, *An Inquiry into the Proper Classification and Treatment of Criminal Lunatics* (London: John Churchill, 1852), pp. 7–8, 17, Appendix, Case XVI. Bucknill served at the Exminster Asylum between 1844 and 1876, and also co-authored the first comprehensive textbook on psychiatry in 1858: Andrew Scull, 'Bucknill, Sir John Charles (1817–1897)', *Dictionary of National Biography* (*DNB*), https://0-doi-org/10.1093/ref:odnb/3874 [accessed 6 May 2020].

[48] Bucknill, *An Inquiry into the Proper Classification and Treatment of Criminal Lunatics*, Appendix, Case VII. The Appendix included numerous similar cases admitted to Exminster Asylum.

[49] Hood, *Suggestions for the Future Provision*, pp. 134–40. See also Richard Hunter and Ida Macalpine, *Three Hundred Years of Psychiatry* (London: Oxford University Press, 1963), p. 1020; Andrews et al., *The History of Bethlem*, p. 502.

of these were received at Bethlem. In a number of cases, no symptoms of insanity had been observed since admission.[50] In 1857 J.P., an 'expert thief', well known to the police in London and the West of England, committed murder in Westminster Workhouse where he was taken suffering from delirium tremens. He was tried and acquitted on the grounds of insanity and removed to Bethlem. At the time of reception, he was, according to Hood, sane and had since shown no symptoms of insanity. An ordinary lunatic asylum was no place for a character with such 'vicious tendencies', who had been in prison eleven times, Hood stressed, but neither was Bethlem. 'Yet though perfectly sane, the doors of every prison are closed against him, and he must remain a tenant of the lunatic asylum, where he produces constant anxiety to those who have the charge of him.'[51] Similar issues were raised concerning cases of convicts admitted to Dundrum during the first five years of its operation. In some instances their sentences had expired, and others were simply deemed to be inappropriate subjects for confinement in Dundrum, such as Mary Sullivan, sentenced to seven years' transportation for larceny, who was described as weak-minded rather than insane. Dundrum's physicians, William Corbett and Robert Harrison, believed that Sullivan, who was unable to speak English, would be better off in an asylum in her native county Kerry, where she would have someone to talk to. Two legal advisors were brought in to provide an opinion on the general situation and concluded that prisoners were entitled to be discharged if recovered, while those still of unsound mind should be restored to the care of their friends or sent to the district asylum.[52]

By the mid-nineteenth century official reports and publications on the challenges of dealing with insane offenders increasingly adopted the terms 'lunatic criminals' or 'insane convicts' to distinguish this group from 'criminal lunatics' who had been found insane prior to or during the trial process. As also reflected in the medical taxonomies discussed in Chapter 3, use of such attributions was by no means consistent, and a crisp division into 'bad' or 'mad' was not strictly adhered to. While plans were put in place to set up a state criminal asylum in England, Bucknill referred to the problems of trying to sift out criminal lunatics and the implications in terms of institutional care, when those 'who have become insane from the long indulgence of criminal propensities' were mixed

---

[50] Hood, *Criminal Lunatics*, p. 16.
[51] Ibid., pp. 14–15. Hood's account provides several examples of similar cases.
[52] Report on the District, Criminal and Private Lunatic Asylums in Ireland, 1857 (1857) [2253], Appendix 1: Cases on Behalf of the Crown as to the Admission of Patients into the Central Criminal Asylum, Dundrum, who have become insane subsequently to their conviction, pp. 71–2.

with 'those who have become criminal for want of timely protection during their insanity'.[53] Further complicating the discussion, he expressed concern that many 'regular insane' confined in public asylums displayed violent, mendacious and immoral tendencies that made them more unmanageable than many categorised as criminal lunatics.[54] He described the present system of classifying criminal insanity as 'arbitrary', depending upon the manner in which the insanity developed and the persons appreciating its nature.[55] The English Commissioners in Lunacy and the Inspectors for Ireland described insane offenders interchangeably as 'criminal lunatics' and 'insane convicts', and the term 'criminal lunatic', far from being reserved for those committed to asylums rather than prisons after being found not guilty by means of their insanity, continued to be widely applied to prison inmates who became insane after committal.[56] Yet there was a push towards differentiating between these two groups in terms of facilities and treatment, Hood urging any new institution to establish rigorous separation between the two classes of patient who had been confined together at Bethlem: 'The criminal lunatic may be a man of education and refinement brought by the deep affliction of insanity to his present position, or he may be a debased character, a hardened villain, who becomes insane while undergoing the punishment which his crimes have deserved.'[57]

Spurred on by continuing pressure from Francis White, with the support of the Lord Chancellor, who also pointed to the benefits in terms of cost and security, Ireland was first to open a specialised state institution, the Central Criminal Asylum at Dundrum in 1850 (Figure 4.1). In 1845 the Central Criminal Lunatic Asylum Act transferred inspection duties from the Inspectors of Prisons to the Inspectorate for Lunacy, who took over responsibility for the oversight and inspection of asylums, and established a central asylum for insane persons charged with offences. Designed by Jacob Owen, architect to the Board of Public Works who also worked with Joshua Jebb on Mountjoy Convict Prison, Dundrum had provision for 120 patients, 80 men and 40 women, and took admissions directly from court as well as from prisons on the authorisation of

[53] John Charles Bucknill, *Unsoundness of Mind in Relation to Criminal Acts* (London: Samuel Highley, 1854), p. 142.
[54] Ibid., p. 144. See also evidence contained in the Report of the Commission to Inquire into the Subject of Criminal Lunacy (1882)[C.3418], Evidence of Dr C. Medlicott and Dr E. Sheppard.
[55] Bucknill, *Unsoundness of Mind*, p. 143.
[56] Report of the Commissioners in Lunacy, 1854, pp. 46, 47.
[57] Hood, *Criminal Lunatics*, pp. 3–4.

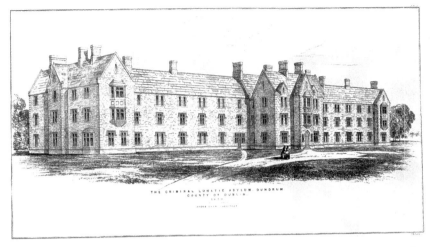

Figure 4.1 The Criminal Lunatic Asylum, Dundrum, Dublin. Transfer lithograph by J.R. Jobbins, 1850, after J. Owen
Credit: Wellcome Collection. Attribution 4.0 International (CC BY 4.0)

the prison surgeon.[58] With its two divisions, the largest group of inmates were those committing offences while 'labouring under insanity', 'where the disease itself depriving their acts of legal or moral responsibility, condones the criminality', while the second, less welcome, group, those becoming insane while in prison, 'not unfrequently bring with them to the Asylum the same obstinacy, impatience of restraint, and perversity of feeling, which had rendered them unmanageable under prison discipline'.[59] In 1856 twenty-four out of 127 inmates at Dundrum were under sentences of penal servitude.[60]

In 1863 England followed suit with the opening of Broadmoor Asylum (Figure 4.2). Built under the direction of Sir Joshua Jebb, Pentonville's architect and Chairman of the Directors of Convict Prisons, it was larger than Dundrum, with provision for 100 female patients and 400 male patients. It was also designed to house two classes of patient – Queen's

[58] Annual Report of Commissioners of Public Works (Ireland), 1847–48 (1848) [983], pp. 15–17; P. Gibbons, N. Mulryan and A. O'Connor, 'Guilty but Insane: The Insanity Defence in Ireland, 1850–1995', *British Journal of Psychiatry*, 170:5 (1997), 467–72; Kelly, 'Poverty, Crime and Mental Illness', p. 315.
[59] Report on the District, Criminal and Private Lunatic Asylums in Ireland, 1874 (1874) [C.1004], Central Asylum Dundrum, p. 104.
[60] Ibid. (1857), Appendix 1: Cases on Behalf of the Crown as to the Admission of Patients into the Central Criminal Asylum, Dundrum, who have become Insane Subsequently to their Conviction, p. 71.

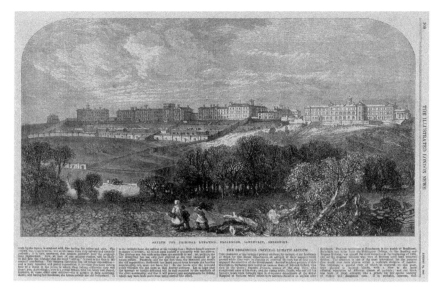

Figure 4.2 Asylum for Criminal Lunatics, Broadmoor, Berkshire, taken
from *Illustrated London News*, 1867
Credit: Wellcome Collection. Attribution 4.0 International
(CC BY 4.0)

Pleasure patients, found insane before or during their trial at a higher
court, and insane convicts, admitted while undergoing penal servitude –
a division reinforced by Dr William Orange, who served as Broadmoor's
second Superintendent between 1870 and 1886.[61]

The first, and by far the more numerous, comprises those unfortunate persons
who, in their various callings, have acquitted themselves blamelessly of their
duties up to the period when they have become insane; then, under the
influence of delusion, and perhaps not watched by those around them, or
under a sudden impulse, they commit a crime. The important point to be
observed is the sequence of events: first insanity, then crime, the crime being
as clearly traceable to the insanity as the effect is to cause. The second class
comprises persons whose histories are widely different. It is made up of those
who for many years have been habitual criminals, have been frequently the
inmates of gaols, whose lives have always been antagonistic to the laws that
govern and restrain the rest of mankind. While in prison, these persons are
difficult to manage, suspicious of those placed over them, impatient of

[61] Shepherd, 'I Am Very Glad and Cheered When I Hear the Flute', p. 475.

discipline, insubordinate, and destructive. Sooner or later they are certified to be insane.[62]

Many of this second class were declared sane or recovered in Broadmoor and were sent back to prison. Those staying in Broadmoor until their sentences expired might be released or moved to another asylum. Following concerns about the number and character of patients transferred from prison and the contamination of the Queen's Pleasure patients, they were subjected to a harsher regime, and spent more time in seclusion. Feigners were often described as a 'third class' of patient, and in both Broadmoor and Dundrum, once identified, moved quickly back to prison. At Richmond District Asylum, which took large numbers of prisoners transferred from Dublin's local prisons, its Superintendent, Joseph Lalor, adopted a similar division to that established at Broadmoor and Dundrum, into the insane but largely honest, whose offences were caused by their insanity, and the habitual criminal, whose offences were largely part of their everyday life. The former might also be treated in district asylums, even though it was acknowledged that there were great disadvantages in mixing the latter with general asylum inmates. Lalor also suggested that 'systematic and skilled education and training are obviously called for in the case of all inmates of asylums, who whether from insanity or criminality may be classed more or less as criminal lunatics, and who are prone to breaches of the moral laws'.[63]

Owing to the pressure on Broadmoor, in 1874 a decision was made to incarcerate male lunatic convicts in a separate wing in Woking Invalid Prison instead of Broadmoor, which it was argued offered 'greater security for safe custody … especially fitted for convicts whose lunacy is sometimes assumed and who are often dangerous'.[64] However, in 1888, following doubts about the legality of housing insane convicts in a prison rather than criminal asylum (Woking was never appointed an asylum under the Broadmoor Act), this decision was reversed and a new block commissioned at Broadmoor especially for convicts.[65] Prisoners becoming insane while incarcerated in county or borough gaols, meanwhile, continued to be sent to county asylums, even though many asylum

---

[62] Anon., 'Criminal Lunatics: Broadmoor and Dundrum', *BMJ*, 1:699 (23 May 1874), 686–7.

[63] Joseph Lalor, 'On the Use of Education and Training in the Treatment of the Insane in Public Lunatic Asylums', *Journal of the Statistical and Social Inquiry Society of Ireland*, 7:54 (Aug. 1878), 361–73, at p. 362.

[64] Commission on Criminal Lunacy (1882), p. 17.

[65] For more details, see Shepherd, 'I Am Very Glad and Cheered When I Hear the Flute', pp. 485–7.

superintendents saw their facilities as unsuitable for dealing with this class of patient.[66]

Dundrum was designed as an institution for lunatics rather than criminals, with the inmates provided first and foremost with asylum facilities and care. Unlike Broadmoor, which imposed a harsher regime on inmates transferred from prison, 'once within the walls of the Central Asylum no distinction is made in regard of the inmates, every just indulgence being alike conceded to all', applying 'those general principles which are now happily established as the foundation of all treatment in cases of mental disease ... we have never recognised the merely legal distinction of their criminality'.[67] Dundrum also quickly became full, and by 1857 was declared 'practically nearly useless for the disposal of lunatic convicts', with prisoners being transferred too late to cure them. Instead, as Dundrum was unable to receive them, they were confined in Philipstown Prison, which housed invalid prisoners, under 'most unfavourable circumstances'.[68] Meanwhile, local prisons in Ireland tended to send insane prisoners to local asylums.

It was claimed in 1874 that while 25 per cent of Broadmoor's inmates had been transferred from a convict prison, at Dundrum the figure was just 10 per cent, a decline from 19 per cent in 1856.[69] The *BMJ* suggested in 1874 that 'lunatic convicts' were found to be troublesome at Dundrum, 'and as the inspectors have a special fondness for this asylum ... they admit as few and send back to prison as many of the convict class as they can'.[70] Dundrum also reported in the same year on the strains resulting from the custody of the convict class, as they required a higher proportion of attendants; 'their admission ... in some instances constitute an unpleasant and unprofitable addition to the ordinary inmates of the institution'.[71] Yet diversions from Dundrum could end badly. In 1872 six prisoners were removed from Spike Island public works prison to the Central Lunatic Asylum, two of whom were

[66] Saunders, 'Institutionalised Offenders', p. 220.
[67] Report on the District, Criminal and Private Lunatic Asylums in Ireland (1857), Dundrum Central Criminal Asylum, p. 19; ibid. (1874), Central Asylum Dundrum, p. 104.
[68] Report of the Directors of Convict Prisons in Ireland (RDCPI), 1857 (1857–58) [2376], p. 10.
[69] Anon., 'Criminal Lunatics and Lunatic Convicts', *BMJ*, 2:705 (4 July 1874), 14–16, at p. 15; Report on the District, Criminal and Private Lunatic Asylums in Ireland (1857), Appendix 1, p. 71.
[70] Anon., 'Criminal Lunatics and Lunatic Convicts', p. 15.
[71] Report on the District, Criminal and Private Lunatic Asylums in Ireland (1874), Central Asylum Dundrum, pp. 104–5.

subsequently sent back to Spike.[72] In the same year, the Director of Spike Island expressed his regret at the murder of a convict by one of these men when they were employed on public works. Convict Mahoney had been confined in Dundrum but then declared sane.[73] Following the murder, Mahoney was retried, acquitted on the grounds of insanity and sent back to Dundrum. He was later declared sane, but would not be moved again: 'There is no doubt danger to be apprehended from the association of such a character with the inmates ... one, however, less than were he again to mix with ordinary convicts.'[74]

Discourses of Guilt and Disease: Psychiatrists, Prison Doctors and Mediating Insanity

Embedded in the issue of where to accommodate criminal lunatics was the complex question of assessing lunacy itself, which built on a long history of negotiations in and around the courtroom between 'discourses of guilt and disease'.[75] This had produced tensions between psychiatry and the law, as the insanity defence became 'an important way for the alienists' claims to expertise and status to be ventured and tested'.[76] Judges questioned the ability of doctors to delve into and understand the minds of defendants, particularly when invoking pleas of temporary insanity or irresistible impulse. Medical witnesses, meanwhile, expressed frustration when judges and juries ignored psychiatric evidence.[77] Psychiatry in general was emerging as a more robust specialism, as the number of asylums expanded in the early and mid-nineteenth century and the volume of writing on medical psychology substantially increased. Disputes drawing on medical discourses and diagnoses to validate insanity, and thus non-responsibility for crimes, became common features of trial proceedings at this time, particularly with regard to serious crimes and capital offences. They were also mirrored in debates between

---

[72] RDCPI, 1872 (1873) [C.731], Governor's Report, p. 20.
[73] Ibid., Director's Report, p. 19.
[74] Report on the District, Criminal and Private Lunatic Asylums in Ireland, 1873 (1873) [C.852], Central Asylum Dundrum, p. 15.
[75] Smith, *Trial by Medicine*, p. 34.
[76] Smith, 'The Boundary between Insanity and Criminal Responsibility', p. 366. See also note 11 for the rich literature on this subject.
[77] Smith, *Trial by Medicine*. For disputes concerning the insanity plea in cases of infanticide, see Hilary Marland, *Dangerous Motherhood: Insanity and Childbirth in Victorian Britain* (Houndmills: Palgrave Macmillan, 2004), ch. 6; Eigen, *Witnessing Insanity*, pp. 147–9; Watson, *Medicine and Justice*, ch. 4; Tony Ward, 'Legislating for Human Nature: Legal Responses to Infanticide, 1860–1938', in Mark Jackson (ed.), *Infanticide: Historical Perspectives on Child Murder and Concealment, 1550–2000* (Aldershot: Ashgate, 2002), pp. 249–69.

magistrates and medical men in local courts in relation to lesser offences where the state of mind of the defendant was in doubt.[78]

However, another set of tensions emerged during this period. As gaol surgeons appeared more frequently as court witnesses after the 1830s, this produced disputes between two sets of 'expert' medical witness, with 'the prison doctor ... clearly in the process of assuming the authority which was later to become a decisive factor in so many trials of the insane'.[79] Just as alienists saw their role as expert witnesses in criminal trials as a means of enhancing their status, so too did prison surgeons, at a time when there was a stepping up of emphasis on mental health as a major component of their work in prisons; through their courtroom interventions, prison doctors had the potential to divert mentally ill offenders away from the prison system. Yet, as Joel Eigen has demonstrated with regard to his analysis of Old Bailey trials in Victorian London, the term 'expert witness' was in itself something of a misnomer. While a number of psychiatrists, like Forbes Winslow, John Charles Bucknill and John Conolly, examined defendants and presented in court on numerous occasions and wrote extensively on criminal responsibility and insanity, other medical witnesses might provide testimony in just one or two cases over the course of their careers. Many of these witnesses would have had no particular knowledge of psychiatry, and much medical evidence continued to be based heavily on the accounts of lay witnesses.[80]

According to even experienced medical witnesses, the problem of assessing prisoners whose mental condition was in doubt began pretrial, with prisoners only being visited a couple of times by physicians for assessment before their court appearance. In cases taking many months to reach court, treatment would also be delayed with disastrous consequences.[81] Additionally, the process 'pitted' doctors against each

---

[78] Cox, *Negotiating Insanity*, p. 103.
[79] Nigel Walker and Sarah McCabe, *Crime and Insanity in England, Volume Two: New Solutions and New Problems* (Edinburgh: Edinburgh University Press, 1973), p. 84.
[80] Eigen, *Witnessing Insanity*, especially ch. 5. See also Cox, *Negotiating Insanity*, pp. 118–19; Marland, *Dangerous Motherhood*, pp. 180–1. See also James Moran, 'The Signal and the Noise: The Historical Epidemiology of Insanity in Antebellum New Jersey', *History of Psychiatry*, 14:3 (2003), 281–301 and Catharine Coleborne, '"His Brain Was Wrong, His Mind Astray": Families and the Language of Insanity in New South Wales, Queensland and New Zealand 1800–1920', *Journal of Family History*, 31:1 (2006), 45–65. For overviews of the careers of Conolly and Bucknill, including their work in medical jurisprudence and as court witnesses, see Andrew Scull, Charlotte MacKenzie and Nicholas Hervey, *Masters of Bedlam: The Transformation of the Mad-Doctoring Trade* (Princeton, NJ: Princeton University Press, 1996), chs 3 and 7.
[81] See, for example, Bucknill, *Unsoundness of Mind*, pp. 145–6.

other in the courtroom, while the medical evidence often failed to provide good guidance for the jury. In Charles Hood's words,

A few hours, perhaps less, are all that is allotted, and he is hurried into the witness-box to state before a learned judge, an astute and adverse counsel, and a perplexed jury, the ground of the opinion he has formed, usually involving some of the more delicate questions of psychological science.[82]

In response to the pressures experienced at Bethlem, Hood also advocated for a more speedy process for moving patients who were found to be no longer insane back into the criminal justice system.[83] Meanwhile, in 1851 Inspectors Francis White and John Nugent questioned the process of acquittal itself in Irish cases involving the insanity plea: 'If there are extenuating circumstances connected with the psychological condition of the accused, they are legitimate subjects to be considered in meting out the after punishment, but certainly not in the first instance for an unqualified acquittal.'[84]

The term 'Criminal Lunatic' itself was also something of a misnomer, running against the principle of not guilty by reason of insanity, and its meaning continued to be debated throughout the second half of the century, complicating the issue of where to place criminals who were also mad.[85] In 1883 William Orange argued that it was impossible to be guilty of a crime and a lunatic at the same time, as the latter could not be held responsible for their criminal act. He added that 'The evils of sentencing persons who are really insane to penal servitude or imprisonment, are much graver than is commonly supposed':

If the punishment is to be carried out in its entirety it necessarily involves much suffering ... whilst if the sentence is not to be carried out thoroughly, but if the understanding is that it is to be modified in its severity, so as to suit the mental condition of the prisoner, it were surely better, in doubtful cases, not to pass sentence until after a satisfactory examination of the mental condition of the prisoner had been made ... every instance in which a prisoner is found, on his trial, to be insane acts as a reminder to the community that, little or much, it has failed in its duty in not having prevented the commission of the crime by placing the prisoner under proper care at an earlier date.[86]

[82] Hood, *Criminal Lunatics*, p. 17.   [83] Ibid., pp. 10–12.
[84] Report on the District, Criminal and Private Lunatic Asylums in Ireland, 1851 (1851) [1387], Central Criminal Asylum, p. 11.
[85] Allderidge, 'Bethlem to Broadmoor', p. 51.
[86] W. Orange, 'Presidential Address, Delivered at the Annual Meeting of the Medico-Psychological Association, Held at the Royal College of Physicians, London, July 27th, 1883', *Journal of Mental Science*, 29:127 (Oct. 1883), 329–54, at pp. 347–8.

Orange went on to suggest that in an ideal society,

> the class of criminal lunatics would disappear, because no-one would be sentenced to punishment without his mental state being ascertained before sentence, instead of, as now so generally happens, afterwards; and, furthermore, because persons known to be insane would then be placed under control before, and not, as now, after they had committed some alarming act of homicide or violence.[87]

He recommended bolstering the process of assessment around the trial and that a prisoner charged with a crime and suspected to be insane should be examined by the prison medical officer, a local asylum superintendent, and additionally by a 'physician of standing', as soon after the crime had been committed as possible.[88]

Prison doctors might dispute the verdicts of psychiatrists based on their observations of prisoners pre-trial, though in other instances they drew the same conclusions concerning the defendant's state of mind. The medical evidence 'intended to show the defendant as sane and responsible' was likely to rely less on deviant acts, but 'simply on an absence of signs of insanity while remanded in prison'.[89] Gilbert McMurdo, surgeon to Newgate Gaol in London, gave evidence in numerous Old Bailey trials between the 1830s and 1850s, making him the most frequent medical witness to testify at insanity trials over that period.[90] McMurdo emphasised that he saw many cases of lunacy and was able to closely observe prisoners suspected of being mentally disordered, having almost daily interactions with them.[91] In 1854, he concurred with the opinion of Dr Forbes Winslow in the case of Hugh Pollard Willoughby, who was accused of wounding with intent to murder, that he was insane and suffering a 'horrible delusion'. In giving evidence McMurdo explained, 'since the day the prisoner was committed to Newgate I have continually seen and conversed with him – I happened to be in the prison immediately after he was taken there, and I saw him then – I am of opinion that he was then, and is now, of

---

[87] Ibid., p. 331; Anon., 'Plea of Insanity in Criminal Cases', *Journal of Mental Science*, 37:157 (Apr. 1891), 260–3, at p. 262.

[88] 'Anon., 'Plea of Insanity in Criminal Cases', p. 262.

[89] Tony Ward, 'An Honourable Regime of Truth? Foucault, Psychiatry and English Criminal Justice', in Helen Johnston (ed.), *Punishment and Control in Historical Perspective* (Houndmills: Palgrave Macmillan, 2008), pp. 56–75, at p. 62.

[90] Eigen, *Witnessing Insanity*, p. 129.

[91] Ibid.; *Old Bailey Proceedings Online* (www.oldbaileyonline.org, version 8.0, 1 Aug. 2019). Gilbert McMurdo was referred to as M'Murdo in the Old Bailey proceedings. See also Joel Peter Eigen, '"I Answer As a Physician": Opinion as Fact in Pre-McNaughtan Insanity Trials', in Michael Clark and Catherine Crawford (eds), *Legal Medicine in History* (Cambridge: Cambridge University Press, 1994), pp. 167–99.

unsound mind.' Willoughby was found not guilty and ordered to be detained.[92]

One year later, however, McMurdo's evidence was key in condemning Luigi Burinelli to death, following his Old Bailey trial for murder. There was a wealth of medical evidence in this case, and while it was agreed that Burinelli had suffered badly from internal piles, which had been treated in Middlesex Hospital, and was acknowledged to be in very poor spirits and melancholic following the death of his second wife in childbirth, McMurdo testified that under his observation at Newgate he had shown no symptoms of aberration of mind, but was suffering from hypochondria. John Conolly, along with other medical witnesses, disagreed, arguing that the defendant was of unsound mind and delusional. McMurdo, while he did 'not profess to be what Dr. Conolly is, set apart to that part of the profession', reaffirmed in giving his evidence his vast experience as prison surgeon:

I have had a great many persons, about whose state of mind inquiry has been made, or was made, under my care during my tenure of office, for a considerable time – I have been surgeon to the gaol of Newgate for twenty-five years, and I have had a great many under my care; some who have been of unsound mind, some who have been thought to be so.[93]

Joel Eigen has argued that unmasking fakery was the primary goal of the prison surgeon.[94] However, beyond that, McMurdo appeared to be very concerned to assert his experience in detecting mental disorder based on daily observation and his lengthy prison career.

By the late nineteenth century the trial hearing had become a key interface where claims of insanity were disputed by prison doctors and psychiatrists working outside of prisons, and the medical press reported avidly on such proceedings. Such reports could be critical of prison surgeons' testimony when this went against that of eminent alienists.[95] Tensions flared, for example, in a case tried in York in 1859, reported

---

[92] *Old Bailey Proceedings Online* (www.oldbaileyonline.org, version 8.0, 1 Aug. 2019), Oct. 1854, trial of HUGH POLLARD WILLOUGHBY (t18541023–1122).

[93] *Old Bailey Proceedings Online* (www.oldbaileyonline.org, version 8.0, 1 Aug. 2019), Apr. 1855, trial of LUIGI BURINELLI (t18550409–464). The trial produced much commentary in medical journals, including 'The Trial and Conviction of Luigi Buranelli for Murder' Plea of Insanity', *Asylum Journal*, 14 (2 July 1855), 209–13. (Burinelli was spelt in different ways in some accounts of his trial.)

[94] Eigen, 'I Answer As a Physician', p. 183.

[95] In 1877 the *Lancet* went so far as to claim that prison surgeons had few resources to draw on in assessing the mental condition of prisoners in an ordinary gaol, and that prison warders – with their day-to-day interactions with prisoners – might be declared more competent to judge such cases: Anon., 'Insane or Lunatic', *Lancet*, 110:2820 (15 Sept. 1877), 401–2. See also Joe Sim, *Medical Power in Prisons: The Prison Medical Service in England 1774–1989* (Milton Keynes and Philadelphia, PA: Open University Press, 1990), ch. 3.

across several issues of the *BMJ* and in the *Dublin Medical Press*, when Mr
Anderson, surgeon of York Gaol, sided with the counsel for the prosecution who had advised the jury to reject the opinions of three eminent
medical witnesses. The three, including Dr Forbes Winslow, claimed the
defendant, James Atkinson, who was charged with murdering his sweet-
heart, was an obvious case of insanity and 'an imbecile' with the intelli-
gence of an eight-year-old child. Anderson declared that he did not think
those gentlemen were better able to give an opinion on questions of
lunacy than himself.[96] In August 1884, in another widely reported trial
taking place in Dublin, the dispute centred on whether James Ellis
French was fit to stand. Several medical men, including Dr Eames,
Medical Superintendent of Cork District Lunatic Asylum (labelled by
the *Lancet* as the 'only specialist'), claimed that he was not in a mental
condition to plead and conduct his defence with due caution. Three
other doctors, including Dr McDonnell, claimed there was nothing
wrong with French physically or mentally, and that he was shamming.[97]

While serving as medical officer at Mountjoy Prison, Dr Robert
McDonnell provided a candid assessment of the difficulties involved in
making such assessments:

There is not a medical officer of a lunatic asylum, or of a prison in this country,
who will not admit that, in many cases, to discriminate with precision between
wickedness and madness is a task too difficult as to be often absolutely
impossible, and that, too, after months of close and careful daily observation.[98]

He added that half of the medical witnesses knew something of the
prisoner and nothing of insanity and half knew something of insanity
but nothing of the prisoner.[99] He was not surprised that many persons of
unsound mind were found in convict prisons. Nonetheless, while the
judge and jury system could not assess such cases 'with the delicacy of a
chemist's balance', and medical witnesses dealt not in certainties but
'probabilities', he pointed out that grave errors had been made, as in the
case of Burton, tried at Maidstone and executed for the horrific murder
of a boy. In McDonnell's view Burton was clearly a madman.[100] Burton
had declared that his only motive was that he wanted to be executed, and

[96] Anon., 'Criminal Responsibility of the Insane', *Dublin Medical Press*, 41:1044
(Jan. 1859), 13; Anon., 'Criminal Responsibility of the Insane', *BMJ*, 2:104 (25
Dec. 1858), 1068; 1:105 (1 Jan. 1859), 17–18.
[97] Anon., 'The Dublin Trials', *Lancet*, 124:3182 (23 Aug. 1884), 347.
[98] Robert McDonnell, 'Observations on the Case of Burton, and So-Called Moral
Insanity in Criminal Cases', *Journal of the Statistical and Social Inquiry Society of
Ireland*, 3:25 (Dec. 1863), 447–56, at p. 450.
[99] Ibid.   [100] Ibid., pp. 450, 454.

it was discovered that his mother was 'a madwoman and his brother of weak intellect'.[101] In this case it was a prison surgeon who had gone 'a long way towards banishing the idea of the prisoner's insanity from the minds of judge and jury'. 'He stated that he had observed the prisoner ever since he had been placed in confinement, that he appeared sane, nor did he observe that he was under any delusion.'[102]

Though psychiatrists working outside of prisons were widely consulted in trial proceedings, in effect it was prison doctors who had most contact with prisoners on remand, many of whom showed symptoms of insanity or were regarded as suicidal. Magistrates sent those suspected of insanity to the local gaol for assessment by prison surgeons and in Ireland prison or dispensary surgeons; the latter were often already familiar with the patient's history.[103] In contrast to the 'expert witness' in court who had seen prisoners just once or twice, prison doctors were 'schooled in multiple observations'.[104] It was particularly in remand prisons (including numerous local prisons in England and Ireland) that prison medical officers built up impressive levels of experience dealing with mentally ill offenders, assessing the state of their minds pre-trial, and taking care of prisoners who had a high risk of suicide.[105] Prison doctors employed in remand prisons were particularly likely to assert their expertise in assessing mental illness, at the same time underlining their heavy workload. At Clerkenwell Prison in London, the medical officers had extensive dealings with suspected cases of insanity and attempted suicides. In 1859 alone a total of 107 attempted suicides were reported, who were placed under close observation by Clerkenwell's surgeon Henry Wakefield.[106] Cases of temporary insanity caused by drinking were frequent that year and additionally thirty cases of suspected insanity were sent from various London police courts, 'calling the surgeon's attention to the state of the Prisoners' mind, and requiring Certificates of his opinion; this duty involves a serious responsibility'.[107] Many prisoners were moved to asylums before their trial or were acquitted on the grounds of insanity and then transferred to asylums. Clerkenwell's prison surgeons worked closely with local asylum superintendents, including

[101] Ibid., pp. 447–8.   [102] Ibid., p. 454.
[103] Cox, *Negotiating Insanity*, ch. 4. As discussed in Chapter 3, in Ireland many prison surgeons held posts as dispensary doctors.
[104] Eigen, *Witnessing Insanity*, p. 130.
[105] See, for English remand prisons, Seán McConville, *English Local Prisons 1860–1900: Next Only to Death* (London and New York: Routledge, 1995), pp. 378–83.
[106] London Metropolitan Archives, MA/G/CLE/114-177/ Item no. 147, Return of the number of prisoners charged with attempting to commit suicide from 1847 to 1859.
[107] Ibid.

Charles Hood at Bethlem and William Sankey at Hanwell, to obtain further assessments on the mental state of prisoners and to organise removals. In February 1860, for example, Elizabeth Livermore was charged with unlawful assault and attempting to stab her victim with a knife. She was acquitted on the grounds of insanity and sent to Clerkenwell to be kept under strict custody, before being removed on the order of the Home Secretary to Colney Hatch Asylum.[108]

II CRIMINAL OR LUNATIC? PRISONER OR PATIENT?: PLACES AND PRACTICES OF CONFINEMENT

Removals between Prisons and Asylums

Decisions concerning the state of mind of prisoners prompted removals back and forth between the prison and asylum, and preoccupied prison and asylum officers throughout the nineteenth century. Processes of removal between institutions were much more than administrative exercises, and a great deal was at stake in determining the placing of lunatics who had committed crimes in terms of the welfare of individual prisoners, institutional wellbeing and management, cost, intraprofessional relationships, the assertion of specialist knowledge and authority, and the very definition of criminal lunacy itself. The ambivalent position taken by asylum doctors has already been referred to, concerned as they were about the impact of mentally ill offenders in asylums, yet also critical of their retention in prisons. Prison doctors too were ambivalent. Along with asylum doctors, they shared a concern to remedy what was increasingly depicted as a disastrous situation for the prison system and the numerous mentally ill prisoners held within it, and, as Robert McDonnell indicated, were likely to find the state of mind of prisoners extremely difficult to assess. However, they were also keen to underline their growing knowledge and expertise, and ability to produce an accurate diagnosis. By the late nineteenth century, as shown in Chapter 3, not just those working in remand prisons, but prison medical officers more generally were expressing confidence about undertaking this work, and were spending a far greater proportion of their time dealing with mentally disordered offenders. In 1869 the Howard Association, expressing concern about 'the *fact*' that many victims of mental disease were exposed to 'penal treatment', quoted figures showing that one in nine prisoners was more or less insane at Perth Prison, while in 1870 Perth's medical officer,

---

[108] Ibid., MA/G/CLE/205–319 [Jan.–Dec. 1860]/Item nos 210, 212, 215, 218.

Dr James Bruce Thomson, estimated that 12 per cent of the Scottish prison population were 'mentally weak in different degrees', noting that similar rates were reported in English and Irish prisons.[109] Dr Charles P. Measor, late Deputy-Governor of Chatham Convict Prison, also claimed in 1869 that his 'experience of convicted criminals induces in me a strong conviction that the amount of mental disease actually existing among them is inadequately appreciated', while he was aware that as many as 5 per cent of inmates of an Irish convict prison were confined in separation under medical observation with a view to ascertaining their mental condition, 'quite exclusive of a large proportion who might be said to have possessed inferior degrees of irresponsibility'.[110]

Managing mentally disordered prisoners, as demonstrated in Chapter 3, was doubtless a significant part of all prison doctors' workloads, particularly as cases were retained in prison when officials were unable to decide – or agree – on their state of mind. If cases of mental disorder were missed at the trial and the prisoner sent to a prison rather than the asylum, this added to the responsibilities of overburdened prison medical officers as they attempted to assess and deal with mental illness in a punitive environment lacking in therapeutic resources. Medical officers were often slow to initiate transfers to asylums, because their heavy workload hindered this, and also as it indicated the failure of the institution to manage the mental health of its prisoners and the detrimental impact of prison regimes on their minds. These factors might vary depending on local circumstances and the type of prison involved, and the weighing up of the disruption such prisoners created against the trouble of moving them. Bucknill observed how,

In the new gaols for separate confinement a noisy lunatic proves such a nuisance, from the reverberation of his cries through the resonant structure of the building, that every effort is sure to be made to have him transmitted to an asylum without delay; but this evil is not felt in the old prisons, nor in the new ones with silent or melancholic patients.[111]

The destinations of many insane prisoners were governed in the first place, not by prison or asylum doctors and administrators, but by the actions of local magistrates. Both the Commissioners in Lunacy and Inspectors complained that lunatics committing minor offences were sent by magistrates to prison, and their insanity ignored, or were passed

---

[109] Modern Records Centre (MRC), University of Warwick, Howard League Papers, MSS.16X/1/7, Annual Reports of the Howard Association, c. 1865–1901, 'Criminal Lunacy', 169–71, at p. 170; J.B. Thomson, 'The Hereditary Nature of Crime', *Journal of Mental Science*, 15:72 (Jan. 1870), 487–98, at p. 492.

[110] MRC, MSS.16X/1/7, 'Criminal Lunacy', p. 170.

[111] Bucknill, *Unsoundness of Mind*, p. 146.

over to the Poor Law authorities, though it was suggested that there was some merit in the latter arrangement, as many such cases were regarded as 'ordinary lunatics' who had not been properly looked after and were rarely of the criminal class.[112] What came to be described as 'magisterial dumping of the insane' was largely prompted by cost considerations, as workhouses and asylums, unlike prisons, were supported by local rates, with maintenance costs in the workhouse being much lower than asylums.[113] Meanwhile, the certification process for asylum admissions was expensive and time-consuming. In Ireland the Prison Inspectors' Report for 1868 described how circulars had been issued in 1807 and then again in 1868, enclosing forms for the committal of lunatics to asylums, yet it was found from returns and on inspections of gaols and bridewells that magistrates still committed insane persons to prison, 'thus, besides the injury inflicted on the individual, seriously interfering with the discipline of the gaols'.[114]

At the local level, a series of cases reported to the magistrates of the West Riding of Yorkshire in 1860 demonstrated how complex the dispersal of prisoners showing symptoms of mental disorder ended up being, involving transfers between prison, asylum and workhouse.[115] In April 1860 James Jenkins, a blademaker, was committed to Wakefield Prison for four months for the theft of steel. His 'friends' reported that he had been leading an 'unsteady' life before he was sent to prison and had showed 'a strangeness of mind indicating insanity'. Once in prison the surgeon came to a similar conclusion. The prisoner's insanity was reported to the Secretary of State, and he was removed in August 1860 to the West Riding Lunatic Asylum.[116] Inquiries into the dispersal of prisoners were also made at the end of their sentences. In May 1860 Robert South was removed to Wakefield House of Correction as a 'disorderly pauper'. At the end of his three-week sentence the prison surgeon, William Wood, reported that, while nothing had occurred during his imprisonment to warrant removal to the asylum, when he was sent on to Sheffield Workhouse the institution's medical officers

---

[112] Anon., 'Criminal Lunacy in 1877. Broadmoor Criminal Lunatic Asylum. Annual Report for the Year 1877. 32nd Report of Commissioners in Lunacy', *Journal of Mental Science*, 24:108 (Jan. 1879), 643–9, at p. 648.

[113] McConville, *English Local Prisons*, p. 290, n. 44; see also Saunders, 'Magistrates and Madmen'.

[114] RIGPI, 1868 (1868–69) [4205], p. xxviii.

[115] The National Archives (TNA), MH 51/754, Insane or Imbecile Prisoners: Duties of Magistrates, 1861. Cases Submitted by West Riding Justices to Mr Atherton 1861. At this time, Wakefield Prison was acting as a local gaol as well as admitting government prisoners.

[116] Ibid. (James Jenkins).

were warned to pay 'special attention to the state of his mind as his Conduct has been such as to create a strong suspicion that he is a Lunatic'. Robert South was transferred a few days later to the West Riding Asylum.[117]

A memo to the West Riding justices a year later explained the 'great inconvenience' resulting from the actions of local magistrates in committing persons charged with offences who were in a state of insanity or mental imbecility to the Wakefield House of Correction. Such persons, the memo complained, caused much trouble to the prison officers, interfered with the discipline of separate confinement, and later put the county to considerable expense and trouble in removing the individuals to an asylum, and obtaining an order of maintenance after establishing which parish was responsible for payment. They urged the magistrates 'where a person was manifestly an idiot or insane at the time of committing felony or indictable misdemeanours' to send them directly to a lunatic asylum.[118] However, as Saunders has pointed out, magistrates were under considerable pressure to make rapid decisions, and the Home Office might have believed that magistrates were sending insane offenders to prison for careful observation by the prison doctor, which would result in a more informed decision about where to send such individuals than their own hasty diagnosis.[119] Both Cox and Saunders have also argued that magistrates might be well informed on the subject of insanity, involved as they were in making arrangements for the medical examination of suspected lunatic prisoners, while many were also members of asylum visiting and management committees, and, as such, aware that local asylums were short of space, security and staff.[120]

The advisability of moving criminals from prison once they were declared insane also divided opinion. Charles Hood proposed that if a criminal became insane after sentencing, 'he should be put into a lunatic ward connected with the infirmary of the prison in which he may be confined, and there treated by the officiating surgeon in the same way as if he were suffering from any other disease'. Though Hood suggested elsewhere that minor offenders who were insane might be sent directly to county asylums, he argued that 'the practice of sending insane prisoners from gaols to county asylums is, in every point of view, objectionable'.[121]

---

[117] Ibid. (Robert South).
[118] Ibid., Memo 11 March 1861, For Justices of WR of Yorkshire, Copy Case as to Committal of Persons to the House of Correction.
[119] Saunders, 'Institutionalised Offenders', p. 244.
[120] Cox, *Negotiating Insanity*, pp. 102–3; Saunders, 'Institutionalised Offenders', pp. 235–6.
[121] Hood, *Suggestions for the Future Provision of Criminal Lunatics*, p. 146.

Hood also observed that 'the medical officers, connected with our public prisons, are men of undoubted professional skill and experience ... fully competent to deal with a disease which may, it is well known, by active treatment, be cut short in its early stages'.[122] Such prisoners, he added, would be closely supervised by the Commissioners in Lunacy whose duties included visiting gaols where lunatics were held.[123]

During an inquiry into the operation of Broadmoor Asylum in 1877, it was also suggested (albeit by means of a minority opinion) that convicts becoming insane after conviction might be better off in lunatic wards in prison, where they would have the possibility of employment, describing the atmosphere in prison as less 'depressing and desponding' and presenting more hope for the future than in an asylum.[124] The conditions for some of Broadmoor's patients appear to have been woeful, with disruptive patients placed in seclusion and several, exceptional for their 'dangerous violence', held for many months in large cages. A number of these had attacked Broadmoor attendants, including W.T., admitted from Millbank Prison in 1867. Sentenced to fifteen years' penal servitude, his conduct in Woking, Portsmouth and Dartmoor was described as 'bad', and he had escaped from Portsmouth Prison in 1865. W.T. had been kept in a strait waistcoat and hobbles for some time before admission to Broadmoor, and in January 1868 he attempted to attack the attendants and take their keys, then in September bit an attendant's leg.[125]

While many claimed expertise in dealing with mental illness, prison surgeons might have a very different perspective on the best place to confine such cases, particularly when prisoners were violent or for those working in poorly resourced local prisons. Surgeon Read, referring in 1862 to the confinement of lunatics in ordinary (local) prisons in Dublin, emphasised how the imprisonment of lunatic prisoners, including 'the violent maniac, the feeble and the imbecile', had been a heavy responsibility for him for the past twenty years:

The consequences are rendered apparent in sanguinary incidents, loss of life, and the most perilous operations of surgery. This blood-stained scene is a blot on humanity, as well as an extravagant impolicy; in fact, an institution for converting derangement into permanent insanity.... Every Board of Superintendence for

---

[122] Ibid., p. 149.   [123] Ibid., pp. 149–50.
[124] Report from a Committee Appointed to Inquire into Certain Matters Relating to the Broadmoor Criminal Lunatic Asylum (1877) [C.1674], Minute of Dissent, F.J. Mouat, MD, pp. 29, 36.
[125] Copy of a Report Made by the Commissioners in Lunacy, on the 14th October 1868 upon Broadmoor Criminal Lunatic Asylum (1868–69) [244], pp. 2–3, 5, Appendix, Table (A), pp. 7–8.

many years has deprecated the principle of committing insane persons to prison, and they have made increasing representations of the violation of prison discipline consequent upon their confinement therein.[126]

There were also resource implications. Over the year 1861 the number of lunatics confined in Richmond Bridewell alone rose from eighteen to thirty-four, making it necessary to employ an additional warder to supervise them.[127]

In effect, by the second half of the century prisons, criminal lunatic asylums and public and district asylums were all housing large numbers of criminal lunatics. In England around 50 per cent of the total were accommodated in public asylums, ensuring that their medical officers had extensive (and often unwelcome) experience of dealing with this group. In 1863, 419 of the total of 877 criminal lunatics were held in custody in county or borough asylums. By 1880, when the total number of criminal lunatics and ex-criminal lunatics in England was 1,288, public asylums held 720 of them.[128] In Ireland the situation differed in a number of respects. Though there were continued complaints about the strains the mentally ill put on both prisons and asylums, the number of criminal lunatics was smaller, and by the 1880s most lunatic prisoners were being moved on to district asylums. In 1866 eight prisons were declared to be the 'most encumbered' with criminal lunatics, with 315 lunatics between them. However, it was suggested that two new asylums at Letterkenny and Castlebar would clear the gaols of most of their lunatics, and with further asylum expansion elsewhere, 'the prisons in Ireland will virtually cease to be as heretofore receptacles for the insane'.[129] In 1868 a total of 69 criminal lunatics were confined in Irish gaols. Of these, twenty-six were moved to Dundrum, twenty-nine to district asylums, five were discharged by the Lord Lieutenant to the charge of their friends, seven, largely committed as vagrants, were discharged by order of the magistrates, and three remained in gaol at the end of the year.[130] Of the 99 lunatics confined in Irish gaols in 1879, eighty-nine were moved to district asylums and ten were discharged by the Lord Lieutenant. This figure included fifty-three who were under sentence of imprisonment or transportation who became insane in gaol,

---

[126] Anon., 'The Board of Superintendence of the City of Dublin Prisons', *The Irish Times*, 16 Jan. 1862.
[127] Ibid.   [128] Commission on Criminal Lunacy (1882), Appendix A, pp. 109–11.
[129] Report on the District, Criminal and Private Lunatics Asylums in Ireland, 1866 (1866) [3721], Gaols, pp. 19–20.
[130] Ibid., 1869 (1868–69) [4181], Gaols, pp. 32–3.

fifty-two of whom were moved to district asylums while one was discharged.[131]

After 1867 county and district asylums had to accept from either state asylums (Broadmoor and Dundrum) or convict prisons certified criminal lunatics whose sentences had expired and could only be detained thereafter as pauper lunatics. This must have been welcome in Broadmoor, which in 1865 had admitted 50 convicts from Chatham, 59 from Portsmouth and 64 from Portland, bringing the total number of lunatic convicts to 266, and in 1868 Broadmoor removed 134 patients whose sentences had terminated to county asylums.[132] Lunatics, however, who had been retained in the prison system without medical certification could be released at the end of their sentences. In October and November 1874 two 'dangerous lunatics' were sent from Millbank Prison to the St George Union Workhouse. Shortly after, one, John Maloney, escaped and the other, Henry Balls, discharged himself. It was reported that neither while in the workhouse showed any symptoms of insanity.[133] The Lunacy Commissioners and Home Office expressed grave concerns about the discharges, underlining the unsuitability of workhouses for confining dangerous lunatics. Rather, the Lunacy Commissioners proposed that 'they should with all possible dispatch be placed in a lunatic asylum', and also questioned why the two men, as dangerous lunatics, were not sent directly to an asylum rather than a prison. The Broadmoor authorities and asylum superintendents, meanwhile, continued to object to the mixing of criminals with lunatics, while Du Cane and the Home Office were keen to retain the penal emphasis with regard to lunatic criminals, and in 1875 the opening of the lunatic wing at Woking appeared to resolve the issue. Male 'prisoner lunatics' were to be retained there, with fewer 'indulgences' than Broadmoor and outside the authority of the Lunacy Commissioners.[134]

---

[131] Ibid., 1880 (1880) [C.2621], Appendix D, Criminal Lunatics, pp. 108–10.
[132] RDCP, 1865 (1866) [3732], p. 238; Copy of a Report Made by the Commissioners in Lunacy, upon Broadmoor Criminal Lunatic Asylum (1868–69), p. 2.
[133] TNA, HO 45/9525, Lunacy: Report on Accommodation at Broadmoor Asylum and Question of Removing Lunatic Convicts from Woking Prison to Broadmoor, 1874–87 (LRAB), 8. Discharge of Insane Convicts, 2 Dec. 1874.
[134] TNA, HO 45/9353/28292, Lunacy. Memos. Concerning Safe Custody of Lunatics at Broadmoor, 1872–78, Du Cane to Home Secretary, 19 Dec. 1873. Cited in Martin J. Wiener, *Reconstructing the Criminal: Culture, Law, and Policy in England, 1830–1914* (Cambridge: Cambridge University Press, 1990), p. 316. See Laura Sellers, 'Managing Convicts, Understanding Criminals: Medicine and the Development of English Convict Prisons, c. 1837–1886' (unpublished University of Leeds PhD thesis, 2017), ch. 3 for more detail on the debates on the use of Woking as a place to confine lunatic prisoners.

In Ireland the 1875 Lunatic Asylums Act confirmed that lunatics removed from prison or from Dundrum to a district asylum were to be treated as 'ordinary patients' and charged to their local district, and were to be subsequently retained or discharged on the authority of the asylum governors.[135] Broadmoor's medical superintendent, William Orange, had suggested in 1870 that such a flow was vital to create space for insane convicts in the specialised criminal lunatic asylums who otherwise would be retained in prison 'not only to their own detriment, but also to the detriment of the sane prisoners'.[136] The 1877 Prison Acts authorised central government to take over the running of local prisons in England and Ireland in addition to their funding, but local ratepayers were to continue to support lunatics and criminal lunatics in asylums.[137] This provided a major incentive for magistrates to keep sending offenders suspected of lunacy to prison, with some 621 being removed to local prisons in England in 1883 on suspicion of insanity, which in most cases in the view of the Prison Commissioners 'was virtually certain'.[138] The prison authorities, they continued, were put in a particularly difficult position when medical officers reported prisoners to be insane but the magistrates declined to provide a certificate for removal to an asylum, 'and it is a question whether in such a case a prisoner should not simply be discharged'.[139] The Prison Commissioners and Inspectors in Ireland protested regularly about this kind of situation, arguing that prison was not a proper place for those whose insanity had been questioned, given the need for special experience and treatment, 'and it cannot be expected that such experience should be available in prisons, more particularly in the small prisons which form the large majority'.[140]

In England the 1884 Criminal Lunatics Act bolstered the role of the Secretary of State in the certification and transfer of criminal lunatics from prisons to asylums.[141] This was in response to mounting pressure from asylum doctors attempting to get rid of dangerous patients, as well

---

[135] 38&39 Vict., c.67, s.10, 12 (1875).
[136] Wellcome Library (WL), *Reports of the Superintendent and Chaplain of Broadmoor Criminal Lunatic Asylum, for the Year 1870* (1871), p. 5.
[137] In 1874 the Irish Treasury introduced a grant-in-aid of 4 shillings per week per asylum patient in Ireland to alleviate the burden on local ratepayers. See Cox, *Negotiating Insanity*, pp. 19–20. A similar arrangement was made in England in the mid-1870s. See Robert Ellis, 'The Asylum, the Poor Law, and a Reassessment of the Four-Shilling Grant: Admission to the County Asylums of Yorkshire in the Nineteenth Century', *Social History of Medicine*, 19:1 (2006), 55–71.
[138] Report of the Commissioners of Prisons, 1884 (1884) [C.4180], p. 7.
[139] Ibid., p. 8.
[140] Ibid., pp. 7–8. See also McConville, *English Local Prisons*, p. 290; Report of the General Prisons Board, Ireland, 1891–92 (1892) [C.6789], p. 19.
[141] 47&48 Vict., c.64 (1884).

as local authorities wanting to be relieved of the burden of maintaining 'quasi-criminal' asylum inmates. It was also prompted by the Home Secretary Sir William Harcourt's concern about the lack of allowance within the criminal justice system for mentally incapable offenders and prisoners, and the 1884 Act extended provision to certify prisoners not just as lunatics, but as suffering from 'imbecility of mind' that made them unfit for penal discipline.[142] This coincided with the stepped-up use and success of the insanity plea more generally, with *The Times* suggesting in 1882 that the notion was spreading that 'there must be something wrong in a man's mental organization before he could have committed a certain crime in certain circumstances'.[143] Harcourt transferred more prisoners than previous Home Secretaries to Broadmoor without trial, and under the 1884 Act all prisoners sentenced to death were to undergo medical examination 'to ensure that no lunatic was executed'.[144] The Act made the Prison Commissioners responsible for the maintenance of prisoners moved to lunatic asylums – prior to that they had only been liable for those for whom a place of settlement could not be ascertained or those committed with very short sentences – and also included provision for interventions in prison regulations on behalf of those suffering 'imbecility of mind', though in practice few prisoners were placed in this category.[145] The 1884 Act encouraged the removal of Broadmoor patients whose sentences had expired to asylums, with twelve transferred in 1885 to English county asylums and ten to Dundrum, for subsequent distribution to district asylums in Ireland.[146] However, it also provided for the retention of criminal lunatics in Broadmoor upon a medical officer's certification that they might be dangerous, care being taken to select for transfer those 'not likely to cause annoyance'.[147]

With costs now borne centrally, magistrates continued to send suspected lunatics to prison for medical observation, and their numbers increased dramatically, from averages of 8.2 and 11.9 per 1,000 committals between 1870 and 1882 to 18.2 per 1,000 between 1884 and 1889,

---

[142] Wiener, *Reconstructing the Criminal*, p. 317; Leon Radzinowicz and Roger Hood, *History of English Criminal Law and Its Administration, Volume 5: The Emergence of Penal Policy* (London: Stevens, 1986), pp. 537–8.

[143] *The Times*, 12 Apr. 1882. Cited in Wiener, *Reconstructing the Criminal*, p. 275. See also Radzinowicz and Hood, *History of English Criminal Law*, p. 684.

[144] Wiener, *Reconstructing the Criminal*, p. 275. See also Walker, *Crime and Insanity in England, Volume One*, pp. 204–10, 228–9.

[145] Wiener, *Reconstructing the Criminal*, pp. 317–18; McConville, *English Local Prisons*, pp. 290–1. See also ch. 3 for changing attitudes to the weak-minded.

[146] WL, *Reports upon Broadmoor Criminal Lunatic Asylum, with Statistical Tables, for the Year 1885* (1887), Superintendent's Report, p. 5.

[147] Ibid.; Wiener, *Reconstructing the Criminal*, p. 320.

with the number for 1889 rising to 22.8.[148] In 1885 Harcourt complained that the common practice 'of using a prison as a place in which a supposed lunatic can be confined in order to ascertain his mental condition certainly calls for alteration', though it was claimed that charging a person with a crime was the only way to keep a person in custody before being 'certified'.[149] It was also regarded as crucial that the prison authorities took on the costs of supporting insane offenders in asylums, in order get rid of a class of prisoners 'who encumber the gaol & interfere with Discipline'.[150] In 1889 the Home Office issued instructions to magistrates to send mentally ill offenders directly to asylums, but this failed to stem the rise in committals to prison, and then subsequent removals to asylums. Between 1890 and 1895 out of a total of 765 convicted lunatics, 334 ended up being converted to pauper lunatics at the end of their sentences.[151] Many mentally ill prisoners, meanwhile, continued to languish in remand prisons. In the year ending March 1893 some 88 cases of insanity were recorded in Holloway Prison, 72 of whom were remand prisoners and 'insane before they came in'.[152] The practice was recognised as a good thing for prisoners and for the public, and difficult to curb, but 'a very inconvenient thing to the prisons'.[153]

The experience for mentally ill prisoners themselves was doubt about the genuineness of their insanity, delays in transfers and, for many, movements back and forth between prison and asylum.[154] Prisoners' own accounts provide valuable, and almost invariably critical, evidence referring to delays in sending insane prisoners to asylums for treatment, and regarded the prison as wholly unsuitable for any form of treatment.

[148] Report of the Commissioners of Prisons, 1889 (1889) [C.5881] [C.5881–1], p. 7. McConville, *English Local Prisons*, p. 231 cites a figure of £4,000 per annum as the additional cost for maintaining these prisoners in asylums in England and Wales after 1884.

[149] TNA, HO 45/9640/A34434, Prisons and Prisoners (4) Other: Medical Examination of Prisoners Unfit for Prison Discipline with a View to Decreasing Number of Deaths in Prisons, 1884–89, 8. Harcourt to Du Cane, Removal of Sick Persons from Prisons, 1 Jan. 1885.

[150] Ibid., 7. Minute on Removal of Persons from Prison, Liddell to Fowler and Du Cane, 16 Dec. 1884.

[151] TNA, HO 45/9955/V10698, Lunacy: Prison Department Reports on Criminal Lunatics Not under Definite Sentence Whose Maintenance Is Chargeable to Prison Vote, 1888–96, 13. Return of the Number of Criminal Lunatics Sent to County and Borough Asylums during the years 1890 to 1895.

[152] Report from the Departmental Committee on Prisons [Gladstone Committee] (1895) [C.7702] [C.7702–1], Evidence of Dr Walker, p. 131.

[153] Ibid., Evidence of Dr Gover, p. 48.

[154] See ch. 3, for more details of the medical management of cases of lunacy and suspected lunacy.

These memoirs, for the most part condemning all aspects of prison discipline, highlighted the poor treatment by doctors of insane prisoners rather than instances of good practice, though occasionally prisoners were positive about their medical care and the prison doctors. One Who Has Endured It described the doctor's visit in Dartmoor as a 'brutal farce', while Susan Fletcher commented that the doctor offered friendly and professional care at Westminster Prison and was as good to her as the prison regulations allowed.[155] Typically the memoirs referred to the inadequate handling of cases of mental breakdown as those afflicted were moved to the punishment cells following displays of violence or infractions of the prison rules, or to the infirmary or padded cell for long periods of observation, pointing out that it was often fellow prisoners rather than the prison medical officers who called attention to cases of insanity. One memoir described the case of a fifteen-year-old boy accused of shamming and found insensible on several occasions. He was treated with blisters to the nape of his neck and a mustard plaster, followed by the stomach pump. Back in his cell, he was found covered in blood, having cut his leg with a broken medicine bottle. He had then eaten the rest of the bottle. Though the doctor confirmed that boy 'was not in his right mind', he was kept in the prison hospital until he supposedly recovered.[156] Another young man described as 'soft' was left in a semi-dark cell without anything to employ his mind. After three weeks 'he took to simply moaning like some dumb beast in mortal agony, and then after another week or so he became perfectly quiet and used to lie day after day stretched on the floor in a half stupefied condition'. He remained in this state for a month until the doctor decided that the boy was insane: 'the necessary papers were signed, and the unfortunate youth transferred to the county lunatic asylum to live at the expense of the ratepayers for the rest of his life'.[157] Florence Maybrick recollected how many female prisoners developed symptoms of insanity over many months or years, adding to the 'ghastliness' of the prison experience and having a harrowing impact on other inmates:

She is kept in the infirmary with the other patients for three months. If she does not recover her reason within that period, she is certified by three doctors as insane and then removed to the criminal lunatic asylum. In the mean time the peace and rest of the other sick persons in the infirmary are disturbed by her

[155] One Who Has Endured It, *Five Years of Penal Servitude* (London: Richard Bentley & Son, 1878), p. 96; Susan Willis Fletcher, *Twelve Months in an English Prison* (Boston, MA: Lee and Shephard; New York: Charles T. Dillingham, 1884), p. 408.
[156] One Who Has Tried Them, *Her Majesty's Prisons: Their Effects and Defects*, vols 1 and 2 (London: Sampson Low, Marsten, Searle & Rivington, 1881), vol. 2, pp. 127–9.
[157] Ibid., pp. 252, 254–5.

ravings, and their feelings wrought upon by the daily sight of a demented fellow creature.[158]

Examples taken from individual convict and local prisons illuminate the day-to-day negotiations and processes involved in removing prisoners to asylums, which were more complex and less clear cut than the legislation would indicate, involving delays and disputes between prison and asylum officers about the destination of prisoners, or uncertainly concerning their mental state. Catherine Murray, described as a 'prostitute', was imprisoned in Mountjoy Prison after she was found guilty of larceny in 1878, following several previous convictions for being drunk and disorderly, and was moved several times between Mountjoy and Dundrum Asylum. During a spell in Mountjoy between March and October 1881 she was reported to be unwell, unfit for strict cellular confinement, badly behaved and violent, showing symptoms of unsoundness of mind and insanity. Murray was removed once again to Dundrum in April 1882.[159] Convicted of murder and sentenced to penal servitude for life, Denis Flanagan was taken from Kilkenny Prison to Mountjoy in December 1887. Two months later he was transferred to Dundrum after attempting suicide. Kilkenny's Governor reported that Flanagan had a severe head wound and, though he spoke rationally, 'from his general conduct and other circumstances I believe him to be suffering from suicidal mania and have no doubt that he will repeat the attempt on his own life at the first opportunity'.[160] Other removals took longer, though it was unclear in many cases precisely when the prisoner was first suspected of suffering mental disorder. Thomas Kearney, sentenced to five years for wounding, spent eighteen months in Belfast Prison, before being removed to Dundrum; Patrick Sheridan, serving five years for robbery with violence, was moved from Mountjoy to Dundrum over two years after he was committed, having been 'under observation while mental state worsened'.[161]

In her study of criminal lunacy in Warwickshire, Janet Saunders noted how 'not only offenders with the less spectacular or obvious mental

[158] Florence Elizabeth Maybrick, *Mrs. Maybrick's Own Story: My Fifteen Lost Years* (New York and London: Funk & Wagnalls, 1905), pp. 82, 177–8. For prisoners' accounts of mental illness, see Hilary Marland, '"Close Confinement Tells Very Much upon a Man": Prison Memoirs, Insanity and the Late Nineteenth- and Early Twentieth-Century Prison', *Journal of the History of Medicine and Allied Sciences*, 74:3 (2019), 267–91.
[159] National Archives Ireland (NAI), General Prisons Board (GPB)/PEN/3/8, Catherine Murray.
[160] Ibid., GPB/PEN/3/58, Denis Flanagan.
[161] Ibid., GPB/PEN/3/30, Thomas Kearney; GPB/PEN/3/34, Patrick Sheridan.

disorders, but also fairly severely disordered "lunatics" and the obviously mentally deficient were being sent to prison'.[162] It was then the onset of spectacular or violent behaviour that was likely to prompt transfers of these prisoners, even though this kind of behaviour might be dealt with for lengthy periods before certification was turned to as a last resort.[163] One man, serving eighteen months for burglary, was sent to the asylum towards the end of his sentence after sixteen months in prison. He had displayed strange behaviour and had been depressed, but it was the onset of excitement and then violence that finally prompted his removal.[164] One case committed to Mountjoy Prison in 1875 attracted the attention of a Commission into Dundrum's management, that, among other issues, was investigating the use of inappropriate restraints.[165] Christina Foster, imprisoned for arson, became insane and was transferred to Dundrum in July of that year, where, after violent outbursts, she was placed in a specially made refractory dress. This subdued her violent outbursts and she was moved back to Mountjoy a year later. In October 1876 she was readmitted to Dundrum, and, after a period of quiet marked by depression, in February 1877 Christina again became violent. She was repeatedly placed in seclusion in the restraining dress, before she was finally removed to Belfast Lunatic Asylum in April 1880, presumably on the expiration of her sentence.[166]

Liverpool Borough Prison has a particularly rich collection of records that, together with local asylum archives, reveal complex histories of conviction, imprisonment and institutional confinement, as well as the importance of locale in a setting shaped by mass migration from Ireland to a port city experiencing in turn prosperity and severe economic downturns and extreme poverty.[167] Despite the insistence of alienists and advocates of specialised asylum treatment that prisons were inappropriate places for the care and treatment of the insane, these prisoner patients were often unwelcome in asylums, and in the Lancashire asylums the problem was also one of scale. Already in 1854 the Committee of Visitors at Lancaster Asylum despaired at the 'rapid influx of admissions', including many vagrant lunatics, via the port of Liverpool, that were filling up Lancashire's asylums with chronic and

---

[162] Saunders, 'Institutionalised Offenders', p. 233.   [163] Ibid.   [164] Ibid., p. 234.
[165] TNA, T 1.13216, Lunacy Commission: Dundrum Criminal Lunatic Asylum Dublin, Report upon Dundrum Lunatic Asylum (printed), n.d. (stamped by Treasury, 20 Feb. 1882).
[166] Ibid., pp. 5–6.
[167] See also, for the harm caused to prisoners by delayed removals and the harsh regime at Liverpool Prison, Catherine Cox and Hilary Marland, '"Unfit for Reform or Punishment": Mental Disorder and Discipline in Liverpool Borough Prison in the Late Nineteenth Century', Social History, 44:2 (2019), 173–201.

incurable cases. They also regretted the lack of a separate asylum for criminal lunatics: 'the inconvenience and evils of their confinement and association with the ordinary inmates of our Asylums, are still suffered to exist'.[168] By 1862 Lancaster Asylum held twenty-four criminal patients though the asylum superintendent, John Broadhurst, insisted that only four or five of these were suitable for removal to the criminal lunatic asylum then about to open at Broadmoor.[169]

Irish patients were perceived as a particular problem, associated as they were with violence, drink, vagrancy, disease, prostitution and high levels of crime as they circulated between prisons and lunatic asylums across England and Ireland, accounting for a large proportion of the inmates of English prisons and asylums, especially in port cities and the northern counties. By 1859 around 14 per cent of prisoners in England were Irish-born.[170] In 1875 it was claimed that 13 per cent of the 446 Irish admissions to Prestwich Asylum were sent from the police courts and gaols of the district.[171] The large number of Roman Catholic prisoners at Portsmouth's public works prison prompted Frederick Richard Falkiner, Recorder of Dublin from 1876 to 1905, to conclude they were 'probably Irishmen'.[172] In the late 1870s the Wakefield Justices estimated that about 16 per cent of their prisoners were Irish-born, and at least an equal number were English-born of Irish parentage.[173] Of the 6,707 Roman Catholic prisoners committed to Liverpool Prison in 1868, 53 per cent were born in Ireland. A small number were repatriated, as in 1874 when an Irish male prisoner, sent back from Rainhill Asylum to Liverpool Prison before the expiration of his sentence, was subsequently transferred to Mountjoy Prison in Dublin, but for the most part Irish prisoner patients remained in Lancashire's asylums and prisons.[174]

[168] WL, *Reports of the County Lunatic Asylums at Lancaster, Prestwich, & Rainhill*, Jan. 1854. *Report of the Committee of Visitors of the County Lunatic Asylum at Lancaster, Jan. 4th 1854*, p. 10.
[169] Report of the Commissioners in Lunacy, 1862 (1862) [417], p. 131.
[170] *Judicial Statistics*, 1859 (1860) [2692], p. xxv.
[171] Liverpool Record Office (LRO), M614 RAI/40/2/3, *Annual Reports of the Lancashire Asylums, 1875–78*. Prestwich Annual Report, 1875, p. 66. See also J.K. Walton, M. Blinkhorn, C. Pooley, D. Tidswell and M.J. Winstanley, 'Crime, Migration and Social Change in North-West England and the Basque Country, c. 1870–1930', *British Journal of Criminology*, 39:1 (1999), 90–112.
[172] F.R. Falkiner, 'Our Habitual Criminals', *Journal of the Statistical and Social Inquiry Society of Ireland*, 8:60 (Aug. 1882), 317–30, at p. 323.
[173] J. Horsfall Turner, *The Annals of Wakefield House of Correction* (Bingley: privately printed, 1904), pp. 246, 252.
[174] LRO, 347 MAG 1/2/2, Proceedings of the Meetings of the Liverpool Justices of the Peace, Minutes 1870–78, Report of Governor, 24 Jan. 1874; Report on the District, Criminal and Private Lunatic Asylums in Ireland, 1886 (1886) [C.4811], Central Asylum at Dundrum, p. 123. Jeremiah O'Connor's passage to Ireland was paid by the Liverpool Discharged Prisoners' Aid Society: LRO, 347 MAG 1/3/3, Proceedings of

Drawing on the minutes of Liverpool Prison's visiting committee, annual reports and asylum casebooks, the transfers of individuals moving between the prison, Liverpool's Rainhill Asylum and other local asylums can be traced.[175] One such individual was Mary Leonard, who was found guilty of burglary at the Liverpool Assizes in December 1868 and sentenced to seven years' penal servitude. After removal to Millbank Prison in London (presumably to confirm her mental state), she was taken to Broadmoor in 1873, and in 1876 at the expiration of her sentence transferred to Rainhill.[176] She was noted to be noisy, incoherent and excitable, and had hallucinations of sight and hearing, believing 'that people enter her room at night and stab her, that poison is put into her food. Says her room is set on fire at night.... Has delusions of an exotic kind and uses obscene language.' Mary Leonard died in Rainhill almost three years after her admission.[177] Irishwoman Catherine Nolan's misdemeanors were noted in the Liverpool prison records in April 1896, when she assaulted a warder and damaged twelve panes of glass. She was handcuffed and put on a no. 1 punishment diet for seven days.[178] A month later she was admitted to Rainhill Asylum, where she was noted to be dangerous to others and intemperate. 'She is subject to outbreaks of violence which usually occur at the menstrual period. At times she is violent, destructive, & abusive.'[179] A year later Catherine Nolan was still described as dangerously excitable, delusional and prone to attack those around her: 'Cannot be left a moment alone owing to her violence.' She continued in this state until October 1898, when her death was recorded as a result of tuberculosis of the lungs and intestines.[180] As the number of admissions to Rainhill increased in the late nineteenth century, its Superintendent, Dr Rogers, despaired at the continual presence of the criminal class 'as they not only give much trouble and interfere with the discipline, but their presence and intercourse have also an injurious and demoralizing effect on the younger patients'.[181]

the Meetings of the Visiting Committee, Liverpool Borough Gaol, Apr. 1878–June 1897, 28 Oct. 1891, p. 191.

[175] Cox and Marland, 'Unfit for Reform or Punishment'.
[176] LRO, M614 RAI/8/7, Rainhill Asylum Female Casebook, Oct. 1873–July 1878, p. 175.
[177] Ibid.
[178] LRO, 347 MAG 1/3/3, Proceedings of the Meetings of the Visiting Committee, Liverpool Borough Gaol, Apr. 1878–June 1897, 29 Mar. 1896, p. 387.
[179] LRO, M614 RAI/8/18, Rainhill Asylum Female Casebook, Oct. 1895–July 1897, p. 85.
[180] Ibid.
[181] LRO, M614 RAI/40/2/4, *Reports of the County Lunatic Asylums at Rainhill, Lancaster, Prestwich and Whittingham, 1879–82*, Report of the Medical Superintendent, Rainhill, 1879, p. 17.

Liverpool Prison, as shown in Chapter 3, was notable for its very high proportion of female inmates, many of whom were Irish and likely to be described as turbulent, prone to drunkenness, violent and as prostitutes.[182] In 1868, 69 per cent of Irish-born prisoners were women.[183] Frances Holden, a thirty-three-year-old single Irish woman, committed on numerous occasions to Liverpool Prison on charges of prostitution, was transferred to Rainhill in July 1873. She claimed that she had been in prison thirty-three times and that 'her child was an officer' there. On admission to the asylum, she was described as suffering from mania and that she was 'at one time … very excited and at others more depressed'. Her behaviour was described as delusional, volatile and destructive. In October 1876 Holden was removed 'unimproved' to Lancaster Asylum.[184] In the case of both male and female prisoners, it was largely violent and disruptive behaviour – rather than a precise medical diagnosis – that prompted removal from the prison to asylum. It was also the case that many of these prisoners became permanent residents at Rainhill, which created long-term problems in terms of the institution's management, resources and ability to admit new cases.

As penal policy in England and Ireland shifted away from reforming and redeeming prisoners towards punishing and deterring repeat offenders in the 1860s and 1870s, prison medical officers were even more likely to transfer troublesome and violent prisoners, typically those with protracted prison careers, characterised by recommittals to prison and repeated breaches of prison discipline and punishments. They were also keen to rid themselves of inmates who were diseased and sick, and prisoners suffering general paralysis of the insane (GPI) were particularly liable to removal. Notably difficult patients, they required extra staff and nursing care and had high mortality rates.[185] These cases were unwelcome in prisons and in asylums, and the movement of prisoners with GPI from Liverpool Gaol to Rainhill and other local asylums reflected what was observed to be a remarkable rise in the disease in Lancashire asylums in the latter decades of the century.[186] By 1896 most of Rainhill's deaths

---

[182] Cox and Marland, 'Unfit for Reform or Punishment'.
[183] LRO, H365.32 BOR, *Reports of the Governor, Chaplain, Prison Minister and Surgeon, of the Liverpool Borough Prison, Presented to the Court of Gaol Sessions, Holden on the 28th Day of October, 1869, Prison Minister's Report*, p. 19.
[184] LRO, M614 RAI/8/6, Rainhill Asylum Female Casebook, Jan. 1870–Oct. 1873, p. 278.
[185] WL, *Reports of the County Lunatic Asylums at Lancaster, Prestwich, and Rainhill, 1855, Report of Superintendent, Rainhill Asylum*, p. 88.
[186] For more detail on the status of Irish asylum admissions, see Catherine Cox, Hilary Marland and Sarah York, 'Emaciated, Exhausted and Excited: The Bodies and Minds of the Irish in Nineteenth-Century Lancashire Asylums', *Journal of Social History*, 46:2 (2012), 500–24, especially p. 516 for cases of GPI.

were cases of GPI, and in that year eighty-nine men and nineteen women in the asylum were afflicted with the condition.[187] These included John Murphy, a thirty-five-year-old married Irish labourer, transferred from Liverpool Prison to Rainhill in December 1896. Typifying cases of general paralysis, he was reported to be 'very noisy and violent and has marked grandiose delusions', and he remained 'in a very restless and exalted state'. Murphy died in Rainhill in January 1899.[188]

Catherine O'Brien, a thirty-year-old Irish woman imprisoned for stealing, was described by her husband on her removal to Rainhill in April 1876 as addicted to drink. Her husband also commented that, while his wife was prone to take things, she did not intend to steal them, a likely indication of one of the commonly reported symptoms of GPI, a tendency to hoard other people's belongings.[189] Dr Henry Maudsley commented critically in 1875 on six 'well-marked' cases of GPI admitted to the West Riding Asylum, '*after having undergone the whole or the greater part of their punishment in gaol* for larceny', that might easily have been diagnosed at the time of imprisonment 'by any medical man who had even the most rudimentary knowledge of the symptoms of general paralysis'.[190] In one case a barrister recognised the disease during the trial, 'yet this unfortunate man remained in gaol for five months before being sent to the asylum; he underwent the punishment of a criminal for five months after a hopeless disease of the brain had begun to make its fatal progress'.[191] The prisoner had become violent and excited in prison, was put into a strait jacket and confined in a padded room during the last three weeks of his imprisonment, after which he was sent to the asylum.[192] While the Lunacy Commissioners expressed concern that such cases were being removed to asylums given the burden they placed

[187] Report of the Commissioners in Lunacy, 1896 (1896) [304], p. 278.
[188] LRO, M614 RAI/11/17, Rainhill Asylum Male Casebook, June 1896–Nov. 1897, p. 105.
[189] LRO, M614 RAI/8/7, Rainhill Asylum Female Casebook, Oct. 1873–July 1878, p. 194. See also Gayle Davis, '*The Cruel Madness of Love': Sex, Syphilis and Psychiatry in Scotland, 1880–1930* (Amsterdam and New York: Rodopi, 2008), p. 90.
[190] Henry Maudsley, 'Stealing as a Symptom of General Paralysis', *Lancet*, 106:2724 (13 Nov. 1875), 693–5, at p. 694 (emphasis in original). Maudsley was a preeminent medico-psychological specialist of the late nineteenth century, his views shaped by positivism and degeneracy theory: see Scull, MacKenzie and Hervey, *Masters of Bedlam*, ch. 8.
[191] Ibid. Maudsley was citing evidence from J. Wilkie Burman, 'Some Further Cases of General Paralytics Committed to Prison for Larceny', *Journal of Mental Science*, 20:90 (July 1874), 246–54. See also J. Wilkie Burman, 'On the Separate Care and Special Medical Treatment of the Acute and Curable Cases in Asylums', *Journal of Mental Science*, 25:111 (Oct. 1879), 315–25; 25:112 (Jan. 1880), 468–80.
[192] Maudsley, 'Stealing as a Symptom of General Paralysis', p. 694.

on the institutions, they were also frustrated at the lack of care in diagnosing them in the first place.

The frequency with which General Paralytics are convicted of larceny and similar offences, and their mental state unrecognised even after a considerable stay in gaol, and who are brought to the asylum either as criminal lunatic or as ordinary cases, some time after their discharge from gaol, is very discreditable to the administration of the law, and deserves more attention, with a view to remedy, than it has received.[193]

Prison medical officers' diagnosis of 'real' or 'genuine' insanity in these and other cases would typically follow prolonged periods of disruptive behaviour by inmates, and the destruction of prison property, suggesting that removal to an asylum was prompted by concerns about management rather than careful judgement, detailed diagnosis or consideration of the prisoners' best interests, bringing into question the claims of prison medical officers to be making decisions on the basis of their expertise in psychiatry. Prison doctors' descriptions of such patients at the point of removal refer to prisoners experiencing 'delusions', or to the 'irritability' or 'excitability' that prompted destructive behaviour; they were less likely to come up with a clear diagnosis or to use labels current in psychiatric practice outside of prisons.[194] This kind of approach magnified the assertions of asylum doctors that prisoners were better off being moved and treated in the asylum by experts in mental disorder, but also confirmed their anxieties about the removal of particularly disruptive patients and their impact on routine and management.

By the late nineteenth century, many asylums in England and Ireland were overcrowded and overstretched, struggling to accept new patients and to effectively maintain regimes of moral management that were based on regularity and order, enhanced diet, work therapy and occupation.[195] They were reluctant to take in insane criminals who were regarded as troublesome, likely to contribute to high mortality rates

---

[193] Anon., 'Criminal Lunacy in 1877', p. 648.

[194] David Nicolson, while medical officer at Woking Prison, described these episodes as 'breaking out' though the term was not used at Liverpool: David Nicolson, 'The Morbid Psychology of Criminals', *Journal of Mental Science*, 19:87 (Oct. 1873), 398–409, at p. 402. See ch. 3 for the unique taxonomy and labelling produced in nineteenth-century prisons, and chs 2 and 5 for instances of breaking out. See also Rachel Bennett, '"Bad for the Health of the Body, Worse for the Health of the Mind": Female Responses to Imprisonment in England, 1853–1869', *Social History of Medicine*, 34:2 (2021), 532–52.

[195] There is an expansive literature on moral management. See e.g. Scull, *The Most Solitary of Afflictions*, ch. 4. For a comparison of the therapeutic regimes at Broadmoor criminal asylum for different classes of inmate, see Shepherd, 'I Am Very Glad and Cheered When I Hear the Flute'.

and who would be a poor and potentially alarming influence on other patients. In 1887, referring to the practice of reclassifying criminal lunatics as pauper patients at the end of their sentences, the Commissioners in Lunacy described how those removed to county asylums

> are a far more dangerous class than those to whom the term is now legally applicable, and if I might devise a name for them, I would call them 'Lunatic Criminals'; implying that they were 'criminals' first and 'lunatics' afterwards. It is by this class that murderous assaults are generally committed.[196]

In addition to concerns about the type of illnesses they brought into the institution and the high mortality rates, there was also the risk of escape.[197] The Superintendent of Somerset County Lunatic Asylum, Dr Charles Medlicott, spoke of the 'contaminating effect' of such admissions, arguing that in most cases 'it is not fair to saddle a criminal who has become insane on our ordinary pauper lunatics', as 'the anxiety and responsibility is endless with a class like that, and the restraint that ought to be exercised in their cases is utterly incompatible with the liberty we wish to give to others where we know that there is a possibility of restoration to reason'.[198]

Turf Wars and Claims of Expertise between Prisons and Asylums

Such challenges to the maintenance of order and institutional wellbeing blighted prisons and asylums throughout the second half of the nineteenth century. At the same time both asylum doctors and prison medical officers continued to assert their unique authority and ability to treat mentally ill offenders, though prison doctors' claims were more likely to be based on ability to recognise, diagnose and manage insanity rather than to treat it. Aside from what appeared to be at times intractable legal and practical issues in reaching decisions on the accommodation of 'prisoner patients', in particular instances discussions on where to place the lunatic prisoner evolved into disputes between prison doctors and the prison commissioners and asylum doctors and lunacy commissioners and inspectors. Prison doctors were lambasted in some of these high-profile cases, for their lack of expertise, knowledge and judgement, as

---

[196] LRO, M614 RAI/40/2/6, *Reports of the County Lunatic Asylums at Lancaster, Rainhill, Prestwich, and Whittingham, 1887–90, Rainhill Asylum Annual Report, 1887, Commissioners in Lunacy Report,* p. 115.
[197] Report of the Commissioners in Lunacy, 1862, p. 133. For criminal patients' escapes from asylums, see ch. 5.
[198] Commission on Criminal Lunacy (1882), Evidence of Charles W.C.M. Medlicott, pp. 72, 1237, 1246.

well as their resistance to transferring cases, and it was argued that prisoners whose mental and physical condition had worsened in prison would have fared better had they been removed to the specialist care available in the asylum.

Many cases were brought to light where mentally disturbed offenders had languished in prison for lengthy periods, as well as of removals of prisoners to asylums who were described as being in a terrible state of mental and physical health, suffering serious abrasions and other injuries, malnourished and in a filthy condition.[199] In 1846 – in the midst of the Famine – the report of Ballinasloe District Lunatic Asylum complained of the terrible condition of the 'poor creatures' transferred from different prisons in the province, 'in a most wretched and deplorable state, with broken down constitutions, and labouring under cachectic disease'. In one week alone, three were admitted in a dying state, including a twelve-year-old child, 'labouring under dementia, epilepsy, and dysentery'. Prisoners were often conveyed in open vehicles, exposed to 'the inclemency of the weather, as well as the gaze of the populace', tied down with ropes or even chains.[200] Prison doctors were still being described in the press in 1867 as not being 'conversant with mental diseases', leaving the quiet lunatic to 'mope in hopeless loneliness'; if turbulent 'he rages in his cell becoming more incurable every hour'.[201] The Irish Prison Inspectors continued to detail the appalling state of many such prisoners held in city and county gaols in their annual reports, such as the 'idiotic' male prisoner discovered in Kilmainham in December 1875, crouched in a corner of his cell, dirty and 'howling like a wild beast'. The man, who was declared 'most unfit for penal treatment in a gaol', had been sentenced to two months' hard labour for stealing but was incapable of any work. He had been regularly admitted to Loughlinstown Union Workhouse, 'and it is to be regretted that he cannot be compelled to remain in it or some other asylum, as the criminal prosecution of someone in his state is not

---

[199] NAI, Government Prison Office (GPO)/Letter Books (LB), Vol. 15, Jan. 1856–Dec. 1856, C.R. Knight to Local Inspector, Spike Island, 19 Jan. 1856; ibid., Walter Crofton to the Inspectors of Lunatic Asylums, 26 Jan. 1856; NAI, GPB/Minute Books (MB)/ Vol. 3, Nov. 1883–Dec. 1886, 22 Jan. 1885, p. 187.

[200] Report on the District, Local and Private Lunatic Asylums in Ireland, 1846 (1847), Ballinasloe District Lunatic Asylum, p. 37. Cachexia is a wasting disorder associated with extreme weight loss and muscle wastage. Dementia during this period denoted a chronic, incurable form of insanity with little expectation of improvement, rather than a disorder specifically related to ageing. See German Berrios and Roy Porter (eds), *A History of Clinical Psychiatry: The Origin and History of Psychiatric Disorders* (London and New Brunswick, NJ: Athlone, 1995), ch. 2; Emily Andrews, 'Senility before Alzheimer: Old Age in British Psychiatry, c. 1835–1912' (unpublished University of Warwick PhD thesis, 2014).

[201] *The Irish Times*, 12 July 1867.

attended with advantage'.[202] In 1885 a complaint was made by the Office of the Inspector of Lunatic Asylums about a prisoner who had been removed from Castlebar Prison; 'as to Insane prisoner Wm. [?Connot] having had serious abrasions on wrists when received in Dundrum Asylum'. The Lunacy Inspector was requested in future to bring such complaints to their notice and Dundrum's medical officer, Dr O'Brien, instructed to deal with the alleged injury.[203]

In many instances, prison officers were accused of causing severe harm or the deaths of insane prisoners, as in a case reported by John Charles Bucknill of an epileptic young man twice imprisoned in the borough gaol owing to his uncontrollable violence. 'I do not know on what principle he was committed to gaol, instead of at once being sent to an asylum. After thirty months' residence he died in a fit.'[204] Nicholas Lawless was committed as a dangerous lunatic to Harold's Cross Prison, south of Dublin, in 1863, at which point the prison surgeon, Dr Ireland, examined Lawless and pronounced him to be mad.[205] After a few months, Lawless's family were informed that he had died. While the cause of death was reported as 'softening of the brain', it appeared that Lawless had died as a result of a 'fearful scalding' when taking a bath. *The Irish Times* criticised the prison for withholding evidence and more generally the practice of committing lunatics declared dangerous to prison.

In a jail there is no provision for the curative treatment of the lunatic; he cannot be isolated from the society of criminals, reckless, it may be, and cruel. The warders are jailers, not attendants upon lunatics; the governor is the ruler of a prison, not the experienced superintendent of an asylum for the insane. No supervision, of the constant and careful kind required for the management of a man devoid of reason, can be exercised in a jail. The very structure of a jail building is unfitted for the safe keeping of lunatics.[206]

The case of Catherine Kelly centred less on her handling by prison officers than on the lack of judgement concerning the timing of her removal. In March 1888 Kelly was brought from Tullamore Prison, King's County to Maryborough District Lunatic Asylum, Queen's County, where she died four days later. Medical Superintendent Dr Hatchell claimed that she had been moved to the asylum in a dying state and that there were marks and bruises on her body. On this occasion the

[202] RIGPI, 1875 (1876) [1497.1], Part II, Appendix, Separate Report on the County and City Gaols and Bridewells, p. 254.
[203] NAI, GPB/MB/Vol. 3, 22 Jan. 1885, p. 187.
[204] Bucknill, *An Inquiry into the Proper Classification and Treatment of Criminal Lunatics*, Appendix, Case XI.
[205] *The Irish Times*, 21 Mar. 1864.   [206] Ibid.

criticism came from the prison rather than lunacy authorities. At the subsequent inquest, the medical member of the General Prisons Board, Dr George P. O'Farrell, concluded that Kelly died of 'extreme exhaustion' and that the prison 'doctor [Dr James Ridley] showed want of judgement in allowing a woman [in such a weak condition] to be removed 18 miles by road'. While Ridley was not accused of wilful neglect, he was criticised by O'Farrell for failing to transfer Kelly to the asylum immediately on reaching a diagnosis of insanity as 'a few hours often make the greatest difference between safety & danger in the removal of Lunatics'.[207]

Revelations and debates about these cases took place against the backdrop of a much broader set of concerns about the high death rates of prisoners in England and Ireland; many prisoners received into custody diseased, exhausted or in a state of insanity died shortly after committal. In 1885 the Prison Commissioners alerted Home Secretary Harcourt to the fact that many prisoners were committed to prison in a 'moribund condition or suffering from serious disease', suggesting that many cases were dying in prison whose condition would have been detected had they been medically examined at their committal.[208] Under Secretary to the Home Office Sir Adolphus Liddell observed that the prison was a place of penal discipline and not 'the proper scene for a Death-bed, and ought not to be converted into a Hospital for Incurables'.[209] Concerned about the number of prisoners suffering from feeble health or serious illness, Harcourt demanded more rigorous medical examinations in prison and insisted that, once identified, such cases should be moved to a workhouse or infirmary as appropriate.[210] In fact, deaths in local prisons declined significantly between the 1860s and 1880s, but still included many cases admitted in an exhausted or dying condition alongside large numbers of lunatic prisoners.[211]

---

[207] NAI, GPB/Incoming Correspondence (CORR)/1888/Item no. 3881, Correspondence relating to inquest on Catherine Kelly, Mar.–Apr. 1888. Dr James Ridley committed suicide in July 1888 during the inquest into the death of the nationalist campaigner John Mandeville, who had been released from Tullamore Prison before Christmas 1887. His family and supporters claimed his treatment in prison had caused his death. See Beverly A. Smith, 'Irish Prison Doctors – Men in the Middle, 1865–90', *Medical History*, 26:4 (1982), 371–94. O'Farrell was appointed Inspector of Lunacy in 1890, see Cox, *Negotiating Insanity*, p. 51.

[208] TNA, HO 45/9640/A34434, Prisons and Prisoners (4), 6. Letter Liddell to the Chairman of Quarter Sessions, 23 March 1885. See also McConville, *English Local Prisons*, p. 291.

[209] TNA, HO 45/9640/A34434, Prisons and Prisoners (4), 7. Minute on Removal of Persons from Prison, Liddell to Fowler and Du Cane, 16 Dec. 1884.

[210] Wiener, *Reconstructing the Criminal*, pp. 318–19.

[211] Report of the Commissioners of Prisons, 1889 (1889) [C.5881], pp. 54, 6. See ch. 3, for conditions in English and Irish prisons.

In England and Ireland, often extensive official investigations were conducted into the deaths of prisoners, which highlighted disputes between prison and asylum officers concerning the actions that had been taken and causes of death. The case of Ferdinand Parker, alias Shortlander, investigated by the Home Office in 1885, centred on the issue of the timing of his removal to an asylum after he had begun to refuse food.[212] Parker had been admitted to hospital in Shepton Mallet Prison in May 1885, on account of his weakness after he declined to eat, declaring the food to be poisoned. By this time the prison surgeon concluded that he was too ill to remove. Though his insanity was said to have commenced on 19 May, he was not certified insane until 5 June. On 11 June he was moved to Somerset and Bath Lunatic Asylum. Examined by the asylum medical officer, Parker was declared to be suffering from mania, was very thin and wasted, and his body scratched and abraded, from what were said to be self-inflicted wounds. He died later that evening after two heart attacks, and the inquest concluded that his death was due to a weak heart and prolonged insufficiency of food. The prison doctors explained that they had been reluctant to force-feed Parker because he had a weak heart, and moreover at times he had taken food.[213] The Commissioners in Lunacy, however, were convinced that he should have been force-fed, adding that

It is the everyday experience of the Commissioners in Lunacy that insane persons who refuse food may be, by proper means, compelled to take sufficient nourishment to keep up their bodily strength till the violence of this phase of insanity has passed.... They see nothing in the circumstance of the present case to have made such a result impossible.[214]

The Medical Inspector of Prisons, Dr Gover, responded that Parker could not have been safely fed by force, stating that the responsible medical officer in charge 'was the best judge'. 'To such an argument it would be quite open to Dr Hyatt [the prison doctor] to reply that the prisoner's heart was not in a condition to bear the strain of forcible feeding, and that but for the attempt made in the asylum he might possibly now be alive.'[215]

---

[212] TNA, HO 144/469/X6313. Lunacy: Removal to Asylum of Prisoners Certified Insane 1885.

[213] Ibid., Warrant of Removal to Asylums under CLA 1884, 10 June 1885; Letter from Somerset and Bath Lunatic Asylum, 15 June 1885 to Commissioners in Lunacy, re Ferdinand Espin Parker alias Shortlander; Letter from Commissioners in Lunacy to Under Secretary of State, 8 July 1885.

[214] Ibid., Letter from Office of Commissioners in Lunacy to the under Sec of State for the Home Dept., 27 Aug. 1885 (emphasis in original).

[215] Ibid., Copy Memorandum by Dr Gover, Medical Inspector on Ferdinand Parker's Case (received HO, 13 Oct. 1886). Prisons, however, were prepared to resort to force-feeding, as illuminated in ch. 3.

Occasionally these cases were more widely publicised, drawing public attention to the failures of the prison system, as in December 1897 when the *Manchester Evening News* reported a 'scandal' at Strangeways Prison involving Edward Cox, an insane prisoner whose ribs had been broken while he was being restrained.[216] Cox had arrived at Prestwich Asylum with severe injuries, but, while the asylum doctors claimed that eight of his ribs had been broken, the officers at Strangeways asserted that all due care had been exercised by the prison medical officers and that 'only one or two ribs' were fractured. The resulting Home Office inquiry revealed that the prisoner had been admitted to Strangeways in April 1897, and the day before his sentence expired on 9 October he became violently insane, assaulting the prison's senior medical officer, Dr Edwards.[217] There was a struggle with five prison officers to move Cox to a padded cell, when the injuries occurred. The discovery of the injuries prompted an extensive investigation into the case with allegations that the prison authorities had withheld relevant information on Cox's mental and physical condition from the Visiting Committee and the certifying magistrate. The Prison Medical Inspector, Dr Smalley, who was asked to examine Cox, criticised the asylum doctors, claiming that they had exaggerated the extent of the injuries. The Chairman of the Prison Visiting Committee, however, insisted that 'his [Smalley's] evidence ought not to outweigh the impartial evidence of the Asylum Surgeons who made careful independent assessments'.[218] It was agreed by all parties that Cox suffered from delusions and was insane. While it was concluded by the Home Office that no unnecessary violence was used against Cox, the prison was criticised for its poor standards of medical care and delays in examining the prisoner.[219]

William Tallack of the Howard Association highlighted the case in a letter to *The Times* in January 1898, reminding readers there had been a similar occurrence in Strangeways eight years previously, when a prisoner had died of injuries that included a fractured breastbone and a number of broken ribs. That case had never been resolved, and Tallack made a strong argument for full disclosure in the public interest in the

---

[216] *Manchester Evening News*, 13 Dec. 1897.
[217] TNA, HO 114/513/X66658. Lunacy: Edward Cox. Injuries to Insane Prisoner Inquiry, 1897–98; ibid./10 To the RH Sir Matthew White Ridley, MP, Principal Secretary of State (HO received 20 Dec. 1897).
[218] Ibid./3, Copy of Report by Dr Smalley ([Prison] Medical Inspector) dated 15/9/97; ibid./2, HM Prison, Manchester to Secretary of State, 18 Nov. 1897 (received HO 20 Nov. 1897).
[219] Ibid./14, Letter Whitehall, 21 Jan. 1898, to R.A. Armitage, Chairman of Visiting Committee of HM Prison, Manchester.

case of Cox as 'a check to the occasional cruelty of warders' and for the protection of prisoners.[220]

Conclusion

While Dr David Nicolson and a few other individuals served long careers that crossed between prisons and asylums, typically moving from posts as assistant medical officer in an asylum to the prison service, in July 1896 the *Journal of Mental Science* asserted: 'Too long have the alienist and the criminologist worked apart.'[221] Responding to the findings of the Gladstone Report of 1895, it was suggested that this distinction in their spheres of labour was 'quite unnatural'. Both our prison colleagues 'and ourselves' had been remiss, it was concluded, in failing to forge common bases for study and collaboration across institutions of confinement.[222] Yet a few years later, Dr David Nicolson himself affirmed that 'Many medical men, including some asylum attendants, who are in every way admirable in their ordinary lunacy work, find themselves not quite at home in the investigation of criminal cases,' given that the methods of examination were often quite different.[223]

Assertions of expertise – which occasionally flared up in hostile exchanges – took place against the backdrop of prison services still facing the pressures of large numbers of lunatic prisoners. This resulted in part from magistrates' persistence in directing such cases to prison, though the increase was also likely to have resulted from prison medical officers' growing willingness to record prisoners as mentally disordered or unfit. Medical Inspector Dr Robert Gover explained how 'In former times

[220] William Tallack, 'Prison Inquiries: To the Editor of the Times', *The Times*, 3 Jan. 1898; William Tallack, 'The Case of Prisoner Gatcliff: To the Editor of the Times', *The Times*, 26 Dec. 1889; 'The Alleged Manslaughter in Strangeways Gaol', *Manchester Guardian*, 27 Dec. 1889. Similar cases had also long been reported in asylums, and Dr Rogers at Rainhill defended his attendants from accusations of foul play in 1870, claiming that patients suffering from broken ribs were often suffering from GPI, who typically were physically weak yet intensely irritating to other patients, leading to quarrels and skirmishes: Occasional Notes, 'Broken Ribs and Asylum Attendants', *Journal of Mental Science*, 16:74 (July 1870), 253–5. See Jennifer Wallis, *Investigating the Body in the Victorian Asylum: Doctors, Patients, and Practices* (Cham: Palgrave Macmillan, 2017), 'Bone', for the wider debate on the softening of ribs in cases of GPI.
[221] Anon., 'Crime and Insanity', *Journal of Mental Science*, 42:78 (July 1896), 602–4, at p. 602. Nicolson was prison medical officer in a number of convict prisons as well as a serving a long stint as Broadmoor's superintendent (1886–96). Dr John Baker worked at Broadmoor before moving to prison posts at Portsmouth and Pentonville.
[222] Ibid.
[223] David Nicolson, 'Can the Reproachful Differences of Medical Opinion in Lunacy Cases be Obviated?', *BMJ*, 2:2020 (16 Sept. 1899), 699–702, at p. 702.

I have no doubt that many prisoners who were insane were dealt with as if they were sane more than now,' with prison medical officers more willing to send insane prisoners on to the asylum in their own interests.[224] In 1893 Gover noted that the number of lunatics proportional to the prison population was larger than any year on record, with eighty-one admissions to local prisons during the year.[225] These ranged from prisoners on very short sentences to those sentenced to ten years' penal servitude, who were recognised to be insane at or shortly after their reception in prison. Most were quickly certified as insane and moved to asylums. 'All were unfit for prison discipline, and many must have been unable to understand why they were placed upon their trial, or the meaning of any of the legal proceedings taken. The insanity was very obvious in most cases.'[226] The Commissioners' Reports also revealed the persistent messiness of dealing with such cases. Of the eleven cases reported in Liverpool Prison in 1893, three were removed to Rainhill Asylum, one to Whittingham Asylum, one was discharged into the care of friends and the rest taken to local workhouses.[227]

The continued admission of the mentally disordered into prisons took place at a time where there was mounting concern about both the high numbers of criminal lunatics more broadly and the rise in lunacy in the population as a whole in England and even more so in Ireland.[228] While the alarming rise in the asylum population of Ireland was widely commented on, the Irish General Prisons Board still referred in 1892 to the 'objectionable and illegal practice prevailing throughout the country, of committing lunatics to gaol, instead of sending them directly to asylums'.[229] A year later the number of asylum transfers had increased to 92: of these, 72 had been found insane on reception, five were imbecile

---

[224] Gladstone Committee (1895), Evidence of Dr Gover, p. 48.
[225] Report of the Commissioners of Prisons, 1893 (1893–94) [C.7197] Part 1, Notes by the Medical Inspector, R.M. Gover, p. 44. See also Wiener, *Reconstructing the Criminal*, pp. 320–1.
[226] Report of the Commissioners of Prisons, 1893, p. 44.   [227] Ibid., pp. 44, 83–6.
[228] In 1874 high numbers of criminal lunatics were reported in Broadmoor with 631 patients, while county asylums housed 93; the total, including a handful in private asylums, was 731: Report of the Commissioners in Lunacy, 1894 (1894) [172], p. 1. For anxieties concerning the rise in lunacy around 1900, see E. Fuller Torrey and Judy Miller, *The Invisible Plague: The Rise of Mental Illness from 1750 to the Present* (New Brunswick, NJ and London: Rutgers University Press, 2002) and, out of many publications in both lay and medical journals, see, for example, Thomas Drapes, 'Is Insanity Increasing?', *Fortnightly Review*, 60:358 (Oct. 1896), 483–93; Thomas Drapes, 'On the Alleged Increase of Insanity in Ireland', *Journal of Mental Science*, 40:171 (Oct. 1894), 519–48; Daniel Hack Tuke, 'Alleged Increase in Insanity', *Journal of Mental Science*, 40:169 (Apr. 1894), 219–34; Daniel Hack Tuke, 'Increase of Insanity in Ireland', *Journal of Mental Science*, 40:171 (Oct. 1894), 549–61.
[229] RGPBI, 1891–92 (1892) [C.6789], p. 19.

or weak-minded and three 'doubtful'.[230] Limerick alone had transferred thirteen male prisoners and six female to asylums, most of whom were insane when committed. Many such prisoners were suffering from dementia or described as imbeciles, and had been imprisoned with short sentences for begging or vagrancy.[231]

Despite the claims of prison doctors, expertise in psychiatry in the context of criminal justice was still often equated with psychiatrists working outside of prisons. In Ireland it was largely lunacy inspectors and asylum superintendents, including Dr Conolly Norman, Medical Superintendent of Richmond Asylum and Dr Moloney of Swift's Hospital (St Patrick's), who were responsible for examining prisoners suspected of being mentally ill. In 1886 the Lunacy Commissioners, as requested by the Secretary of State, compiled a list of persons residing near each English prison who were fitted for the role of examining persons charged with capital offences reported to be of unsound mind or in whose case the defence of insanity was likely to be advanced. The list was largely composed of asylum superintendents. Dr Orange and Dr Gover had been relieved of their duties in this regard, Orange owing to his poor health, Gover because he was over-committed; Du Cane also argued that Gover's appointment was incompatible with his role as Medical Inspector of Prisons. Dr Henry Bastian, formerly an Assistant Superintendent at Broadmoor, was appointed to deal with cases in the metropolitan area, with a list of reserves including two eminent psych-iatrists, Dr George Fielding Blandford and Dr Henry Maudsley, along with Dr Edgar Sheppard, retired Medical Superintendent of Colney Hatch Asylum, for a hefty fee of five guineas for a day's examination or for providing evidence.[232]

By the late nineteenth century many asylum doctors and some doctors working in the prison service itself argued that prison medical officers needed to be exposed to a period of training in lunacy outside of the prison, in order to deal with those prisoners who required special care. While such views, which were also strongly voiced in evidence given to the Gladstone Committee in 1895, can be construed as pointing to the continuing inadequacy of prison medical officers in dealing with mental disorder, they could also represent recognition of the reality of their roles and ambition to have their increasing experience and knowledge of the field enhanced and given more authority. 'That candidates for medical

---

[230] RGPBI, 1892–93 (1893–94) [C.7174], p. 8.   [231] Ibid., p. 9.
[232] TNA, HO 45/9632/A26128: Lunacy: Salaries of Drs. Gover and Orange. Arrangements and Fees for Examinations of Prisoners on Capital Charge, as to Insanity, 1883–86.

appointments should be required to show that they have given special attention to lunacy' also indicated that their heavy workload in this area of practice was being acknowledged.[233] The Medical Superintendent of Wakefield Asylum recommended that prison medical officers should spend six months attached to a large county asylum, as 'the difficulties of diagnosis are very great'. He also argued that the number of medical officers should be doubled in London's receiving prisons, given the huge workload that often necessitated (over)rapid diagnosis.[234] By the 1890s, David Nicolson was advocating asylum training and secondments for prison medical officers, at the same time suggesting that while prison doctors could enhance their skill sets, asylum doctors might be uncomfortable with criminal cases.[235] Nicolson went on to chair a committee of inquiry in Ireland in 1905 examining the issue of 'borderland' cases transferred between prisons and asylums, and it was recommended that candidates for appointment as medical officer in convict prisons be required to produce testimony of special experience among the insane in asylums.[236]

During the latter part of the nineteenth century there was growing concern that while 'sane criminals' were finding their way into the criminal lunatic asylums of Broadmoor and Dundrum, as well as other asylums, the sanity of many of those imprisoned for their crimes was also being called into question. The Gladstone Report concluded with a memorandum 'Insanity in Prisons' that, while denying that the prison system produced mental breakdown, concluded that the number of cases of insanity had greatly increased since the prison system had been centralised twenty years previously. The Medical Inspector of the Prisons Board claimed that the practice of sending insane persons to prison contributed to this increase, while the Commissioners in Lunacy argued that many individuals were only dealt with as lunatics after they had committed an offence and thus found their way into prison, while more cases of insanity were actually being identified in prison.[237] Prison administrators and prison doctors were increasingly reproached for their failure 'to realise how slender and impalpable is the border-line between

[233] Anon., 'Crime and Insanity', p. 602.
[234] Gladstone Committee (1895), Evidence of Dr Bevan Lewis, p. 306.
[235] Ibid., Evidence of Dr David Nicolson, p. 312; Nicolson, 'Can the Reproachful Differences', p. 702.
[236] NAI, Chief Secretary's Office Registered Papers/1905/12904, *Report on the Committee of Inquiry into certain Doubtful Cases of Insanity amongst Convicts and Person Detained*, 1905, pp. 10, 16.
[237] Notes and News: 'Report of the Departmental Committee on Prisons, 1895', *Journal of Mental Science*, 42:178 (July 1896), 666–7.

crime and insanity ... the proper inmates of an asylum are too frequently treated with the penal discipline of a prison'.[238] The Report, however, at a point where medical men – working in prison and outside of it – were gaining in professional authority and experience in dealing with criminal offenders, finally opened up the possibility of cooperation between the asylum and prison, 'which cannot but make for a better understanding of the sources and relationships of crime and insanity'.[239]

[238] J.J. Pitcairn, 'The Detection of Insanity in Prison', *Journal of Mental Science*, 43:180 (Jan. 1897), 58–63, at p. 58.
[239] Anon., 'Crime and Insanity', p. 602.

5   'He Puts on Symptoms of Incoherence'
Feigning and Detecting Insanity in Nineteenth-Century
Prisons

In November 1889, Dr R.M. Gover, Medical Inspector of Prisons, travelled to Derby to investigate the case of two prisoners who had allegedly feigned insanity, 'acted the lunatic', in Nottingham and then Derby Prison. The case would trigger heated exchanges between the Commissioners of Lunacy and Prison Commissioners regarding the mental state of convict George Hamsley, apparent ringleader of the two-man attempt to escape the grim conditions of the prison for the milder regime of the asylum. Hamsley's determined efforts to achieve this were described to Gover on his visit to Derby Prison by his then repentant accomplice, fellow-prisoner, Oliver Porcia. Porcia explained to Dr Gover that he had met Hamsley in Nottingham Prison while at exercise. The two were put in adjacent dark cells for being noisy and agreed to make a noise all night. 'If', Hamsley advised Porcia, 'we act the lunatic, we shall both be sent to the asylum, and should then get plenty of good food.'[1] The pair continued with their disruptive behaviour, smashing the cell ventilators, laughing and 'footstepping'. The Governor had Porcia put in irons, but, egged on by Hamsley, he went on with the violence and noise, Porcia recollecting how 'I hankered after the good diet, the cricket playing and talk of the Asylum,' though he dared not 'go partner with him in tearing up my clothes, as I was afraid of a flogging'.[2] Both were moved in due course from Nottingham, not to the asylum, but, to their intense disappointment, to Derby Prison. There they continued to feign insanity but without the desired effect. On the day of his discharge, however, Hamsley finally got his wish granted. Furious at the absence of the gratuity and set of clothes that he had anticipated on leaving prison, he marched directly from the prison to Derby Town

---

[1] The National Archives (TNA), HO 144/477/X22478 4a, Lunacy: Prisoner admitted to Lunatic Asylum on the Day Following his Discharge from Prison, 1889 (1897). Copy report by Dr Gover, Medical Inspector, dated 11 Nov. 1889. (The case appears to have been filed almost a decade later.)
[2] Ibid.

Hall where he talked incoherent nonsense to the policeman on duty. He was duly seen by the police surgeon and removed to Derby Borough Asylum. The Superintendent of Derby Asylum and his colleague at Leicester Asylum, where Hamsley was subsequently taken, were convinced of Hamsley's madness and that he was a 'genuine lunatic', much to Inspector Gover's exasperation.[3]

Unusual in its detail and in Porcia's confession that the two men were indeed feigning insanity, this case provides rich evidence of prisoner agency and knowledge of the prison system. While Hamsley and Porcia did not succeed in their aim of being transferred to an asylum, through their assertive actions they were able to disrupt the regimes of two prisons, create a good deal of work for the prison officers and prompt a top-level inquiry. The case also highlights a common assumption, held by both prison officers and prisoners themselves, that in stark contrast to the deprivations and harsh regime of the prison, the asylum offered a milder discipline, good diet, comfortable surroundings and a variety of amusements. Dr Tennyson Patmore, Medical Officer at Wormwood Scrubs Convict Prison, affirmed that criminals 'appear to graduate with highest honours in malingering ... which may procure for the "insane" adept the genial luxuries of asylum life with its tobacco, cricket, dances, and so on'.[4] 'The temptation to feign insanity in order to become subject to the necessarily milder discipline here must be great,' noted George Revington, Resident Physician and Governor at Dundrum Criminal Lunatic Asylum, in 1898. Convicts returned from Dundrum to prison, he explained, 'convey exaggerated ideas of the comforts of Dundrum to their fellow-prisoners'.[5]

Prisoners would go to great lengths to be moved to an asylum, though they then risked long-term or permanent incarceration. 'The man who feigns madness is playing with very dangerous tools,' asserted one prisoner observer. Once labelled 'balmy' or 'weak-minded', prisoners could lose their chance of remission and find themselves not on a brief respite visit to Broadmoor Criminal Lunatic Asylum but a permanent stay.[6] The concerns of prison administrators were somewhat different; they feared that removal to an asylum would offer prisoners who successfully feigned mental illness opportunities for easy escape, as well as enabling them to

---

[3] Ibid.

[4] Tennyson Patmore, 'Some Points Bearing on "Malingering"', *British Medical Journal*, 1:1727 (3 Feb. 1894), 238–9, at p. 239.

[5] Report on District, Criminal and Private Lunatic Asylums in Ireland, 1898 (1898) [C.8969], Appendix B: Central Criminal Asylum Dundrum: Report of the Resident Physician and Governor, p. 73.

[6] Jabez Spencer Balfour, *My Prison Life* (London: Chapman and Hall, 1907), p. 77.

avoid their due punishment. While conditions for insane convicts at Broadmoor were inferior to the Queen's Pleasure patients, those found insane prior to or during their trial, they were still superior to prison regimes. At Dundrum Criminal Lunatic Asylum convict patients were differentiated from those admitted at the Lord Lieutenant's pleasure; regarded as tainted by their criminality, when viable in the frequently overcrowded asylum, they were separated from the other patients. However, they still were subject to the same conditions of treatment as other Dundrum inmates, that is, first and foremost as asylum patients rather than criminals. Meanwhile, prisoners transferred to public asylums in England and Ireland were likely to be treated in a similar way to ordinary pauper patients.[7]

This case also reflects the more widely felt uncertainty in determining the authenticity of cases of mental disorder among prisoners. The evidence suggested that Hamsley was feigning. That at least is what Porcia claimed. But we can question how seriously we take his account, given that Porcia may not have been the most reliable of witnesses, and was keen when he spoke to Inspector Gover to both attribute blame and express regret for his own actions. Porcia asserted that he had been persuaded, duped, by Hamsley into acting the fool. He convinced Gover, who declared that he had no reason to disbelieve Porcia; he had dropped his attempts at imposture and was behaving well. Gover noted, meanwhile, that Hamsley was an 'inveterate schemer' and 'old prison hand'. He had been in Leicester Prison eight times as well as reformatories at Worcester and Birmingham.[8] The prison chaplain and doctor at Nottingham also concluded that Hamsley was not suffering from insanity, and indeed he had been flogged for his feigning attempts shortly before he left Derby Prison, an action that infuriated the Lunacy Commissioners who believed (based apparently on information they received after Hamsley entered the asylum) that he was insane. In the end, Hamsley managed to convince not one but two asylum medical

---

[7] Jade Shepherd, '"I Am Very Glad and Cheered When I Hear the Flute": The Treatment of Criminal Lunatics in Late Victorian Broadmoor', *Medical History*, 60:4 (2016), 473–91, at p. 475; National Archives of Ireland (NAI), Chief Secretary's Office Registered Papers (CSORP)/1905/12904, *Report on the Committee of Inquiry into Certain Doubtful Cases of Insanity Amongst Convicts and Person Detained*, 1905, p. 15. Insane convicts transferred from prisons were retained in Broadmoor and Dundrum until their sentences expired, when they were discharged to another asylum or released, or were declared sane and sent back to prison until the end of their sentences. Prisoners removed to public asylums whether from prisons or from criminal lunatic asylums could remain there indefinitely if considered uncured. See ch. 4 for details of transfers of prisoners between prisons and asylums.

[8] TNA, HO 144/477/X22478, Lunacy: Prisoner admitted to Lunatic Asylum, 1889 (1897).

superintendents of his insanity, doctors experienced in assessing mental disorder and presumably cautious about admitting ex-prisoners and malingerers to their already over-packed institutions. Finally, the case underlines the extent to which prison staff, and particularly prison medical officers, claimed that they and they alone had developed a special knowledge and practical ability to detect and unveil cases of feigning.

> The Superintendent of the Derby and Leicester Lunatic Asylums believe Hamsley to be a genuine lunatic, but it is to be remarked that the Superintendents of Asylums have no great experience of imposture and are not so well qualified to judge a case of this character as a shrewd and skilful Medical Officer to a Prison, like Dr Greaves of Derby. The opinion I have formed, after careful consideration and inquiry, is that the man Hamsley is a crafty impostor – reckless, ill-tempered, ill-conditioned and idle; and that the Visiting Committee and other authorities of Derby Prison treated him according to his deserts.[9]

Feigning in Prison

The prison has loomed small in terms of historical scholarship on feigning. While the phenomenon of malingering has been subject to widespread investigation in the context of military medicine, there has been little historical analysis of feigning within the prison system and few attempts to draw on evidence from individual prisons.[10] The prison was also largely absent from debates and moral anxieties, ongoing at the turn of the twentieth century about the growing prevalence of feigning and its increasing visibility. In January 1905 the *Lancet* declared that

---

[9] Ibid.

[10] For malingering in military contexts, see Roger Cooter, 'Malingering in Modernity: Psychological Scripts and Adversarial Encounters during the First World War', in Roger Cooter, Mark Harrison and Steve Sturdy (eds), *War, Medicine and Modernity* (Stroud: Sutton, 1999), pp. 125–48; Joanna Bourke, *Dismembering the Male: Men's Bodies, Britain, and the Great War* (Chicago: Chicago University Press, 1996); Ted Bogacz, 'War Neurosis and Cultural Change in England, 1914–22: The Work of the War Office Committee of Enquiry into "Shell Shock"', *Journal of Contemporary History*, 24:2 (1989), 227–56; Matthew Ramsey, 'Conscription, Malingering, and Popular Medicine in Napoleonic France', in Robert Holtman (ed.), *The Consortium on Revolutionary Europe, 1750–1850: Proceedings, 1978* (The Consortium on Revolutionary Europe: Athens, GA, 1978), pp. 188–99; R. Gregory Lande, *Madness, Malingering, and Malfeasance: The Transformation of Psychiatry and the Law in the Civil War* (Washington, DC: Brassey's, 2003). For feigning and resistance to work in asylum contexts, see Sarah Chaney, 'Useful Members of Society or Motiveless Malingerers? Occupation and Malingering in British Psychiatry, 1870–1940', in Waltraud Ernst (ed.), *Work Therapy, Psychiatry and Society, c. 1750–2010* (Manchester: Manchester University Press, 2016), pp. 277–97. Nichol has explored malingering in the context of convict protest in early nineteenth-century Australia: W. Nichol, '"Malingering" and Convict Protest', *Labour History*, 47 (1984), 18–27.

'shamming disease' or 'malingery' had 'reached a high point of perfection ... the rewards of proficiency are great'.[11] Referring to soaring levels of dependence on begging and charity, and pointing to the extraordinary lengths that feigners would go to elicit pity, assistance and admission to hospitals and convalescent homes, the article attributed this to widespread moral decay and reluctance to work. Meanwhile, in the army and navy 'strenuous exertions', including the self-infliction of severe injuries, were undertaken to avoid service and unpleasant duties.[12] The *Lancet* article made no mention of the context of the prison, and when Sir John Collie published what was to become a landmark text on malingering in 1913 he included only a handful of references to prisons.[13]

Yet for prison doctors working in both convict and local prisons feigning was far from a new phenomenon. It had preoccupied them since at least the early nineteenth century, and high levels of malingering were depicted as one of the main challenges of their already arduous roles. Alongside other disruptive and threatening behaviour – refusal to work, hunger strikes, violence and rioting – malingering challenged the maintenance of order in prisons, and added to the difficulties prison medical officers faced in maintaining prisoners' health while supporting the disciplinary regime of the prison.[14] Prisoners were notorious for their talent and persistence in shamming, and detecting, reporting and, on many occasions, authorising the punishment of alleged cases of feigning – involving physical self-harm, suicide attempts, feigned disease or insanity – pitted prisoners against prison medical officers keen to assert their skills in uncovering deceit. Prison archives and official reports allude extensively to the trouble caused by feigning, one Salford prison surgeon, Henry Ollier, declaring in his quarterly report for winter 1831, that 'as usual much of the Surgeon's time has been occupied in judging between feigned and real sickness'.[15] Many prison officers were recruited to prisons following army service, and might well have had experience of

---

[11] Anon., 'Malingery', *Lancet*, 165:4245 (7 Jan. 1905), 45–7, at p. 45.

[12] Ibid., pp. 45–6.

[13] Sir John Collie, *Malingering and Feigned Sickness* (London: Edward Arnold, 1913). A much-extended edition was produced in 1917, again with little on prisons. See also Anon., 'Recent Works on Malingering', *Dublin Journal of Medical Science*, 144:2 (Aug. 1917), 119–21.

[14] For prisoner agency and prison riots, see Alyson Brown, *English Society and the Prison: Time, Culture and Politics in the Development of the Modern Prison, 1850–1920* (Woodbridge: Boydell, 2003); Alyson Brown, *Inter-war Penal Policy and Crime in England: The Dartmoor Convict Prison Riot, 1932* (Basingstoke: Palgrave Macmillan, 2013).

[15] Lancashire County Record Office, QGR/4/31: Surgeons' Report: Salford House of Correction, Michaelmas 1831. Cited Peter McRorie Higgins, *Punish or Treat? Medical Care in English Prisons 1770–1850* (Victoria, BC: Trafford, 2007), p. 132.

malingering in military contexts; some concluded that prisoners – after all already practised in deception and subterfuge – were generally more adept and determined in their feigning efforts than soldiers.[16]

It was claimed that prisoners resorted to a variety of exploits to avoid transportation, punishment or heavy labour, to have prison discipline moderated, to get themselves transferred to the prison infirmary, where they could rest up and enjoy a better diet, or to prompt their removal to an asylum. These included eating soap or soda to fake disordered digestion or inserting copper wire or worsted to poison flesh to the much more extreme tactics of crushing limbs or self-maiming. In 1837 the prison surgeon at Coldbath Fields reported instances of scraping lime from the walls to cause skin inflammation and sores, forced vomiting and simulating the spitting of blood from the lungs. Prisoners also feigned madness and threw themselves off treadwheels in pretended fits.[17] At Salford House of Correction prisoners were reported in the same year for injuring their legs and eyes, simulating dysentery by mingling their evacuations with blood and itch by pricking their fingers with pins.[18] Former soldiers were said to be frequent offenders and passed on their knowledge to other prisoners, though it was observed of transfers of former soldiers from prison to Dundrum Asylum that these frequent malingerers might well 'overdo' their efforts and be easily detected.[19] At Mountjoy Prison an attempted suicide had been preceded by the prisoner faking dysentery stools by mixing stirabout with blood from his nose, and cutting himself with tin and glass while confined in Down County Gaol. One convict at Spike Island, who subsequently committed suicide, complained of a skin eruption on his chest, which the medical officer believed was self-inflicted, as a series of pin scratches. Other prisoners claimed to be suffering from numbness and pain, and some refused

---

[16] Major Arthur Griffiths (1838–1908), Inspector of Prisons and deputy governor of several prisons, had served in the army between 1855 and 1870, seeing active service in the Crimean War, and had run the convict establishment in Gibraltar before joining the English prison service: Bill Forsythe, 'Griffiths, Arthur George Frederick (1838–1908)', *Dictionary of National Biography* (*DNB*), https://0-doi-org/10.1093/ref:odnb/33581 [accessed 3 Jan. 2018]. Dr Robert McDonnell (1828–89), Medical Officer at Mountjoy Convict Prison from 1857 to 1867 and member of the Royal Commission on Prisons in Ireland, 1883–84, was stationed during the Crimean War at the British Hospital at Smyrna. From 1855 he served as civil surgeon at the General Hospital, Sebastopol: C.A. Cameron, *History of the Royal College of Surgeons in Ireland* (Dublin: Fanin and Company, 1916), pp. 496–9.

[17] Higgins, *Punish or Treat?*, p. 134.

[18] Report of the Inspectors of Prisons of Great Britain, Northern and Eastern District, 1837 [89], p. 71.

[19] Report on the District, Criminal and Private Lunatic Asylums in Ireland, 1873 (1873) [C.852], Central Asylum Dundrum, p. 14.

food.[20] The medical officer of Chatham Prison reported for the year 1872 that out of 358 injuries and contusions, 163 had been 'wilful', including many attended with danger to life, and 27 fractures had been 'purposely produced', 16 resulting in immediate amputation. There had been 163 cases where objects were placed under the skin to create sores and 62 instances of mutilation or attempted mutilation.[21] So eager were Chatham's prisoners to avoid hard labour that in 1877 it was reported that they would carry out assaults on officers 'probably for the sole purpose of obtaining a skulk in the punishment cells'.[22]

In the latter decades of the century feigning was increasingly associated with anxieties about heredity, degeneration, recidivism and criminal-mindedness, and gained more coverage in medical journals, criminological publications and forensic texts, and formed part of the curriculum of lecture courses on psychiatry.[23] It also remained a prominent feature of prison doctors' day-to-day workload, the medical officer of Portland Prison complaining in 1870 that 'The unpleasant topic of malingering will, I fear, always have its place in the medical return of a convict prison.'[24] Prison medical officers, observed the *Lancet* in 1877,

have to deal with malingering of every shape and form. The art, in fact, is practised among convicts with refinement that baffles description, and seems attainable only by cunning thieves and lazy wretches, who prefer preying on society to earning an honest livelihood, and who for the most part occupy our prisons. All this adds considerably to the difficulties of their work.[25]

The Medical Officer at Mountjoy Prison, Dr Robert McDonnell, remarked in 1863, on the difficulties of discriminating between

---

[20] NAI, Government Prison Office (GPO)/Incoming Correspondence (CORR)/1851/ Mountjoy/Item no. 74, Correspondence relating to the attempted suicide by Convict Brennan in Mountjoy, 23 Jan. 1851; Royal Commission into Penal Servitude Acts, Minutes of Evidence [Kimberley Commission] (1878–79) [C.2368] [C.2368–I] [C.2368–II], Evidence of Dr O'Keefe, pp. 875–7. See ch. 2 for a fuller account of Brennan's case.

[21] Report of the Directors of Convict Prisons (RDCP), 1872 (1873) [C.850], p. 293.

[22] Seán McConville, *A History of English Prison Administration, Vol. 1, 1750–1877* (London, Boston and Henley: Routledge & Kegan Paul, 1981), pp. 398–9. See Philip Priestley, *Victorian Prison Lives: English Prison Biography, 1830–1914* (London: Pimlico, 1985), pp. 131–3 for hard labour at Chatham.

[23] For feigning in prison in the late nineteenth century, see Jade Shepherd, 'Feigning Insanity in Late-Victorian Britain', *Prison Service Journal*, 232 (2017), 17–23; Stephen Watson, 'Malingerers, the "Weakminded" Criminal and the "Moral Imbecile": How the English Prison Officer Became an Expert in Mental Deficiency, 1880–1930', in Michael Clark and Catherine Crawford (eds), *Legal Medicine in History* (Cambridge: Cambridge University Press, 1994), pp. 223–41.

[24] RDCP, 1869 (1870) [C.204], Portland Prison: Medical Officer's Report, p. 144.

[25] Anon., 'The Medical Department of the Convict Service', *Lancet*, 110:2810 (7 July 1877), 18.

'wickedness and madness ... a task so difficult as to be often absolutely impossible, and that, too, after months of close and careful daily observation'.[26] Dr John Campbell, Medical Officer at Woking Invalid Prison, described in 1884 the challenges of dealing with 'impostors of the most determined description' in an establishment where the officers were already heavily burdened with managing serious and fatal diseases on an everyday basis.[27] In the same year, a number of prison surgeons reporting to the Royal Commission of Prisons in Ireland, including Dr P. O'Keefe at Mountjoy, commented that feigned madness was common among convicts. Former Chairman of the Directors of Irish Prisons, Sir Walter Crofton, observed that feigning, alongside genuine incidences of mental excitement, accounted undoubtedly for 'the most trying cases' that a medical officer had to deal with.[28]

It is with the feigning of insanity that this chapter is primarily concerned. Harder to adjudicate than cases of physical self-harm or feigned sickness, prison medical officers grappled to reach a conclusion on the authenticity of a prisoner's mental disorder in an environment where a great many prisoners were presenting with symptoms of insanity or weak-mindedness. Prison medical officers were required on a regular basis to reach decisions about whether prisoners were attempting to dupe the prison authorities in order to improve the circumstances of their confinement or were genuinely mad and in need of treatment or removal to an asylum. 'No case', as Dr Conolly Norman, Medical Superintendent of Richmond Asylum in Dublin and one of several consultants on lunacy for the General Prisons Board in Ireland, succinctly put it, 'is more calculated to try the judgement of the most skilled specialist than one in which there is reason to fear the possibility of feigned insanity.'[29]

The task of adjudicating such cases fundamentally shaped prison practice and assisted in developing particular approaches in prison psychiatry, which emphasised skill in detection and the ability to discriminate between the true and pretended lunatic. In a period when, as seen in Chapter 4, there was broad agreement outside of the criminal justice system (and some reservations within it) that the insane did not belong in prison and doubts expressed about the fitness of prison medical

---

[26] Robert McDonnell, 'Observations on the Case of Burton, and So-called Moral Insanity in Criminal Cases', *Journal of the Statistical and Social Inquiry Society of Ireland*, 3:25 (Dec. 1863), 447–56, at p. 450.

[27] John Campbell, *Thirty Years' Experience of a Medical Officer in the English Convict Service* (London, Edinburgh and New York: T. Nelson and Sons, 1884), p. 65.

[28] Royal Commission on Prisons in Ireland, Vol. 1. Reports, Digest of Evidence, Appendices: Minutes of Evidence, 1884 (1884–85) [C.4233] [C.4233–I], pp. 94, 505.

[29] NAI, General Prisons Board (GPB)/CORR/1888/Item no. 13247, Correspondence in relation to the fee of Dr Norman, consulting lunacy case, Kilmainham, Dec. 1888.

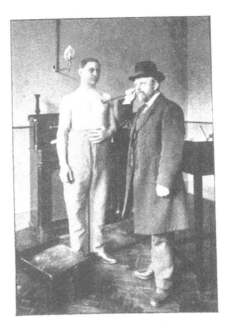

The Doctor

Figure 5.1 Doctor examining prisoner, Wormwood Scrubs, c. 1891
Credit: Archives Howard League for Penal Reform, Modern Records Centre,
University of Warwick

officers to intervene effectively to deal with mentally ill inmates, prison doctors retaliated, in a similar way to Medical Inspector Dr Gover in the Hamsley case, to claim that in effect they had a better and deeper knowledge than asylum doctors of the particular challenges of diagnosing mental disorder in prison.[30] The detection of feigning was an important element in putting forward a case that their special knowledge and practical experience made prison doctors alone fit to assess mental illness in the prison context.

---

[30] See ch. 4 for disputes between prison medical officers and asylum superintendents concerning the placing of insane offenders and delays in removing patients to asylums, and for proposals on how to extend prison medical officers' experience of dealing with mental illness towards the end of the century. See also Seán McConville, *English Local Prisons 1860–1900: Next Only to Death* (London and New York: Routledge, 1995), p. 300.

Roger Cooter has argued that studies of feigning need to be set within the broader context of forensic framing and detection that increasingly typified science and medicine as it became more analytical in the late nineteenth century.[31] This had a particular resonance in prisons as medical officers, as seen in Chapter 3, set about the task of producing a new taxonomy of mental disorder applicable to their prisoner patients, that coincided – but was discrete from – the production of new classificatory systems in asylum practice. One aspect of this production of new categories and definitions connected feigning, mental illness and criminality as a form of hybrid mental disorder, in an approach that spoke to wider concerns about habitual offenders, shirkers who were morally weak, unable and unwilling to reform and to earn an honest living. Watching out for prisoners' attempts to feign insanity also served as a check on the recommendations of expert medical witnesses, including psychiatrists working outside the prison service, who assessed prisoners suspected to be mentally ill prior to their trial. If found mad and, therefore, not responsible for their actions, prisoners would be removed to a criminal lunatic asylum. If found sane, they were sent to prison.[32] The role of the prison medical officer, therefore, was not only to discover shamming but also to weed out cases of true insanity missed around the trial and before sentencing and committal. Prison doctors were also warned that, by placing too much emphasis on detection, cases of real illness, real mental breakdown, might be missed. Prisoners adept in feigning were able, argued Tennyson Patmore, to facilitate their removal to the asylum or 'the Elysian delights of the prison infirmary', improve their diet or obtain relief from work, but he also warned: 'Be ready for malingering by all means; but first look for real disease; and, having found malingering, still look for real disease, as the two may coexist.'[33]

Feigning under the Separate System

While the practice and detection of feigning was part and parcel of prison work well before the introduction of separate confinement in the mid-

---

[31] Cooter, 'Malingering in Modernity', p. 128. Cooter draws on John V. Pickstone, 'Ways of Knowing: Towards a Historical Sociology of Science, Technology and Medicine', *British Journal for the History of Science*, 36:4 (1993), 433–58.

[32] For the role of medical men in determining insanity prior to and during trials, see ch. 4 and, for example, Roger Smith, *Trial by Medicine: Insanity and Responsibility in Victorian Trials* (Edinburgh: Edinburgh University Press, 1981); Joel Peter Eigen, *Witnessing Insanity: Madness and Mad-Doctors in the English Court* (New Haven, CT: Yale University Press, 1995); John Peter Eigen, *Mad-Doctors in the Dock: Defending the Diagnosis, 1760–1913* (Baltimore, MD: Johns Hopkins University Press, 2016).

[33] Patmore, 'Some Points Bearing on "Malingering"', p. 239.

nineteenth century, feigning insanity took on a new meaning as it threatened to undermine the separate system of prison discipline while it was being established and rolled out across Britain and Ireland. It is difficult to assess whether instances of feigning actually increased in response to the introduction of the separate system but prison officers appear to have become particularly alert to it and to prioritise its detection. Under the conditions of extreme isolation imposed by separate confinement, the mental breakdown of prisoners, as we saw in Chapters 2 and 3, was to become a major preoccupation for prison officers. So too was feigning insanity with its associated noise, disruption and chaotic behaviour; it came to represent the antithesis of the order, obedience and containment demanded by separate confinement.

In Pentonville Model Prison, where separate confinement was first imposed in its most rigorous form in 1842, its Commissioners downplayed incidences of mental illness and resisted transfers to Bethlem Asylum, associating those cases of mental breakdown that they did acknowledge to previous instances of mental illness or to 'mental weakness' among the prisoners rather than to the regime itself.[34] Prison staff also argued that many cases of apparent mental disorder were attributable to attempts to feign insanity, particularly as the convicts were said to quickly learn and understand that weakness of mind might be interpreted as an inability to withstand the rigours of separation, resulting in a mitigation of the discipline, removal to an asylum or another prison, or even discharge on medical grounds.

Our prisoners are occasionally guilty of gross imposition, and, like prisoners in general, can simulate mental as well as physical pain with much dexterity. Some of them have been well acquainted with the opinion commonly prevailing out of doors, that the separate system produces insanity, and they have on more than one occasion told me so. It thus not unfrequently happens, that they will make allusions to the state of their memory, and to sensations in their heads, talking in a manner which, though it may prove totally inconsistent with mental disease, yet often succeeds in impressing careless observers with a fear that they are showing indications of unsoundness of mind.[35]

Under a system designed to test the prisoner's mind, moral rectitude and capacity to improve and reform, the stakes were high when it came to discovering cases of feigning, which revealed the opposite and

---

[34] See Catherine Cox and Hilary Marland, '"He Must Die or Go Mad in This Place": Prisoners, Insanity and the Pentonville Model Prison Experiment, 1842–1852', *Bulletin of the History of Medicine*, 92:1 (2018), 78–109.

[35] Report of the Commissioners for the Government of the Pentonville Prison (RCGPP) (1847–48) [972], Annual Report of the Physician to the Pentonville Prison, p. 52.

undesirable traits of moral weakness, sloth and craftiness. In the late nineteenth century feigning dovetailed with mounting concerns about high levels of recidivism among convicts when 'ideas regarding habitual criminality were supported by theories of mental and bodily degeneration'.[36] However, the detection of feigning was certainly a key aspect of the work of prison medical officers in the early decades of the separate system. In Pentonville, the process of assessing whether a prisoner was shamming was characterised by lengthy deliberation and differences of opinion among the prison's officers. The chaplains, influential and self-appointed authorities on matters of the mind at Pentonville during the 1840s, were liable to challenge the opinions of the medical officers. In 1847 Chaplain Joseph Kingsmill, in what appeared to be a jibe at the prison doctors, as well as an acknowledgement of the difficulties of detecting shamming, declared that 'it must be exceedingly difficult to medical men to discriminate between those of this class who simulate mental disease, and those who may be in a slight degree affected already, and may be counterfeiting more'.[37]

Seen in the context of the total number of offences recorded in official accounts, at first glance feigning appears to be insignificant. The Annual Report of the Pentonville Commissioners for 1845 noted only three cases of shamming to commit suicide and three cases of simulating madness and imbecility out of a total of 245 offences, the vast majority of which related to prisoners' attempts to communicate with each other, and in other years even smaller numbers of cases were listed.[38] Yet the entries in the Medical Officer's journal for just one month of that year, June 1845, exemplify the extent of suspected feigning (as well as the rich descriptive language associated with it) and its day-to-day impact on prison work.

That Reg. No. 486 Ockden had stated that, he was under an impression that castration formed part of his sentence ... prisoner possesses a low cunning which leads him [the Medical Officer] to suspect dissimulation, & that he probably is inclined to impose ... That, he has no doubt Reg. 683 was shamming insanity ... that he had been called to Reg. 641 Wm. Kent, who had suspended [hung] himself, & who had evidently shammed the attempt to obtain indulgences.... That, he had particularly examined Pr Jas. Graham Reg. 635 who is very hypochondrical that he has no hallucination & that his intellect appears just what it was when first received into the Prison.[39]

[36] Shepherd, 'Feigning Insanity', p. 17. See ch. 3 and also Neil Davie, 'The Role of Medico-legal Expertise in the Emergence of Criminology in Britain (1870–1918)', *Criminocorpus, revue hypermédia* [Online], *Archives d'anthropologie criminelle* and related subjects, 3 [11 Oct. 2010] criminocorpus.revues.org/316; Watson, 'Malingerers, the "Weakminded" Criminal and the "Moral Imbecile"', pp. 227–31.
[37] RCGPP (1847) [818], p. 41.   [38] RCGPP (1846) [751], p. 25.
[39] TNA, PCOM 2/85, Pentonville Prison, Middlesex: Minute Books, 1845–46, 7 June 1845, pp. 5–6.

William Kent had staged his 'insincere' suicide attempt 'by suspending himself by means of his hammock girth, at a moment when he knew an officer was near his cell', a frequent ploy according to prison doctors. He was punished by confinement in the dark cell along with prisoner No. 683 who was given '3 days dark cell punishment diet, for refusing to work at his trade, & to go to bed at the appointed hour, & also for writing nonsense on his waste paper, his object being to create a belief that he is imbecile'.[40]

Such cases, recorded in the prison's minute books and journals, not only prompted debate and disputes, sometimes spread over several weeks or months, but in some instances remained unresolved. In October 1847 Joshua Craig (Convict No. 1166) was noted to be showing symptoms of excitement. While Assistant Chaplain John Burt, supported by the testimony of the schoolmaster, became increasingly convinced that Craig's insanity was genuine, Pentonville's medical officer, Dr Rees, did not share this view, suggesting that Craig 'puts on symptoms of incoherence and that he does not consider him the subject of mental disease in any form'.[41] In November Craig was placed in a dark cell, despite the chaplain's continuing concerns, which were rebuffed by Rees and the Prison Governor Robert Hoskins, who also believed that Craig was feigning. Rees concluded that Craig 'invents nonsense, said he was the Saviour, but considers he was not impressed with the idea, as his conduct & manner are not that of an insane person, but impertinent'. Finally in December 1847 Craig was removed to the *Justitia* prison hulk by order of the Secretary of State, the Governor and Rees still claiming that Craig was feigning insanity, and Rees certifying that he was 'free from mental affection'.[42] Craig's case, for Pentonville's officers, typified prisoners' 'unfitness' for the regime and the discipline of separation, their intrinsic weakness blamed on bad character or 'incorrigibility', and, like Craig, such prisoners were punished by confinement in the dark cell, by dietary restrictions or were beaten.[43]

Just as cases of mental disorder appeared rapidly after the opening of each new prison or as older prisons were adapted for the implementation of separate confinement, so too did allegations of feigning, in a

[40] Ibid., pp. 3–4.
[41] TNA, PCOM 2/353, Pentonville Prison, Middlesex: Chaplain's Journal, May 1846– Mar. 1851, 9, 11 and 15 Oct. 1847, pp. 83, 85; TNA, PCOM 2/87, Minute Books, 1847, 23 Oct. 1847, p. 74.
[42] TNA, PCOM 2/87, Minute Books, 1847, 6 Nov. 1847, p. 83, 22 Nov. 1847, pp. 92, 93, 18 Dec. 1847, pp. 111, 113 (emphasis in original).
[43] TNA, PCOM 2/85, Minute Books, 1845–46, 7 June 1845, pp. 3–4.

phenomenon that challenged both convict and local prisons. Dublin's Mountjoy Prison opened in 1850 and, as outlined in Chapter 2, adopted the Pentonville system of separate confinement with some modifications. In 1854 Medical Officer Francis Rynd reported a cluster of feigned suicide attempts, intermingled with cases of weak intellect, depression of spirits and debility of constitution, which pointed to many convicts' unfitness for the system of separate confinement.[44] Edmund Fitzmaurice was reported for a feigned attempt to commit suicide by cutting his throat 'very slightly' with a knife, and Rynd pronounced him 'quite well'. The Deputy Governor concluded that Fitzmaurice was trying to effect his removal from Mountjoy: 'his sentence is 6 years' servitude for highway robbery and violence and he came here with a bad character'.[45] For prisoners confined in Philipstown, an associated labour prison and invalid depot, feigners were accused of being workshy and trying to avoid the general discipline of the prison. Prisoner Michael Burke, who had been transferred from Dublin's Newgate Prison in 1855, was described in correspondence to the Directors of Convict Prisons as violent and dangerous, 'a furious maniac'.[46] Two days later, in a follow-up letter, the Philipstown Governor had changed his opinion regarding Burke's behaviour, which he now attributed to his bad character. Burke had 'assumed a recklessness approaching to insanity; but I only considered this as a trick to evade the regular work and routine discipline of the prison'. During his imprisonment at Philipstown, Burke had been in hospital four times for inflammation of the eye, 'for having worried himself into a fit in a passion when reported for fighting and disobedience', for a fever, and lastly for 'simulating insanity'.[47] However, two months later Medical Attendant Jeremiah Kelly reported that while Burke's general health was much improved, he was of 'unsound mind' and not fit to be kept in Philipstown. He needed constant watching, day and night, and Kelly recommended that he be removed to an institution specialising in the alleviation of mental disease.[48] The prison officers bemoaned the fact that Burke had been removed from Newgate as an 'invalid' and that the Newgate authorities had masked his bad character. As certificates were

---

[44] NAI, GPO/CORR/1854/Mountjoy/Item nos. 14–162.
[45] Ibid./Item no. 162, Letter from the Deputy Governor Mountjoy to the Director of Convict Prisons, 2 Dec. 1854.
[46] Ibid., 1855/Philipstown/Item no. 18, Letter from Governor to the Directors of Convict Prisons, 11 Jan. 1855.
[47] Ibid., 13 Jan. 1855.
[48] Ibid./Item no. 63, Letter from Jeremiah Kelly, Medical Attendant, to the Directors of Convict Prisons, 9 Mar. 1855.

drawn up to facilitate his removal to a lunatic asylum, it is hard to assess whether Burke was genuinely believed to be mentally ill or being removed because he was so disruptive, and whether his feigning attempt had succeeded or if the Philipstown prison officers were willing to go along with it to get rid of such a difficult prisoner.

At the old Liverpool Borough Gaol feigned suicide was largely associated with prisoners' efforts to avoid transportation or punishment, the Governor's journal recording one such case in July 1845 of a prisoner making two successive – and, in the Governor's view, feeble – attempts:

July 26. – J. B., 779, a prisoner who had been sentenced to 10 years' transportation, feigned an attempt to hang himself this afternoon by means of a band of oakum ... which he had fastened to one of the window bars. When found he was lying upon the floor apparently in a fit, and the band, which it was absurd to suppose would bear the weight of a man, broken ... I directed him to have a shower-bath immediately, which was administered to him by Jones, the surgeon's assistant.

A day later, the prisoner 'made another feint to hang himself', using a strip torn from his blanket. After fiercely resisting the shower-bath, the prison officers threw some water over him in the yard, and he was put in 'lunatic restraints'.[49] The Governor concluded

These attempts, or feigned attempts, at suicide on the part of this prisoner, it appears to me, are barefaced attempts at imposition, practised in order to excite commiseration, with a view to get off transportation. It would be absurd to suppose that he could have succeeded in his ostensible object by the means he used on either occasion.[50]

By 1855, Liverpool had a large new prison designed for separate confinement, transportation had been for the most part abandoned, and attempts to feign insanity were now attributed to efforts to seek mitigation of the new discipline, to avoid work or to secure removal to the asylum. In a visit to the recently opened prison, Inspector Herbert P. Voules reported that 'six ... prisoners' had 'feigned attempts to hang themselves, with a view to procure their removal from separate confinement'.[51] In Liverpool, those attempting suicide were handcuffed in long irons, placed on a 'reduced', punishment diet and secluded in a 'dark cell' subject to the approval and sometimes recommendation of the medical officer. In assessing such cases, prison medical officers carefully

[49] Report of the Inspectors of Prisons of Great Britain, Northern and Eastern District, 1845 [675], p. 91.
[50] Ibid.
[51] Report of the Inspectors of Prisons of Great Britain, Northern and Eastern District, 1857–58 [2373], p. 22.

noted the timing of suicide attempts, the proximity of the prison officers, and the prisoners' determination and resolve, evidence of their cunning and contrivance.

When Brixton Prison opened in 1853 and Mountjoy Female Prison in 1858, it was the volatility of women, their tendency to 'break out', that was commonly remarked upon.[52] This contrasted with male prisoners who were regarded as being more likely to feign insanity, inspired by a direct motive and typified by cunning, deceit and planning, though in practice male prisoners too were subject to breakouts and were frequent instigators of cell smashing. Male cases also provided the vast majority of examples of feigning in prison records, forensic textbooks and journal articles on the subject. However, like feigning, breaking out involved disruption of prison discipline, insubordination and oftentimes reflected the desire of the women to achieve an improvement in their conditions. Observing the conduct of women at Millbank Prison, part of the English female prison estate after 1816, Arthur Griffiths described how it was 'often difficult to draw the line between madness and outrageous conduct; and the latter is sometimes persisted in in order to make good a pretence of deranged intellect'. He added that cases of '"trying it on," or "doing the barmy," which are cant terms for feigning lunacy, used to be frequent, but diminished as long experiences protected prison doctors increasingly from deception'.[53] Despite Griffiths' claim, breaking out was a persistent phenomenon. Women might also join forces or share knowledge in presenting themselves as mentally weak, as noted by the Medical Officer of Castlebar Prison, county Mayo, in 1888: 'I have remarked for many years that a number of female prisoners committed from Ballina for Drunkenness or begging have apparently entered into a conspiracy to declare when they enter this Prison that they suffer from epileptic fits.' New admissions from the town were carefully watched and information collected from the local constabulary about the women's previous conduct.[54]

[52] See ch. 2 for the implementation and adaptation of separate confinement for women and their tendency to break out. See also Neil Davie, '"Business as Usual?" Britain's First Women's Convict Prison, Brixton 1853–1869', *Crimes and Misdemeanours*, 4:1 (2010), 37–52; Rachel Bennett, '"Bad for the Health of the Body, Worse for the Health of the Mind": Female Responses to Imprisonment in England, 1853–1869', *Social History of Medicine*, 34:2 (2021), 532–52; Beverly A. Smith, 'The Female Prisoner in Ireland, 1855–1878', *Federal Probation*, 54:4 (1990), 69–81, at p. 75.

[53] Arthur Griffiths, *Memorials of Millbank, and Chapters in Prison History* (London: Henry S. King & Co., 1875), p. 208.

[54] NAI, GPB/CORR/1888/Item no. 6679, Correspondence re epilepsy, malingering, Extract Medical Officer's Journal, Castlebar Prison, 13 June 1888.

Instances of breaking out frequently involved self-harm and attempts at self-destruction, as in the case of Bellina Prior, confined in Armagh Prison in 1888, who, when questioned as to why she had attempted to cut her throat with a piece of glass replied 'it was only a bit of fun'.[55] Dr David Nicolson, while working as Medical Officer at Woking Prison, referred more generally to 'doubtful attempts' at suicide – 'half real, half sham and mostly impulsive' – where the prisoner 'in some reckless way appears to seek self-destruction'. He concluded that these were most common in female convicts, 'many of whose senseless and impulsive acts have a periodicity, which serves to remove them from the category of actual pretences'.[56] He referred to one such female prisoner, showing signs of 'real despondency' who tried to strangle herself with her hand-kerchief, 'and told me that she did it because she was unable to read'.[57] Some women prisoners who attempted suicide or self-harmed were transferred to asylums, including a woman who had been held in Cork Prison where she repeatedly inserted pins and needles into her breast, doing herself 'most serious injury'.[58] A year later, after her transfer to the newly opened Mountjoy Female Prison, she was removed to Dundrum Criminal Lunatic Asylum.[59]

Though prison officials dreaded suicides for their impact on the dis-cipline of the prison and its management and because they resulted in extensive inquiries by the Prison Commissioners and Inspectors, reporting of what were concluded to be feigned suicides – as in the Liverpool example above – could take on an almost cavalier tone. Prison officers widely agreed that many suicide attempts were feigned; David Nicolson suggested the figure could be as high as three out of four.[60] In Pentonville in 1869, four feigned suicide attempts were dis-missed as efforts to excite sympathy or create alarm, 'and are undeserving of notice'; in Portland in the same year those feigning suicide had the aim, according to the governor, of evading labour or trying to get into the

---

[55] NAI, GPB/CORR/1888/Item no. 4991, Correspondence re Bellina Prior, HMP Armagh, Apr. 1888, Letter from J.A. Chippendale, Governor to Chairman of the GPB, 30 Apr. 1888.

[56] David Nicolson, 'Feigned Attempts at Suicide', *Journal of Mental Science*, 17:80 (Jan. 1872), 484–99, at p. 487.

[57] Ibid.

[58] Report of the Directors of Convict Prisons in Ireland (RDCPI), 1857 (1857–58) [2376], p. 118.

[59] RDCPI, 1858 (1859) [2531], p. 94.

[60] Nicolson, 'Feigned Attempts at Suicide', pp. 487–8. When working at Millbank Prison, Dr Gover calculated that in the three years ending in 1869 there had been 50 attempts at suicide. One was successful, 13 serious or doubtful and 36 feigned (cited by Nicolson).

infirmary.[61] Attempts by prisoners to strangle themselves with scraps of oakum or knotted handkerchiefs (the technique apparently most often used by women), or by 'scratches' to the throat, were mocked for the feebleness of their efforts. When a prisoner has decided to feign suicide, Nicolson observed, he then had to make some calculations, 'and as a rule he arranges that the performance shall be in full play when his cell-door is opened at one or other of the accustomed visits of the officer'.[62]

Prisoner James Slavin staged his suicide attempt in the water closet of Galway Prison, knowing, according to the prison officers, that other prisoners would be passing by, his object being to secure removal to a lunatic asylum.[63] At Mountjoy Prison feigned suicide attempts were particularly prevalent, constituting the most common form of feigning, and the prison's medical officers claimed that prisoners staged their suicide attempts to ensure timely discovery. Dr O'Keefe insisted one such prisoner who had succeeded in committing suicide was not of unsound mind but had feigned a suicide attempt expecting to be interrupted while O'Keefe was on his round of cell visitations. O'Keefe was delayed on this particular day and discovered the prisoner when he had been dead for ten minutes.[64] Other accidental deaths were attributed to miscalculations in timing or method. For the most part, Nicolson argued, 'convicts do not seek death ... their whole aim seems to lie in the direction of self-preservation, and to the same end point almost all their scheming devices and impostures'.[65] 'The feigner proportions his attempt to the amount of personal inconvenience and risk which he thinks he can stand, but takes good care generally not to hurt himself much.'[66] However, things could go wrong for the feigner; 'it is an awkward thing for anyone to try experiments with his neck in a noose; and it is not to be wondered at if now and again the impostor is caught in his own trap'.[67]

The detection of feigning placed an enormous strain in other ways on prison medical officers who were also dealing with cases of 'real' insanity and 'determined' attempts at suicide. At Limerick Prison among the prisoners who had been confirmed as insane or deemed to have made serious attempts at suicide in 1867, was prisoner M.M.G., under a two-year sentence, who was initially reported by Prison Inspector Dr John

---

[61] RDCP, 1869, Appendix, pp. 17, 98.
[62] Nicolson, 'Feigned Attempts at Suicide', p. 491.
[63] NAI, GPB/CORR/1891/Item no. 10985, Inquiry, by Joyce, 10 Oct. 1891, at Galway Prison into attempted suicide of James Slavin.
[64] Kimberley Commission (1878–79), Evidence of Dr O'Keefe, p. 877.
[65] Nicolson, 'Feigned Attempts at Suicide', p. 488.   [66] Ibid., p. 499.
[67] Ibid., p. 496.

Lentaigne as being excited but likely to be feigning insanity. This was confirmed in a note from the medical officer of the prison, who was of the opinion that 'he is a schemer'. Yet the man was later removed to the district asylum where he remained 'a confirmed lunatic'.[68]

I now refer to this case, because it illustrates a class of those sometimes met with in separate cellular prisons, especially among prisoners under long sentences of one and two years. In such prisons sometimes, without the greatest care and judicious treatment, the intellect and reason of the prisoner becomes affected, he loses his power of self-control, and a man is believed to be malingering who is passing through the stages of incipient insanity.[69]

Convict W.D. was also reckoned to be an 'imposter' when first admitted to Millbank in 1869. He was described as being sly and suspicious and showed a lack of consistency in his symptoms. The surgeon at Leeds Borough Gaol had, however, directed special attention to the case before he was moved to Millbank and he was placed under special observation. He was filthy in his habits, noisy and violent, and believed himself endowed with supernatural powers. It was eventually concluded that W.D. was suffering from 'impending dementia' and he was removed to Broadmoor.[70]

Prisoner Susan Fletcher, confined in Westminster Prison in 1881, asserted that while 'the cunning may deceive even a very clever physician ... the really sick and suffering may possibly ... be neglected' and real cases of mental illness might be missed by the medical officer. This was confirmed by prisoner B.2.15 [R.A. Castle] in his account of prison life, who noted that the passage of prisoners into a 'tragic mental state' could pass unnoticed by the chaplain and medical officers on their flying visits around the prison.[71] Despite his apparently cynical approach to suicide attempts, David Nicolson, his experience built up as Medical Officer at Woking, Portland, Millbank and Portsmouth prisons before he took up the post of Deputy Superintendent at Broadmoor in 1876, underlined the need for caution in prison practice: 'we have to be ever on our guard lest, on the one side, deception is being practised upon us; and lest, on the other, we be carried away, in our mistrust, to a hasty

[68] Report of the Inspectors General of Prisons in Ireland, 1869 (1870) [C.173], p. 400.
[69] Ibid., pp. 400–1.   [70] RDCP, 1869, Appendix, p. 51.
[71] Susan Willis Fletcher, *Twelve Months in an English Prison* (Boston, MA: Lee and Shephard; New York: Charles T. Dillingham, 1884), p. 330; B.2.15 [R.A. Castle], *Among the Broad-Arrow Men: A Plain Account of English Prison Life* (London: A. and C. Black, 1924), p. 164. For prisoners' accounts of mental illness, see Hilary Marland, '"Close Confinement Tells Very Much Upon a Man": Prisoner Memoirs, Insanity and the Late Nineteenth- and Early Twentieth-Century Prison', *Journal of the History of Medicine and Allied Sciences*, 74:3 (2019), 267–91.

treatment of real manifestations as being false and due to imposture'.[72] Similarly, James Murray, Assistant Medical Officer at Wakefield Prison, emphasised that

The medical officer has a double duty to perform in his official capacity, and has to keep an open unbiased mind on his daily rounds, and on each separate case, so that on the one hand a 'skulker' may not by his means escape his due punishment by feigning disease, and on the other hand that proper medical care and treatment may be granted to those who are really ill and require medical attention.[73]

The Lure of the Asylum and the Prison Doctor as Detective

The attempts of prisoner George Hamsley, whose case opened this chapter, to prompt his transfer to the promised utopia of the asylum would have come as little surprise to prison governors, medical officers and experts in legal medicine. Hamsley had a powerful motive, a vital clue in detecting feigners in prison. 'We do not meet with feigning in ordinary private practice', Dr G. Fielding Blandford, lecturer on psychological medicine at St George's Hospital, London, asserted, 'but if any of you become surgeon to a jail or to the army, you will not seldom be called to see malingerers who adopt this as a means of getting to comfortable asylum quarters, or obtaining a discharge from duty.'[74] Major Arthur Griffiths, appointed Deputy Governor of Millbank Prison in 1870, at a point when Millbank was functioning as a repository for lunatics from other prisons, noted that while 'ordinary people' had little to gain by being considered mad, for convicts this could greatly improve their conditions.[75]

A further benefit of removal to the asylum was the relative ease of escape or even release, facilities that prisoners who successfully orchestrated their relocation utilised effectively. The push to reduce escapes was one of the driving factors behind campaigns for the establishment of criminal lunatic asylums at Dundrum and Broadmoor, where security would be tighter than in county and district asylums.[76] After their establishment, however, Dundrum and

---

[72] David Nicolson, 'The Morbid Psychology of Criminals', *Journal of Mental Science*, 21:94 (July 1875), 225–50, at p. 242.

[73] James Murray, 'The Life History of a Malingering Criminal', *Journal of Mental Science*, 36:154 (July 1890), 347–54, at p. 347.

[74] G. Fielding Blandford, *Insanity and Its Treatment: Lectures on the Treatment, Medical and Legal of Insane Patients* (Edinburgh: Oliver and Boyd; London, Simpkin, Marshall, Hamilton, Kent, and Co., 1892), p. 443.

[75] Griffiths, *Memorials of Millbank*, p. 191.

[76] In 1846, for example, of the fifteen prisoners received from gaols into Clonmel District Lunatic Asylum, three attempted to escape. Report on the District, Local and Private

Broadmoor also regularly referred to escape attempts and successful escapes in their annual reports, notably in cases where feigning was suspected. In 1873 four inmates made attempted escapes from Broadmoor, all of whom were male convicts; one, who had been convicted of murder and his death sentence commuted to penal servitude, violently attacked a male attendant before escaping.[77] In order to reduce the incidence of escapes, in 1879 Irish Lunacy Inspectors John Nugent and George Hatchell, inspired by a similar scheme in Pennsylvania, proposed establishing a depot, specifically for the containment of prisoners 'attacked, while under confinement, with actual or pretended mania'. They had long felt that 'the simulation of madness exercises a baneful influence on prisoners, inducing them to attempt a similar course in the hope of removal to an asylum, where restraint being less, the chances of escape become greater'.[78] Such a measure was never implemented, and escapes continued to take place. In 1890, prisoner F.J. (formerly known as A.J.) was admitted for the third time to Dundrum. Noted to be 'a habitual criminal' and former soldier, who had been discharged from the army with heart disease, he was transferred from Maryborough Prison after being sentenced to seven years' penal servitude for housebreaking. 'A cunning, ill-disposed, malevolent criminal, insanity possibly counterfeited. He succeeded in effecting his escape from here in the year 1863, and made an unsuccessful attempt of a daring character in 1879.'[79]

Meanwhile in county and district asylums, prisoners transferred on the grounds of insanity continued to make their escapes. In England, some thirty-eight criminal lunatics escaped from county asylums and evaded recapture between 1856 and 1862, and sixty-nine between 1863 and 1878.[80] Rainhill Asylum, near Liverpool, recorded numerous escapes by prisoners transferred from prisons and Broadmoor or on remand. In March 1873 William Moore was transferred from Kirkdale Prison to Rainhill while awaiting trial for stealing lead. In June he escaped as the patients were coming out of church '& has not since been heard of'.[81] John Flanaghan

Lunatic Asylums in Ireland, 1846 (1847) [820], Appendix: Clonmel District Lunatic Asylum, p. 43.

[77] Wellcome Library, *Reports of the Superintendent and Chaplain of Broadmoor Criminal Lunatic Asylum, For the Year 1873* (1874), Superintendent's Report (W. Orange), p. 5.

[78] Report on the District, Criminal and Private Lunatic Asylums in Ireland, 1879 (1878–79) [C.2346], Central Criminal, or Dundrum Asylum, p. 15.

[79] Report on the District, Criminal and Private Lunatic Asylums in Ireland, 1890 (1890) [C.6148], Appendix G: Central Asylum Dundrum: Report of the Resident Physician [Isaac Ashe], p. 118 (no. 796).

[80] Report of the Commission to Inquire into the Subject of Criminal Lunacy (1882) [C.3418], Appendix 12, p. 143.

[81] Liverpool Record Office (LRO), M614 RAI/11/5, Rainhill Asylum Male Casebook, May 1870–Dec. 1873, p. 211.

was brought in June 1874 to Rainhill by Kirkgate Prison's jailor prior to his trial for burglary. It was noted that he had been in and out of gaol since 1853. Flanaghan first escaped in September and was picked up in Blackburn selling a stolen pair of trousers, and again in December, when he was found asleep at the roadside. He was reported to be constantly fighting with the other patients and was finally removed to Broadmoor in January 1876.[82] In 1881 the Superintendent of Somersetshire County Asylum referred to the case of a military prisoner brought from Taunton Gaol, who he suspected of malingering. The prisoner was removed to the infirmary, 'and in a very short time it was reported to me that this man when he went out used to call in at public-houses'. When the prisoner was told that it was against the rules, he escaped 'and put it into the heads of others to endeavour to escape. Altogether I had a great deal of trouble with that man.'[83]

Dr Alex Robertson, Physician to the City Parochial Asylum and Hospital in Glasgow, who had extensive experience of receiving prisoners suspected of feigning, suggested that once in the asylum such individuals might then be able to negotiate release, 'if after maintaining his deceit for such a period as would allay suspicion, he should seem to his guardians to have become gradually restored to reason'.[84] One such case was that of convict Ball, convicted of robbery in 1851 and sentenced to transportation. Following removal to Millbank Prison, Ball convinced the prison medical officer that he was insane, and was transferred to Bethlem. He remained in Bethlem for two years before receiving a ticket-of-leave. Five years later the same prisoner was convicted of housebreaking, and, following his trial and committal, again simulated madness. Though his deception was revealed by another prisoner just before his removal to an asylum, by that time he had convinced three visiting justices and two medical men of his insanity.[85]

Many prisoners accused of feigning insanity had complex careers of crime, imprisonment and asylum care. In 1864 the Governor of Wexford Gaol wrote to the Lunacy Inspectors inquiring into the case of Bridget McGrath, who had been transferred as a lunatic from Mountjoy Female Convict Prison to Dundrum in April 1863 and who had subsequently

---

[82] LRO, M614 RAI/11/6, Rainhill Asylum Male Casebook, Dec. 1873–July 1877, p. 58; Lancashire Archives, QAM 4/2, Register of Class 1 Lunatics, Covering Admissions 4 Feb. 1869–15 Feb. 1893, p. 111.

[83] Commission on Criminal Lunacy (1882), Evidence of Charles W.C.M. Medlicott, 18 Mar. 1881, pp. 72, 74.

[84] Alex Robertson, 'Case of Feigned Insanity', *Journal of Mental Science*, 29:125 (Apr. 1883), 81–5, at p. 85.

[85] Alfred Swaine Taylor (the late), *The Principles and Practice of Medical Jurisprudence*, 6th edn (London: J. & A. Churchill, 1910), vol. 2, p. 901; Anon., 'Feigned Insanity', *Chambers's Journal*, 20:1034 (20 Oct. 1883), 657–9, at p. 658.

escaped. She had been rearrested and was being tried for stealing, and the Governor requested information to ascertain whether she was considered recovered and sane, and thus fit to be recommitted under a sentence of penal servitude, or still to be dealt with as a lunatic.[86] Alfred Jones, who also went under the aliases of Edward Bowler and Thomas Browne, was transferred from Spike Island Prison to Dundrum on 26 August 1863 after being certified insane. Several weeks later he escaped. In May 1865 he was found in Cork County Gaol on a new charge of burglary and robbery and sentenced in July to ten years' penal servitude, before escaping from the local bridewell the day after his conviction. In September when Jones reappeared under a new sentence in Mountjoy Prison, the medical officer concluded that he was weak-minded.[87]

The detection of feigning among offenders became as much a preoccupation for the staff of asylums as for prison medical officers. In 1864 the relative calm of Broadmoor Asylum was broken by two inmates, who had been removed from Millbank Prison and who were being held in seclusion. They were reported to be causing a serious disturbance and to be extremely noisy. Broadmoor's Superintendent, Dr Meyer, 'much doubted their insanity' and they were quickly removed with an order of the Secretary of State back to Millbank.[88] Keen to keep the admission of the convict class to a minimum, efforts were made to reveal instances of malingering quickly at Dundrum Asylum and to send such cases back to prison. It was anticipated that removals from prisons were very likely to include cases of 'reputed insanity', given that Dundrum's existence and 'mode of life in it' was well known to convicts.[89] At Castlebar Asylum two cases of 'feigned insanity' were admitted from the county gaol in 1872, but on admission were told that they were not insane and must complete the full term of their five-month imprisonment. The two men determined on a sham attempt at suicide, believing it would ensure a short stay in the asylum and then a free discharge. One of them slashed

[86] NAI, GPO/Letter Books (LB), Vol. 20, Jan. 1863–Dec. 1864, Letter no. 808, Patrick Murray to Inspector of Lunatic Asylums, Dublin Castle, 19 Mar. 1864.
[87] NAI, GPO/LB, Vol. 7, Jan. 1865–Dec. 1867, Letter no. 156, 11 Aug. 1865, Case of Convict Alfred Jones (in Wexford Gaol) for instructions as to his disposal; NAI, GPO/LB, Vol. 21, Jan. 1865–Dec. 1866, Letter no. 262, P.J. Murray to Dr Corbett, Dundrum, 29 May 1865, Letter no. 502, unknown to Inspectors, Lunatic Asylums, 14 Sept. 1865.
[88] Report of Commissioners in Lunacy on the Present Condition of Broadmoor Criminal Lunatic Asylum and its Inmates (1864) [216], p. 2.
[89] Report on the District, Criminal and Private Asylums in Ireland, 1862 (1862) [2975], Central Asylum Dundrum, p. 28; Report on the District, Criminal and Private Asylums in Ireland (1873), Central Asylum Dundrum, p. 28.

his throat, resulting in a bloody but harmless incision; the other resorted to a mock strangulation. Both were declared to be irredeemable drunkards, and one had been convicted forty-seven times. 'After a residence of a month', the medical officer declared, he 'got rid of two of the most accomplished schemers I ever met with.'[90] In many instances feigning was attempted on more than one occasion. In 1886, while undergoing his sentence in Downpatrick Gaol, labourer W.M., serving five years for arson, was stated to be delusional, believing his food was poisoned and that everyone was watching him, and he was moved to Dundrum. There he was declared sane and returned to prison. On his return to prison he violently assaulted the warders who were escorting him, and 'so successfully feigned insanity that he again imposed on the authorities of the gaol' and was returned to Dundrum, where he confessed that 'he had again feigned insanity for the purpose of obtaining the greater freedom and indulgence accorded here'.[91]

Some of those feigning mental illness, however, found the asylum to be a challenging environment, despite the better conditions, and requested transfers back to prison. At Dundrum it was reported that malingerers were subdued by being made 'special objects of suspicion and vigilance' and as a result sought a return to penal servitude.[92] In other cases they objected to association with lunatics: 'The malingerer after a time gets tired of his condition, the conversation and the monotonous language of his associates.'[93] It was reported that many of those certified insane quickly became amenable and even useful after removal to Dundrum. They remonstrated against association with lunatics, and demanded to be returned to gaol, also aware that they were losing their modest payments for labour when remaining in Dundrum.[94]

Many cases of suspected feigning were reckoned to be particularly perplexing, even after extensive investigations. In 1858 distinguished psychiatrists John Charles Bucknill and Daniel Hack Tuke selected two local cases – both men lived in Devon at this point – to include in their *Manual of Psychological Medicine*, the first comprehensive textbook on

---

[90] Report on the District, Criminal and Private Asylums in Ireland, 1872 (1872) [C.647], Gaols, p. 14.
[91] Report on the District, Criminal and Private Asylums in Ireland; with Appendices, 1887 (1887) [C.5121], Central Asylum Dundrum, p. 138.
[92] Report on the District, Criminal and Private Asylums in Ireland; with Appendices (1873), Central Asylum Dundrum, pp. 15–16.
[93] Report on the District, Criminal and Private Asylums in Ireland; with Appendices, 1875 (1875) [C.1293], Central Asylum Dundrum, p. 22.
[94] Report on the District, Criminal and Private Asylums in Ireland; with Appendices, 1888 (1888) [C.5459], Central Asylum Dundrum, p. 30. For more on transfers between prisons and Dundrum, see ch. 4.

insanity.[95] Prisoner Warren, convicted at Devon Assizes and sentenced to fourteen years' transportation, had been declared insane after three months in gaol and removed to Devon County Asylum, where Bucknill was Medical Superintendent. Eight months later he was returned as recovered to prison, but within an hour of his readmission was 'apparently affected with a relapse of his mental disease'. He refused to answer questions, walked to and fro in his cell, muttering to himself and sometimes howling, refused food for days together, beat the door of his cell and turned his bedclothes over constantly. Though a dunking in a near-scalding bath, authorised by the prison governor, was claimed to cure him of his dirty habits, for two years he maintained all other symptoms of insanity. Then, suddenly, Bucknill and Tuke reported, his resolution weakened, and he requested removal to the government depot for convicts in preparation for transportation. 'In this remarkable case, the perseverance of the simulator, his refusal to converse, or to answer questions, and the general truthfulness of his representation, made it most difficult to arrive at a decisive opinion.'[96]

The second persistent example of feigning noted by Bucknill and Tuke was that of John Jakes, convicted in 1855 of 'pocket-picking' at Devon Easter Sessions and sentenced to four years' penal servitude. On hearing the sentence, Jakes was reported to have fallen down in the dock, as if in fit of apoplexy, and when removed to gaol it was concluded that he was hemiplegic and apparently demented, though his filthy behaviour and consumption of his own excrement raised doubts about whether his case was genuine. His insanity was, however, certified by the surgeon of the gaol and a second medical man, and he was moved to the asylum. The convicting magistrates, who were familiar with the prisoner's character and track record, were convinced he was feigning. Bucknill and Tuke were brought in and carefully examined Jakes. In their opinion, he had all the symptoms of hemiplegia:

if they were feigned, the representation was a consummate piece of acting, founded upon accurate observation. In the asylum, the patient was ... apparently demented. He had to be fed, to be dressed, to be undressed, and to be led from place to place; he could not be made to speak; he slept well.[97]

[95] For Bucknill, see Andrew Scull, Charlotte MacKenzie and Nicholas Hervey, *Masters of Bedlam: The Transformation of the Mad-Doctoring Trade* (Princeton, NJ: Princeton University Press, 1996), ch. 7, and for Daniel Hack Tuke, see Anne Digby, 'Tuke, Daniel Hack (1827–95)', *DNB*, https://doi.org/10.1093/ref:odnb/27804 [accessed 7 May 2020].

[96] John Charles Bucknill and Daniel Hack Tuke, *A Manual of Psychological Medicine Containing the History, Nosology, Description, Statistics, Diagnosis, Pathology, and Treatment of Insanity, with an Appendix of Cases*, 2nd edn (London: John Churchill, 1862), pp. 374–5.

[97] Ibid., pp. 375–6. Hemiplegia is a condition caused by a brain injury that results in weakness, stiffness and lack of control in one side of the body.

Then on 17 August Jakes escaped, confirming for the magistrates that their conclusions had been correct and that several medical men had been deceived. Jakes converted the handle of his tin cup into a false key, unlocked a window guard, escaped at night into the garden and then scaled a high door and wall. He was never heard of again. Even then, however, Bucknill and Tuke posed the question of whether Jakes could have deceived medical men forewarned of deception or if, as an accomplished housebreaker, 'that things impossible to other lunatics might have been accomplished by him'.[98]

As in the examples of Warren and Jakes, expert opinion was sought in cases of feigning, by and large from psychiatrists working outside of prisons. This certainly occurred from time to time in Pentonville, as in 1847 when Drs Edward Thomas Monro and John Conolly, two of London's foremost alienists and medical witnesses, and respectively physicians at Bethlem and Hanwell asylums, examined Convict H. Jones, 'declining to give any certificate of insanity without further evidence, but recommended a continuance of care and watching'.[99] Ireland's longest-serving Lunacy Inspector of the nineteenth century, Dr George Hatchell, was brought into several prisons to adjudicate on individual cases of feigned insanity and to assess 'batches' of prisoners to help staff differentiate between those feigning insanity, the weak-minded and the truly insane.[100] Such practices can be interpreted in different ways. They can be taken as signifying professional collaboration and exchanges of expert views on psychiatric matters, an area where up until the late nineteenth century few prison medical officers claimed much in the way of special training. But potentially they undermined prison medical officers' claims of expert knowledge in the detection of feigning acquired through long experience of working with prisoners.[101] A number of alienists explicitly urged prison medical officers to rely on

---

[98] Ibid., p. 376.

[99] TNA, PCOM 2/86, Minute Books, 1846, Medical Officer's Journal, 19 June 1847, p. 304. (The entry dates do not align consistently with the dates of the minute books.)

[100] NAI, GPO/CORR/1860/ Mountjoy (Male) Prison, Item no. 6, Letter from Robert Netterville, Governor Mountjoy to Directors, Convict Prisons, 30 Dec. 1859; NAI, GPO/CORR/1872/Government/Item no. 484/11, Letter from Under Secretary to Spike Island, 11 Jan. 1872; /Item no. 1084/48, Letter from Under Secretary to Spike Island, 3 Feb. 1872; /Item no. 1084/56, Letter from Under Secretary to Spike Island, 17 Feb. 1872.

[101] John Campbell at Woking was keen to explain in his evidence to the Kimberley Commission that he had only once asked for the advice of the medical superintendent of the neighbouring Brookwood Asylum in the case of two men who he believed to be sane: Kimberley Commission (1878–79), Evidence of Dr John Campbell, 2 July 1878, p. 573.

them in diagnosing convicts.[102] They pointed out that prison medical officers did not have the time to carry out detailed and prolonged examinations of criminals suspected of feigning, and, responsible as they were to the government and prison authorities, the public, and prisoners and their families and associates, it was suggested that they might occasionally err 'in the prisoners' favour'.[103] Jade Shepherd has argued that by the late nineteenth century Broadmoor's medical officers and superintendents had stricter standards in diagnosing insanity than prison medical officers and were keen to return convicts back to prison. Meanwhile, as attitudes towards them hardened, some prisoners were disappointed about their treatment at Broadmoor, and quickly confessed their imposture.[104] In 1868 the Lunacy Commissioners commented on the grim conditions at Broadmoor, its prison-like appearance and the cheerlessness of its wards, the lack of opportunity to work and particularly to the confinement of dangerous and violent inmates in seclusion in cells or even cages (with several convict prisoners reportedly held in cages in that year), conditions unlikely to recommend themselves to prisoners feigning insanity.[105]

The observation cell, as Stephen Watson has pointed out, was to become an important tool in the detection of malingerers in prison. These were modified cells, sometimes with an iron railing instead of a door, or extra spy holes, and often padded or lined with thick rope. They came into increasing use after the 1880s across England and Ireland when magistrates began to send cases to prison on remand to confirm their mental state.[106] A series of checks was also put in place before prisoners were removed to asylums, and, while alienists might have argued that prison doctors did not devote enough time to their

---

[102] Conolly Norman, 'Feigned Insanity', in Daniel Hack Tuke (ed.), *A Dictionary of Psychological Medicine: Giving the Definition, Etymology and Synonyms of the Terms Used in Medical Psychology with the Symptoms, Treatment, and Pathology of Insanity and the Law of Lunacy in Great Britain and Ireland* (London: J. & A. Churchill, 1892), pp. 502–5.

[103] John Charles Bucknill and Daniel Hack Tuke, *A Manual of Psychological Medicine: Containing the Lunacy Laws, the Nosology, Aetiology, Statistics, Description, Diagnosis, Pathology, and Treatment of Insanity: with an appendix of cases*, 4th edn (London: J. & A. Churchill, 1879), p. 469; Anon., 'The Medical Department of the Convict Service', p. 18.

[104] Shepherd, 'Feigning Insanity', pp. 22–3.

[105] Copy of a Report Made by the Commissioners of Lunacy, on the 14th October 1868 upon Broadmoor Criminal Lunatic Asylum (1868–69) [244], pp. 2–5.

[106] Watson, 'Malingerers, the "Weakminded" Criminal and the "Moral Imbecile"', p. 228. For example, a padded cell was installed at Kilmainham Gaol in 1885. NAI, GPB/CORR/1885/Item no. 7489. See ch. 4 for assessments of remand prisoners by prison surgeons and medical witnesses.

investigations, prison medical officers would assert that the checks were both lengthy and rigorous. In Irish prisons it was common when there was uncertainty about a prisoner's mental state to place them under observation in the padded cells that were specially installed from the 1880s onwards.[107] This provided the opportunity to distinguish between the 'mannerisms' of the 'imposter' and 'insane person', and 'the facilities afforded for prolonged observation ... away from the main block ... help towards a settlement as to the proper mode of disposal'.[108] By the late 1870s prisoners believed to be insane in the English prison system were removed to Millbank, where observation cells had been used routinely after the 1860s. At Millbank prisoners were kept in association, but only after they were thoroughly checked and found to be cases of 'genuine insanity'. Dr Gover concluded, 'It is very inadvisable to avoid placing an imposter in association, for that is the very object which he has in view.' However, it was estimated that two-thirds of prisoners sent to Millbank with suspected mental disorders were 'actually insane'.[109] In that case, they were transferred to the lunatic wing at Woking Invalid Prison. However, even before they reached Millbank, prisoners would have been checked to ensure that they were genuine cases. In Pentonville this involved being placed in the observation cell, where they were kept until the medical officer was satisfied that they were not simulating insanity.[110] Campbell asserted his confidence in evidence presented to the Kimberley Commission in 1878 in the rigorous procedures that ensured that few imposters reached Woking, as the prisoners were under observation at other prisons for a considerable time 'by men of a good deal of experience'. However, in the book reflecting on his career that was published a few years later, he devoted an entire chapter to the subject of malingering at Woking, 'by impostors of the most determined description'.[111] Campbell also reported that numerous prisoners sent with bodily ailments to Woking evinced impairment of the mental faculties, and many of these were also suspected of feigning, particularly the younger men,

---

[107] NAI, GPB/CORR/1888/Item no. 1365, Papers relating to padded cell, Castlebar Prison; NAI, GPB/CORR/1886/Item no. 7036, Documents referring to the restraint of prisoner William Steele at Londonderry Prison, May 1886; NAI, GPB/CORR/1887/ Item no. 13757, Papers relating to the removal of Prisoner Julia Hourihan to Cork Lunatic Asylum from HM Female Prison Cork, 1887.

[108] NAI, CSORP/1905/12904, Minute from Geo. Plunkett O'Farrell and E.M. Courtney, Office of Inspectors of Lunatics, to Under Secretary 10 June 1904, p. 15.

[109] Kimberley Commission (1878–79), Evidence of Captain W.T. Harvey and R.M. Gover, pp. 71, 129.

[110] Ibid., Evidence of V.C. Clarke, p. 141.

[111] Ibid., Evidence of Dr John Campbell, p. 573; Campbell, *Thirty Years*, ch. V, at p. 65.

though others were found to be genuine cases and removed to asylums after a period of observation in the infirmary.[112]

It was agreed by prison doctors and alienists alike that prisoners would work hard to 'act' the lunatic, and to overcome the various obstacles to successful transfers out of the prison system. How good they were at this and how good doctors were in detecting them was open to different interpretations. The high quality of such performances was noted in a number of prison memoirs. One prisoner suggested that it was difficult for doctors to assess cases of malingering, 'for many old convicts are such accomplished actors they are able to imitate the peculiarities of idiocy with wonderful correctness, until the habit becomes second nature'.[113] However, an increasingly expansive literature on forensic psychiatry suggested that feigners were relatively easy to uncover (aside from such exceptional cases as described by Bucknill and Tuke). Blandford described most feigners as 'clumsy performers' and 'doubtless they who have the insane ever before their eyes will most readily detect the sham disorder'.[114] 'There are', he went on, 'cases on record where skilful cheats have deceived for a long period even alienist physicians, but such are rare.'[115] Feigned insanity was 'overacted in outrageousness and absurdity of conduct', usually by 'ignorant and vulgar persons'; 'the person generally talks a quantity of bosh from ignorance of the true characteristics of the disease which the skilled medical man have never heard a really insane person indulge in'.[116] Presentations of feigned insanity, according to the *Lancet*, 'usually resemble the popular stage idea of insanity rather than the true products of mental alienation. It is not uncommon for the malingerer to combine two forms of insanity and this may be of value in detection.'[117] Alongside over-acting, one clue to watch for was that the malingerer would eventually tire himself out and go to sleep, while a genuine lunatic would be unable to rest. In a lecture course on mental illness directed at general practitioners that was likely to have attracted future prison medical officers, Conolly Norman pointed to the difficulties of pretending incoherence, 'a characteristic of the maniacal state.... It used not be uncommon for persons feigning insanity to feign acute mania. Although apparently easy nothing is more difficult

[112] RDCP, 1863, Appendix, Woking Prison, p. 263.
[113] W.B.N., *Penal Servitude* (London: William Heinemann, 1903), p. 150.
[114] Blandford, *Insanity and its Treatment*, p. 442.   [115] Ibid., p. 448.
[116] Bucknill and Tuke, *A Manual of Psychological Medicine*, 2nd edn, pp. 370, 372; Lyttelton S. Winslow, *Manual of Lunacy: A Handbook Relating to the Legal Care and Treatment of the Insane*, with a preface by Forbes Winslow (London: Smith, Elder & Co., 1874), p. 295.
[117] Anon., 'Malingery', p. 46.

to feign than incoherence.'[118] L. Forbes Winslow described how the feigner would exaggerate his symptoms, especially when he believed he was being watched; he would also be distinguished by the absence of bodily symptoms present in true lunatics – disordered digestion, headache, sleeplessness – and the desire of the truly insane to appear intelligible and to mask their mental disorder.[119]

Whereas alienists and forensic experts claimed that prisoners were bad actors, easily unmasked by those who were used to working with lunatics, prison medical officers were likely to suggest that prisoners were not only determined but also rather good actors, and that the prison medical officer was uniquely placed to act as detective and differentiate between real cases of insanity and attempts to feign. 'Only the lynx-eyed prison medical officer, backed by long experience', declared Major Griffiths, 'sooner or later detects the flaw.'[120] Dr McDonnell at Mountjoy reported that convict David Simmons (no. 5192) was one of the most 'obstinate malingerers that has ever come before me'. He had injured himself severely on two occasions, first 'by scratching with his nails some spots of psoriasis scattered over his body', and second by 'scraping some marks tattooed upon his arm so as to produce extensive ulceration of it'. He subsequently confessed his feigning to McDonnell and the prison officers, but McDonnell was afterwards 'informed that he has lately again assumed the manners of a maniac but in my presence he has not since his readmission to this prison played the lunatic'.[121] By the late nineteenth century the detection of malingerers was deemed so important by prison doctors that, according to Stephen Watson, it was 'invariably mentioned in pleas for better pay and conditions of service'.[122]

Even so detection in some cases was not straightforward. 'There is a method in all madness,' declared barrister J.H. Balfour-Browne:

The very close observation of mental disease by one of a sufficiently powerful intellect thoroughly to understand and appreciate its manifestations, might lead to such a deceptive reproduction of a number of symptoms as to puzzle many

---

[118] Royal College of Physicians of Ireland, Heritage Centre, Conolly Norman Lectures, 1905–07, CN/1, First Series, Mar.–May 1905, Lecture, 'The Maniacal State', 3 Mar. 1905. Irish medical practitioners tended to draw on and publish in English textbooks and forensic literature during the late nineteenth and early twentieth centuries, though notably Norman wrote the entry on feigned insanity in Tuke's 1892 *Dictionary of Psychological Medicine*.

[119] L. Forbes Winslow, *Mad Humanity: Its Forms Apparent and Obscure* (London: C.A. Pearson, 1898), pp. 80–1.

[120] Griffiths, *Memorials of Millbank*, p. 191.

[121] NAI, GPO/CORR/1860/Mountjoy (Male) Prison/Item no. 47, Correspondence from Robert Netterville, Governor Mountjoy to Directors of Convict Prisons, 15 Feb. 1860.

[122] Watson, 'Malingerers, the "Weakminded" Criminal and the "Moral Imbecile"', p. 227.

individuals, not trained to distinguish between very fine shades of expression, as indicative of varying springs of action.[123]

Balfour-Browne went on to explain that a physician well acquainted with mental disease would be hard to deceive. Yet even though prisoners would not on the whole be regarded as in any way in possession of a powerful intellect, they still were able to produce doubt in the minds of many prison medical officers. Dr John Campbell described the 'consequent trouble, anxiety, and responsibility devolving on the medical officer which cannot be well realized by those who have not experienced them'. While acknowledging that cases of feigning were also found in the military and naval services, Campbell noted that among convicts 'the imposition is carried out with almost incredible determination'.[124] This added to the strain of working with the many prisoners admitted to the lunatic division at Woking Invalid Prison who were 'of a doubtful character, and took the most active part in the violent, outrageous, and disgusting acts which were for a time of rather frequent occurrence' and made feigned attempts at suicide.[125] Many prisoners also expressed 'great disappointment' at being brought to Woking rather than a lunatic asylum.[126]

Mad, Bad and the Benefits of Diagnosis

Describing his tenure at Mountjoy between 1857 and 1867, McDonnell claimed that he had to deal with 'a good many cases' of feigning, but also asserted that under his management and with close observation of individuals, there were far fewer incidences.[127] Similarly, in 1870, Dr E.S. Blaker, medical officer at Portland Prison, declared that feigning insanity had wonderfully decreased, 'and I am sincerely glad to be able to say so, as it demands in the detection an exercise of great care and judgement, and it is often a long time before the mind can be fully satisfied as to the real or feigned aspect of the case'.[128] Given the wealth of evidence in terms of the attention paid to malingering in medical and forensic literature and official reports and inquiries during the last quarter of the century, as well as the number of cases noted in prison and asylum records – including McDonnell and Blaker's own prisons – their confidence appears to have been misplaced. However, Blaker also went on to

---

[123] J.H. Balfour-Browne, 'Feigned Insanity', *Medical Press and Circular*, 10 (19 Oct. and 2 Nov. 1870), 301–5, 345–7, at p. 345.
[124] Campbell, *Thirty Years*, p. 70.   [125] Ibid., p. 100.   [126] Ibid., p. 87.
[127] Kimberley Commission (1878–79), Evidence of Robert McDonnell, p. 459.
[128] RDCP, 1869, Appendix, p. 145.

suggest that feigning presented an interesting abstract question for psychologists:

whether a man who can simulate insanity is really at the time perfectly *mens sana in corpore sano*.... Insanity and crime are, I have no doubt, often very closely allied, and we may hope that psychological science will at some future time be able clearly to define a line of demarcation.[129]

This demarcation line, the question of what came to divide insanity and sane behaviour, madness and badness, and indeed the issue of whether feigning itself was a form of mental disorder preoccupied prison medicine in the latter part of the century. Indeed optimism about the decline in feigning might indicate that feigning had been absorbed into broader taxonomies of criminality and madness, with madness and badness 'so intermingled that observers cannot determine which it is that regulates their conduct'.[130]

By the 1860s and 1870s, as seen in Chapter 3, prison regimes had become harsher with emphasis on punishment rather than reform. A cluster of prison acts were directed towards the centralisation of the prison system, making conditions and discipline as uniform as possible. These acts also provided for the weekly regular inspection of all prisoners, which, as Martin Wiener has pointed out, gave the doctor the power to declare a prisoner fit or unfit, mentally or physically, and thus remove him from ordinary prison discipline and from the category of 'responsible moral agent'.[131] As doctors' powers apparently increased, they had the potential to be at odds with the prison administration, yet many, though not all, supported the imposition of rigorous and harsh discipline and in particular cast doubt on prisoners showing signs of insanity or mental weakness. In the shift from a reformist approach to more penal regimes prison officers remained on high alert for instances of shamming, even though the objectives of prison discipline had shifted. Whereas malingering was once seen as an affront to the system of separate confinement and obstacle to reform, it was now interpreted increasingly as the efforts of the workshy and crafty to evade the tough discipline of the prison. One observer noted in 1863 that doctors feared the risk of being deceived and 'many really mad are regarded with suspicion ... and are treated like the rest of the prisoners if their conduct be not too glaringly outrageous'.[132]

---

[129] Ibid.   [130] Blandford, *Insanity and its Treatment*, p. 446.
[131] Martin J. Wiener, *Reconstructing the Criminal: Culture, Law, and Policy in England, 1830–1914* (Cambridge: Cambridge University Press, 1990), p. 122.
[132] [Frederick Robinson], *Female Life in Prison*, vol. I (London: Hurst & Blackett, 1863), p. 239. Cited Wiener, *Reconstructing the Criminal*, pp. 125–6.

The precise, skilful and protracted process of reaching an assessment on feigning emphasised in the medical literature could also break down into practices involving cruelty and forced confessions. The evidence of the 1878–79 Kimberley Commission, particularly of ex-convict Harcourt and Medical Officer Francis Askham, as well as testimony given by Dr Patrick O'Keefe at Spike Island, demonstrated that medical officers could react brutally to what they concluded was persistent malingering. O'Keefe reported to the Commission that prior to his appointment at Spike the prisoners might have taken advantage of the medical officers' inexperience and frequently reported sick. This came to an abrupt halt following the appointment of O'Keefe, whose response to the feigning of pains and sickness was to apply the galvanic battery to give 'light electric shocks, and it had the effect of curing them'.[133] O'Keefe also described a prisoner who had committed suicide disparagingly as 'rather of a low type'. The man had claimed to have a skin eruption that was caused by self-inflicted scratching, but, according to O'Keefe, was not of unsound mind.[134] At Dartmoor, Harcourt was kept by Askham, who regarded him as a malingerer, for extended periods on a bread and water diet and 'treated' with a galvanic battery. Harcourt was also, he claimed, subjected to brutal treatment at Portland, where Askham was again his medical officer, following an accident.[135] While Askham claimed that he did not use the galvanic battery to detect malingering, after applying it to treat Harcourt's loss of muscular power and nervous energy, he concluded that he was indeed 'a malingerer'.[136] Askham was also accused of applying blisters and of excessive use of restraint in irons in cases where prisoners were showing symptoms of mental disorder.[137] He denied that prison caused a deterioration in prisoners' mental condition and when asked if persons might become mad owing to the treatment – one convict had claimed that prisoners were strapped down, provoked into madness, and then punished – Askham replied, 'It is utterly impossible. No such thing could possibly take place.'[138] Michael Davitt described in his prison memoirs of 1885, based on his experiences of Millbank, Dartmoor and Portsmouth prisons, how prisoners wounded themselves, smashed their cells or covered themselves in their own filth

---

[133] Kimberley Commission (1878–79), Evidence of Patrick O'Keefe, p. 875.
[134] Ibid., pp. 875–6.
[135] Ibid., Evidence of H.F. Askham, pp. 726–31. See also Anne Hardy, 'Development of the Prison Medical Service, 1774–1895', in Richard Creese, W.F. Bynum and J. Bearn (eds), *The Health of Prisoners* (Amsterdam and Atlanta, GA: Rodopi, 1995), 59–82, at p. 76.
[136] Kimberley Commission (1878–79), Evidence of H.F. Askham, p. 727.
[137] Ibid., pp. 733, 737.   [138] Ibid., p. 742.

in order to feign insanity, or to 'put on the barmy stick', though would-be feigners of insanity would be put under special surveillance, 'which made it well neigh impossible for an imposter to deceive his warders for any length of time'. He also referred to the practice in one prison of prisoners suspected of feigning insanity being fed their own excrement in the dinner-tin; those who ate it were declared insane.[139]

Punishment was meted out to many suspected feigners, and, alongside observation, became part of the process of reaching a decision on whether insanity was true or shammed; whipping was also recommended by some prison medical officers as a remedy for feigning. Provision was made in the 1877 Prison Acts in England and Ireland for prison medical officers 'to apply any painful test to a prisoner to detect malingering or otherwise', with the authority of an order from the visiting committee of justices or a member of the Prison Commissioners in England and General Prisons Board in Ireland.[140] According to Dr James Murray at Wakefield Prison, flogging was not only an important tool in the detection of feigned diseases, but also a potential cure.[141] The regime at Liverpool Borough Gaol appears to have been particularly harsh, its medical officer very willing to impose discipline. In June 1891 James Bibby was charged with refusing the wheel [treadwheel] and of violence towards a prison officer. The prisoner claimed to have had sunstroke and to feel giddy and noted that he was unable to control his temper. Dr Hammond was satisfied that the prisoner was feigning insanity in a very clumsy way, and he was punished with twenty-four strokes of the birch rod.[142]

In 1894 prisoner Frank O'Brien was charged with misbehaviour and feigning insanity and refused to speak. The prison officers expressed the unanimous opinion that he was shaming insanity. One warder described how on 13 June:

I went into the cell of the prisoner and found him standing on the table he had taken a sheet and tied it to the bar of a window and had tied it round his neck. He saw me and I sent out to call assistance and as I did so he kicked the table away from under him and as I re entered the cell with assistance I found him swinging by his neck.

---

[139] Michael Davitt, *Leaves from a Prison Diary; Or, Lectures to a 'Solitary' Audience* (London: Chapman and Hall, 1885), reprinted with introduction by T.W. Moody (Shannon: Irish University Press, 1972), vol. 1, pp. 144–5, 142–3.

[140] 36&37 Vict., c.49, s.52 (1877); 40&41 Vict., c.21, s.42 (1877).

[141] Murray, 'The Life History', pp. 352–3.

[142] LRO, 347 MAG 1/3/3, Proceedings of the Meetings of the Visiting Committee, Liverpool Borough Gaol, Apr. 1878–June 1897, 24 June 1891, p. 179.

Dr Hammond agreed that this was a case of malingering, and that O'Brien was dirty, had done no work and was pretending to be insane, and had this opinion confirmed by another doctor. The prisoner was closely watched, adding further evidence of his imposition, and he was ordered to be birched.[143]

Alongside the cruder methods of beating and starving suspected feigners, or placing them in a dark cell, 'hints for the detection' of feigned insanity advocated use of the actual cautery to blister the skin (the sight of its preparation might suffice, some prison officers claimed), while the stomach pump might make a man take his food. A dose of tartar emetic (a powerful vomit), opiates and cold shower baths were also recommended, 'but probably nothing is as efficacious as the application of a galvanic battery'.[144] John Campbell at Woking had used galvanic treatment in cases of feigned paralysis with remarkable effect and noted that malingerers had a 'perfect horror' of galvanism.[145] Dr Murray, Medical Officer at Sligo Prison, when managing the repeated suicide attempts of prisoner Michael Costello in 1886 – he tried to hang himself several times – ordered the 'Straps & muff to be applied ... [the prisoner] to be placed in padded cell and to be visited frequently during the night. To get a cold douche bath twice daily.' When Costello then refused to eat and speak, Murray commented in his journal: 'I would wish to have a good powerful Electric Machine supplied to this prison for such cases.' He tried to force the 'ruffian' to eat, using a jaw opener and soft tubes. Costello relented, eating 'Bread 3 Eggs battered up with 1 quart of milk'. Murray observed in his journal entry that 'Costello is evidently the worst possible character, but I hope he is now tamed for some time at least.' Although he continued to keep Costello in a padded cell and under observation, Murray remained 'fully persuaded that his motive was removal to a Lunatic Asylum, where he would have a better chance of escape'.[146]

Recidivists, by nature lazy and incapable of sustained exertion, according to A.R. Douglas, Deputy Medical Officer at Portland, were still capable of making it 'their business to give as much trouble as they can' and were 'often malingerers of a high order'.[147] Meanwhile, weak-minded prisoners were also referred to as 'doubtful' cases, adding further complexity in determining 'whether a man is insane, or weak-minded, or

---

[143] Ibid., 27 June 1894, p.293.   [144] Blandford, *Insanity and its Treatment*, p. 447.
[145] Kimberley Commission (1878–79), Evidence of Dr J. Campbell, p. 580.
[146] NAI, GPB/CORR/1888/Item no. 1365, Papers relating to padded cell at Castlebar Prison, 1886–88.
[147] A.R. Douglas, 'Penal Servitude and Insanity', *Journal of Mental Science*, 44:185 (Apr. 1898), 271–7, at pp. 274–5.

whether he is shamming'. A number of such cases ended up at Woking, including one prisoner sent on from Chatham, who had been flogged and kept on a bread and water diet, which as John Campbell acerbically remarked, were actions 'not likely to improve' his weak-mindedness.[148] Yet Campbell, concerned about the build up of weak-minded cases at Woking, also commented that 'utmost caution is required to discriminate between the really weak-minded and those cunning miscreants who feign mental peculiarities as a cloak for their misdeeds. These men belong to the worst description of criminals, and are proper subjects for the most deterring punishments.'[149]

Prison psychiatry moved to resolve such blurring by producing new categories and descriptors that allowed for this. David Nicolson contended that feigned insanity, a crucial aspect of the psychological states of prisoners, was a 'hybrid condition ... where we have certain external appearances and manifestations which are more or less like those of insanity, but which are nothing but the promptings of a sane mind behind the scenes'.[150] 'The detection of feigned insanity is, and ever will be, difficult,' asserted Blandford, 'when we have to examine men and women in whom madness and badness are so intermingled that observers cannot determine which it is that regulates their conduct.' Many criminals who were perpetual inhabitants of gaols were 'so silly in their motiveless fury, and childish in mind, that we may call them imbeciles or insane ... such there will ever be on the border-land of insanity'.[151] For many feigners their previous lives 'have been one continuous history of deception, and of shifty devices for living without work'.[152]

James Murray cited a complex and enduring case of malingering, involving various pains, fits, self-inflicted wounds, hypochondria and excessive grumbling, that led to extensive periods in the prison hospital at Wakefield, but was only marked by one instance where the prisoner's mental condition was questioned, when he was reported to be 'weak-minded and under observation'.[153] Yet the case was described as intriguing as a 'psychological study'. The prisoner's 'hereditary acquirements are unsound, mentally and morally', and he was the product of 'a neurotic father, and a more immoral mother'. 'From the beginning

---

[148] Kimberley Commission (1878–79), Evidence of Dr J. Campbell, pp. 572–3, 571, 580.
[149] Campbell, *Thirty Years Experience*, p. 82.
[150] Nicolson, 'The Morbid Psychology of Criminals', p. 242. See also ch. 3 for the creation of specific prison taxonomies.
[151] Blandford, *Insanity and Its Treatment*, p. 446.
[152] William A. Guy and David Ferrier, *Principles of Forensic Medicine*, 7th edn, rev. William R. Smith (London: Henry Renshaw, 1895), pp. 259–60.
[153] Murray, 'The Life History', p. 353.

of his prison-life he shows marked disinclination to settled labour or restraint of any kind, and finding that the only means of escaping his irksome duties is by personal defect, he mutilates himself and continues to do so whenever occasion requires.'[154] In this case, all elements of 'moral instability and depravity' were present, and, citing psychiatrist Henry Maudsley, Murray suggested that the man was a 'natural criminal', with a 'defective mental organization … a specially manufactured article of an anti-moral and anti-social type – sprung from a family in which insanity existed'. 'If we add to this a considerable amount of low cunning and dogged persistence in striving to avoid legally-imposed labour, we are enabled to distinguish the mental conditions under which he became a confirmed criminal and a successful malingerer.'[155] Thus malingering was itself, in the view of Murray, a form of mental disorder.

The practical problem of making distinctions between sane feigners and the truly insane, however, persisted, and in 1904 the Inspectors of Lunacy in Ireland expressed concern about a group of patients held in Dundrum Criminal Lunatic Asylum who had been transferred from Marybrough Invalid and Convict Prison as insane, but who were regarded to be of sound mind by Dundrum's medical officers. They took advantage of the visit of David Nicolson, by then one of the Lord Chancellor's Visitors in Lunacy and the Home Secretary's referee in cases of doubtful insanity, to serve on their committee of inquiry into the question of how to reach a decision and lay down some general principles on this matter, including the length of observation necessary in cases they described as 'borderland' and who were 'constantly being transferred from Prison to Asylum, and from Asylum to Prison, to the serious detriment of discipline in both institutions'.[156] The remainder of the Committee was composed of Dr Woodhouse, Medical Inspector of the General Prisons Board, and Inspectors of Lunatics George Plunkett O'Farrell and E.M. Courtney. The report commented on the difficulties of making assessments, framing their inquiry in terms of the broader challenges of 'criminalmindedness', 'moral obliquity, criminality, and general viciousness of conduct': 'the absence of well-established delusions and the predominance of insane-like, but not necessarily insane, conduct … have the effect of causing some confusion as to the meaning

---

[154] Ibid.   [155] Ibid., p. 354.
[156] NAI, CSORP/1905/12904, Minute from Geo. Plunkett O'Farrell and E.M. Courtney, Office of Inspectors of Lunatics, to Under Secretary, 10 June 1904, Minute from Inspectors of Lunatics, 13 June 1904, Minute from Sir Frederick Cullinan to Assistant Under Secretary, 22 June 1904.

or value of the term "insanity"'.[157] By 1904 Marybrough had devoted one small block to accommodate those refractory and weak-minded prisoners unfit for prison discipline, and it was pointed out in the report that 'where the delusion or other token of mental disease is either obscure, ambiguous or suspicious, the case often requires prolonged observation and study'. This happened in separate cells where the medical officer could take his time assessing the prisoner with a view to his potential removal.[158] In terms of laying down categorical instructions concerning the removal of convicts to Dundrum, however, the report was unable to offer much specific guidance. It pointed out the need for prolonged observation, for thorough acquaintance with the prisoner's history, character and circumstances, including his social class, and that much depended on 'professional knowledge and experience'. It was also recommended that candidates for appointment as medical officer in convict prisons be required to produce testimony of special experience among the insane in asylums, and in cases of doubtful insanity, an advisory board should be appointed to hold an inquiry.[159]

Conclusion

Dr Gover was to claim special insight into the case of Hamsley that opened this chapter; his acquired knowledge of Hamsley's back story as a criminal and his broader understanding of prisoners' minds, predilections and behaviour enabled him to confirm that he was feigning insanity. Travelling from London to Derby to examine the evidence, take witness statements and to detect the truth in this case, Gover fully enacted his role as 'Inspector' as well as underlining the expertise of the prison medical officer. Experienced prison doctors, such as David Nicolson, John Campbell, John Baker and Robert McDonnell, stressed the importance of looking carefully at individual cases, arguing that they were uniquely placed to differentiate between feigned and 'real' cases of insanity, their skills gained through being 'acquainted with prison life'.[160] Their knowledge of both insanity and criminality distinguished them from psychiatrists and other medical witnesses whose expertise was different, limited and partial.

---

[157] Ibid., *Report on the Committee of Inquiry into certain Doubtful Cases of Insanity amongst Convicts and Person Detained*, 1905, p. 10.
[158] Ibid., p. 11.   [159] Ibid., pp. 14–15.
[160] John Baker, 'Some Points Connected with Criminals', *Journal of Mental Science*, 38:162 (July 1892), 364–9, at p. 364.

Yet, at the same time, prison medical officers acknowledged the difficulties of adjudicating such cases, the 1904 Report into Doubtful Cases of Insanity in Ireland noting that the question 'ever utmost' in the thoughts of prison medical officers was whether the 'insane-like behaviour' of prisoners was genuine or feigned:

No special act or kind of act will decide this question. In the prison arena refusal to work, insubordination, violence and destructiveness may each in turn be the role of the mere criminal or of the lunatic: while delusions, incoherence, and imbecility may be that of the lunatic or imposter feigning insanity. Again, attempts at suicide, refusal of food, self-torture in any form, nudity, setting fire to cell or furniture, noisy raving, gross filthiness or indecency are not in themselves indications of insanity, although they figure largely as stock performances in the would-be lunatic's repertoire.[161]

Feigning in prison constitutes an important – and hitherto relatively neglected – part of the history of malingering more broadly, bringing into question Simon Wessely's conclusion that malingering only moved resolutely into the sphere of medical expertise in the early twentieth century when progressive social legislation facilitated financial rewards for malingering.[162] This chapter has demonstrated that interest in feigning was already deeply embedded in prison practice and it was seen as a crucial aspect of the prison doctor's role by early in the nineteenth century. The challenge feigning posed to the ethos of the separate system was as significant as its fusion with fears about recidivism and the criminal mind later in the century. The feigners' objective of avoiding work and prison discipline – whether it was the moral work of reform and improvement or hard labour – confirmed their shiftlessness, idleness and constitutional weakness.

For prison medical officers the stakes were high – in terms of actual day-to-day workload and their reputation within the prisons where they were employed, as well as professional standing. There was considerable interest in the mental state of prisoner feigners, and in framing new labels to describe them, suggesting that the 'psychologization' of malingering became well established during the nineteenth century.[163] The phenomenon of feigning in the view of prison doctors was associated with the

---

[161] NAI, CSORP/1905/12904, *Report on the Committee of Inquiry into certain Doubtful Cases of Insanity*, p. 15.

[162] Simon Wessely, 'Malingering: Historical Perspectives', in P.W. Halligan, Christopher Bass and David A. Oakley (eds), *Malingering and Illness Deception* (Oxford: Oxford University Press, 2003), pp. 31–41, at p. 31.

[163] Rather than during the First World War as Roger Cooter has suggested. Cooter, 'Malingering in Modernity'. This is supported in the context of the asylum by Sarah Chaney, 'Useful Members of Society or Motiveless Malingerers'.

workings of the criminal mind and constituted in itself a particular form of mental disease.[164] So while prison medical officers denied the genuineness of the insanity on display, often punishing these prisoners, they also recategorised feigners as having 'a defective mental condition', which had not only caused them to feign but also to become a confirmed criminal in the first place – 'anti-moral' and 'anti-social' with a 'depraved moral tendency', 'low cunning', and 'dogged persistence'.[165] As such, for the prison doctor, feigners represented a combination of inbuilt criminality, a desire to avoid labour, a determination to get what they wanted despite the risk of punishment and of inflicting upon themselves physical or mental harm. Feigners were a persistent challenge for the prison doctor yet also increasingly acted as a locus through which doctors asserted their specific expertise and differentiated themselves from psychiatrists working in the asylum system.

[164] Murray, 'The Life History', p. 348.   [165] Ibid., p. 354.

6   Conclusion
The Decline of the Separate System, the Prisoner Patient and Enduring Legacies

---

> The greater number of the cells are tenanted all day long, except for the little respite of chapel and exercise, and you may partly tell by the pallor of the tenant's face how many days, weeks, or months of his sentence he has worked out in changeless solitude. If the doctor – whose duties, by the way, are infinitely the most responsible in the prison – has certified him fit for labour ... he is put at once upon a purely penal task, which is generally as unprofitable as it is unpleasant.... They depress, irritate and degrade men of any feeling and intelligence.[1]

Towards the close of the nineteenth century English and Irish prisons still contained and retained large numbers of mentally ill inmates, a situation acknowledged and deplored by the prison services in both countries. Prisons were declared inappropriate for the incarceration and treatment of mentally disordered prisoners as well as the increasing numbers of weak-minded inmates, who disrupted their management and were unable to bear or profit from the discipline. Prison officials and prison medical officers, however, were far less willing to attribute mental disorder to prison regimes and conditions, clinging to the mantra that most insane inmates were already suffering from mental illness when they entered prison. In contrast, critics of late nineteenth-century prisons, reform groups and former prisoners, drew attention to the apparent failure of prisons in terms of their cruel and ineffective discipline, the high rate of recommittals and their poor governance, with Edmund Du Cane, responsible for both local and convict prisons in England, the subject of particularly robust criticism.[2] They also

---

[1] London Metropolitan Archives, ACC/3588, Burt J. (Warder at H.M. Prison, Wormwood Scrubs), Reminiscences of Twenty-Nine and Half Years as an Officer in H.M. Prison Wormwood Scrubs. Extract from 'Scenes from the Prison World' by Tighe Hopkins, 5 Oct. 1895. Hopkins published extensively on English and French prisons and prisoners of war, including *The Silent Gate: A Voyage into Prison* (London: Hurst & Blackett, 1900).

[2] See W.J. Forsythe, *Penal Discipline, Reformatory Projects and the English Prison Commission 1895–1939* (Exeter: University of Exeter Press, 1991), ch. 2; Victor Bailey, 'English Prisons, Penal Culture, and the Abatement of Imprisonment, 1895–1922', *Journal of British Studies*, 36:3 (1997), 285–324.

highlighted the high incidence of mental breakdown in prisons, which they attributed directly to severe prison regimes. As shown in the quotation above, novelist and penal reformer Tighe Hopkins emphasised in 1895 how prison discipline degraded, irritated and depressed, adding his voice to those of many prison writers who described the eroding of mental energy, the bleakness and misery of prison systems designed to isolate and dehumanise their inmates. In particular, campaigners lobbied for the end of the separate cellular system that had dominated prison policies and practices since the 1840s.

Prison Psychiatry and Campaigns for Reform

By the 1890s this pressure, which via the press, novels and periodical articles increasingly built public support, prompted a reassessment of deterrent penal policies. The Howard Association, as seen in Chapter 4, intervened in cases highlighting poor treatment or brutality in prisons. The Association's Secretary William Tallack had long been a critic of Du Cane, and had given evidence to the Kimberley Commission in 1878, pointing to the neglect of prisoners and instances of cruelty. The Humanitarian League, meanwhile, publicly stated that the prison system was 'pitiless, indiscriminate and needlessly and culpably severe'.[3] In January 1894, the *Daily Chronicle* published a series of articles, 'Our Dark Places', presumed to have been written by Reverend W.D. Morrison who was associated with the Humanitarian League, but more likely authored by the newspaper's assistant editor H.W. Massingham, who had toured a number of prisons shortly before the articles appeared.[4] The articles described prisons as gloomy, severe and obsolete, and referenced the 'nervous strain of a prisoner's life', with prisoners subjected to silence and morbid introspective hopelessness.[5] Coinciding with a wider spiritual revival and growing concern about urban conditions in England, penal practices and conditions were also criticised by the Salvation Army. Many discharged convicts came under their care, 'mentally weak and wasted', suffering a loss of identity, and incapable of pursing ordinary occupations.[6]

---

[3] The National Archive (TNA), PCOM 7/38-1. Cutting from the *Daily Chronicle*, 1 Feb. 1894. Cited Forsythe, *Penal Discipline*, p. 23.
[4] Bailey, 'English Prisons, Penal Culture, and the Abatement of Imprisonment, 1895–1922', p. 288.
[5] *Daily Chronicle*, 23 and 25 Jan. 1894.
[6] *The Nation*, 8 May 1909; Report from the Departmental Committee on Prisons [Gladstone Committee] (1895) [C.7702] [C.7702–1], Evidence of Col. Barker, pp. 274–83. See also William James Forsythe, *The Reform of Prisoners 1830–1900* (London and Sydney: Croom Helm, 1987), pp. 219–24.

In Ireland it was the 1884 Royal Commission on Irish Prisons that highlighted the flaws in the treatment of prisoners, including the confinement of those suffering mental illness. In the 1880s, the imprisonment of leading nationalists, including Charles Stewart Parnell and John Dillon, had brought Irish prisons to the public's attention, prompting the establishment of the Royal Commission. It was concerned with assessing whether the Irish prison system was administered with 'intentional or systematic harshness'.[7] Much of the Royal Commission's criticism focused on unsanitary conditions in prisons, particularly at Omagh Prison, where the Governor had died of typhoid in 1882. The Report also highlighted the excessive punishment of refractory prisoners whose 'mental condition may be described as the borderland between sanity and insanity', and recommended the appointment, in a similar way to England, of a Medical Inspector or Superintending Medical Officer.[8] In general the Royal Commission was critical of local prisons in Ireland, and of the management of the prison estate, with allegations that Charles F. Bourke, Chairman of the General Prisons Board from November 1878 until 1895, was dictatorial in his style and his relationship with the prison inspectors was acrimonious.[9] While less critical of convict prisons, the Commission oversaw the closure of Spike Island in 1884, as recommended by the 1878 Kimberley Commission.[10]

While Ireland did not hold an equivalent to the Gladstone inquiry, its Royal Commission aired similar concerns about the deleterious effects of punitive prison discipline. Meanwhile, Irish political prisoners added powerful voices to the mounting criticism of the English prison system where many had served time, giving evidence to both the Kimberley Commission and the Departmental Committee on Prisons (Gladstone Committee) in 1895. Chiefly focused on the situation in English prisons, Gladstone can be regarded as emblematic of the change in tone in both England and Ireland and growing public distaste for prison policies and practices. The 1895 inquiry, chaired by the Liberal Herbert Gladstone, Parliamentary Under Secretary at the Home Office between 1892 and 1894, included three other members of parliament – the Liberal and lawyer, Richard Haldane, Conservative Sir John Dorington, who had experience as a lunacy commissioner, and Irish nationalist member, Arthur O'Connor – along with the magistrate to the London police

---

[7] Beverly A. Smith, 'The Irish General Prisons Board, 1877–1885: Efficient Deterrence or Bureaucratic Ineptitude?', *Irish Jurist*, 15:1 (1980), 122–36, at p. 128.
[8] Royal Commission on Prisons in Ireland, Vol. 1. Reports, Digest of Evidence, Appendices; Minutes of Evidence, 1884 (1884–85) [C.4233] [C.4233–1], pp. 14, 20.
[9] Smith, 'The Irish General Prisons Board', p. 131.
[10] Royal Commission on Prisons in Ireland, 1884 (1884–85), p. 37.

courts, Albert De Rutzen, Dr J.H. Bridges and an expert on women's labour questions, Miss Eliza Orme. The Committee heard a wide range of evidence from witnesses based within and without the prison system, and visited six convict prisons and seventeen local prisons.[11] They also drew parallels with conditions in Irish prisons, referencing the findings of the influential 1884 Royal Commission.[12]

One issue that emerged strongly in the evidence presented to the Gladstone Committee was the excessive rate of mental disorder among prisoners and the equally excessive demands this imposed on prison medical officers. While far from being a typical prison, the detailed inquiry into Holloway Prison, shone a light on the stresses in both prison systems. Magistrates in England and Ireland were still remanding in custody large numbers of prisoners whose mental state was suspect, and as Holloway replaced Clerkenwell as London's chief remand prison in 1886 it bore the brunt of these admissions in England. As Medical Inspector Dr Robert Gover pointed out, 'in London the sending of insane persons to prison under sentence is in great measure prevented by making use of Holloway Prison as a place in which accused persons can be observed and tested'.[13] In 1889, 401 prisoners of 'doubtful insanity' were remanded there for observation, and of these 215 were declared sane, 107 of weak or impaired intellect and 85 were reported to be insane.[14] The Gladstone inquiry also underlined Holloway's huge turnover of prisoners, a situation mirrored only in one other English prison, Liverpool, which had around 18,000 admissions per annum by the mid-1890s.[15] In 1893–94, 12,467 males and 9,701 females passed through Holloway Prison, and its medical officer, Dr George Walker, had to examine between 20–30 and 80–90 prisoners each day.[16] Medical inspections were by necessity brisk, given Walker's many other duties. However, reporting on the mental state of prisoners was highlighted by Walker as a task requiring 'great care' and the 'most important duty' of a prison medical officer, and he pointed out that making these assessments might require two to three examinations per prisoner.[17] In 1894 Walker claimed to have examined 1,056 such cases, some remanded by the magistrates for observation, while others had committed a serious crime or were suicidal and regarded by the medical staff as 'special cases'.[18]

---

[11] Forsythe, *Penal Discipline*, p. 25.   [12] Gladstone Committee (1895), pp. 39–40.
[13] Ibid., J.H. Bridges, 'Memorandum on Insanity in Prisons', p. 48.   [14] Ibid.
[15] Ibid., Evidence of Dr Walker, p. 133. For the pressure on Liverpool Prison, see chs 3 and 4.
[16] Ibid., pp. 128–9. See also Seán McConville, *English Local Prisons 1860–1900: Next Only to Death* (London and New York: Routledge, 1995), pp. 298–9.
[17] Gladstone Committee (1895), Evidence of Dr Walker, p. 129.   [18] Ibid., p. 131.

As with the 1884 Royal Commission on Irish Prisons, the evidence presented to the Gladstone Committee revealed an ongoing reluctance to acknowledge the impact of prisons in producing mental disorder, which, as Chapter 2 has shown, was already very evident in the 1840s as the separate system was being established. In the year ending March 1893 some 88 cases of insanity were recorded in Holloway, 72 of whom were remand prisoners and 'insane before they came in'. Their insanity, Walker declared, had nothing to do with their imprisonment in Holloway, and a great many had been in asylums before and some frequently in prison.[19] It was also claimed that of 354 cases of insanity in local prisons in England for the year ending March 1894, in only 60 cases was insanity noted a month or more after admission.[20] However, finally, if somewhat grudgingly, it was concluded, that the statistics showed 'the fact that among the prison population the ratio of insanity arising among persons apparently sane on admission is not less than three times as that amongst the general population of corresponding ages'.[21] It was also agreed this figure was shaped by the fact that 'Insanity and crime are "simply morbid branches of the same stock"' and 'that they do so dovetail into each other conditions of mental enfeeblement, insanity, and crime'.[22] This mingling of medical and criminal theories on the nature of the criminal mind, discussed in detail in Chapter 3, can be located time and again in prison medical officers' discussions on the nature of insanity and weak-mindedness in the prison context from the 1860s onwards.

A number of witnesses presenting to the Gladstone Committee referred to Walker's excessive workload at Holloway. Dr David Nicolson, then Superintendent at Broadmoor, explained that he had the relative luxury of having between one and two hours to interview and assess a patient, highlighting the contrast with prisons and the pressure faced by prison doctors.[23] The report also underlined the extensive experience and ability of prison doctors in making difficult judgements on a prisoner's mental state that required great skill, particularly in cases of murder. Nicolson emphasised that the work was heavy and taxing but that prison medical officers were competent to do it: 'Everything that one can bring to bear upon it was required, more particularly in the way of approaching and of knowing the individual.'[24]

---

[19] Ibid.   [20] Ibid., Bridges, 'Memorandum on Insanity in Prisons', p. 48.
[21] Ibid., p. 49.
[22] Ibid., Evidence of Dr Bevan Lewis, p. 303; Bridges, 'Memorandum on Insanity in Prisons', p. 49.
[23] Ibid., Evidence of Dr David Nicolson, p. 312.   [24] Ibid.

However, he conceded that prison doctors needed experience of dealing with 'actual lunatics', and one of the recommendations of the final report was that evidence of this should be required for prison medical appointments.[25] The inquiry also revealed the extent to which observation and 'testing' still dominated the practices of prison medical officers. Dr Tennyson Patmore, Medical Officer at Wormwood Scrubs, remarked that the detection of delusions might take several visits over several months. He also wished to bring the attention of the committee to the fact that prisons still contained a large population who endeavoured to 'malinger insanity' and the duty of the medical officer was to ensure, through long observation, 'the ends of justice are not defeated by our being taken in by the malingerer'.[26]

Among several witnesses to the Gladstone Committee who had experienced imprisonment, Michael Davitt, Fenian and land reformer, provided extensive evidence. He had served almost nine years of penal servitude in Millbank, Dartmoor and Portland prisons, and had also given evidence to the Kimberley Commission in 1878. Alongside his condemnation of prison discipline, conditions of labour, dietary and medical care, Davitt criticised the nine months of solitary imprisonment and urged it to be abolished or reduced to short periods at the beginning and end of sentences, as it was a horrific experience for first-time offenders, while 'old lags' had no fear of it and used it for malingering purposes to avoid hard labour.[27] 'I believe that solitude must necessarily tend to injure all minds. To be shut up for 23 hours out of every 24 for nine months, and not allowed to speak except in the instances I have given, is a fearful ordeal for any human being to go through.'[28] Davitt argued there was a great deal more of insanity and weak-mindedness among prisoners than was recorded in official reports and statistics, and noted a large increase in the incidence especially among prisoners who had been in prison on several occasions.[29]

Irish prisons received less condemnation from the Gladstone Committee and individual English prisons were compared unfavourably with them. Captain Frank Johnston, Governor at Dartmoor Convict Prison, was quizzed on why the death rate at Dartmoor was twice that of Irish prisons and why corporeal punishment, which had not been implemented in Irish convict prisons for over a year, was still used

---

[25] Ibid., p. 34.
[26] Ibid., Evidence of Dr T.D. Patmore, p. 208. See ch. 5 for medical officers' efforts to combat malingering.
[27] Ibid., Evidence of Michael Davitt, pp. 382–94, especially pp. 383, 384.
[28] Ibid., p. 389.   [29] Ibid., p. 390.

there.[30] The Prison Commissioner, Robert Sidney Mitford, could not account for the notable differences in rates of punishments and deaths, though it was suggested by the Commissioners that discipline in Irish prisons was enforced less vigorously than in England.[31] William Murphy has argued that owing to the pressures exerted by political prisoners on Irish prisons, rules and discipline were relaxed somewhat, and in 1889 new regulations gave the General Prisons Board discretion to further ameliorate conditions.[32] This gradual winding down of the rigour of the discipline coincided with the departure of Bourke as Chair of the General Prisons Board in March 1895.[33] By that time, the average daily number of prisoners was 2,323, with mentally ill prisoners generally removed swiftly to asylums when necessary. Nonetheless, despite criticism by the 1884 Royal Commission on Irish Prisons of prison medical officers' failure to acknowledge the high rates of mental disorder among prisoners, prison doctors continued to insist that the prison regime was not at fault. In its Report for 1895, the General Prisons Board, noted that 75 prisoners were transferred to asylums, of whom 61 were reported to be insane on admission, one weak-minded and one 'doubtful'. Among the remaining twelve prisoners, four were reported sane while in prison, but were found to have been insane at the time when their offences were committed. The Board therefore concluded that only eight prisoners became insane in prison; one became ill three days and another twelve days after committal.[34] While William Tallack of the Howard Association had little good to say about English prisons, he was more positive about the Irish prison regime. During 1895 he visited a number of Irish prisons and was impressed at the variety of labour and the conditions. He also stressed the excellent results produced in Irish medical departments and the influence of their medical officers. He conceded, however, that the level of mental disorder in Irish prisons was still a concern, with some insane prisoners still retained in prison to save rates; some 82 insane prisoners were admitted in 1893–94, though it was claimed that only eight of these became insane in prison.[35]

---

[30] Ibid., Evidence of Frank Johnson, p. 297.   [31] Ibid., pp. 359, 360.

[32] William Murphy, *Political Imprisonment and the Irish, 1912–1921* (Oxford: Oxford University Press, 2014), p. 8.

[33] Report of the General Prisons Board (Ireland) (RGPBI) 1895 (1894–95) [C.7806], p. 12.

[34] RGPBI, 1895–96 (1896) [C.8252], p. 7.

[35] Modern Records Centre, University of Warwick, Howard League Papers, MSS.16A/7/1/ William Tallack: Manuscript Notebook Recording Visit to Ireland and Inspections of *Irish Prisons*, June 1895; William Tallack, 'Irish Prisons', *The Times*, 24 June 1895.

The issues of detecting malingerers, prison medical officers' workload and the nature of insanity and weak-mindedness in prisons were at the core of the work of the 1904 Committee of Inquiry into Doubtful Cases of Insanity Amongst Convicts in Ireland. Originally appointed to assess whether a group of prisoners, transferred from Maryborough Prison to Dundrum Lunatic Asylum, were 'really insane' and to agree on a set of principles for prison and asylum medical officers when dealing with such cases, the Committee conducted a detailed review of each case and of the management of weak-minded prisoners at Maryborough Prison. The Report of the Committee emphasised the importance of 'skilled observers', whose 'common sense' and 'practical experience' in 'individual cases' helped them detect malingers and prisoners who sought 'entrance to the haven of asylum life'.[36] The Committee noted the burden on prison staff of transferring 'backwards and forwards, from Prison to Asylum, and from Asylum to Prison, of persons of this class ... and [the] inconvenience and expenses to the Public Service'. While the number of mentally ill inmates in Irish prisons was not as high as in English prisons, the Committee's survey of the life-histories of each prisoner under review highlighted the persistence of the problem as significant numbers of the mentally ill were still sent to Irish prisons despite efforts to divert them.[37]

While the Gladstone Report was welcomed as 'the beginning of a beneficent revolution', its impact has been questioned, as has its status as a real turning point, though its publication did result in Du Cane's immediate, albeit reluctant, resignation.[38] As noted above, in Ireland the full rigour of penal discipline had eased somewhat in response to the demands of political prisoners. The Gladstone Committee recommended individualised treatment to develop prisoners' moral instincts, to train them in orderly and industrial habits, and to improve their mental and physical health. It also advocated the separation of prisoners into types, including first offenders, habitual prisoners, the feeble-minded and drunkards, to be dealt with by special programmes. And finally it recommended the reform of the separate system, and a renewed emphasis on productive, collective labour and recommended the

[36] National Archives of Ireland, Chief Secretary's Office Registered Papers/1905/12904, *Report on the Committee of Inquiry into Certain Doubtful Cases of Insanity Amongst Convicts and Person Detained*, 1905, p. 10.
[37] Ibid.
[38] Sidney and Beatrice Webb, *English Prisons under Local Government* (London: Longmans, Green and Co., 1922), p. 220; Christopher Harding, '"The Inevitable End of a Discredited System"? The Origins of the Gladstone Committee Report on Prisons, 1895', *The Historical Journal*, 31:3 (1988), 591–608.

abolition of penal forms of labour, including the treadwheel and crank. On its recommendations, the Borstal Institution for male juveniles aged between sixteen and twenty-one was established at Rochester in Kent in 1901, and the Committee influenced the opening in 1906 of the Clonmel Borstal in Ireland. As Gladstone's recommendations were encoded into regulations in England, the rules for Irish prisons were 'assimilated' to the English model, with the implementation of a new set of rules for local prisons in 1902.[39]

The Gladstone Committee also rearticulated the expertise of prison medical officers, notably in the detection of malingering and weak-mindedness, and pointed to their ability to understand the relationship between criminality and mental deterioration. It has been regarded as a watershed moment for prison medical officers who were accorded increased authority. Yet, as shown in Chapters 3–5, prison medical officers in England and Ireland had been claiming this particular form of expertise from the 1860s onwards as they sought to navigate the demands of their role as physicians and enforcers of prison discipline. Their expertise was rooted in their ability to deal with mental illness in criminal justice settings, and through the production of new taxonomies that applied in prison contexts. The detection of malingering had been a key part of the prison medical officer's role from early in the nineteenth century. However, Gladstone reaffirmed the significance of the prison doctor in dealing with mental illness, as well as the substantial part this played in making up their workload. As reformatory aspirations had diminished, the prison medical officer had overtaken chaplains in medi-ating on matters of the mind.[40] Though the spiritual revival and individ-uals such as Reverend Morrison were no doubt important in the build-up to the Gladstone inquiry, the era of the chaplain's dominance in diag-nosing and mediating mental disorder, as outlined in Chapter 2, was long gone by 1895.

Locale, as our study demonstrates, was also a key factor in terms of the particular pressures facing prisons and in relation to the way power was brokered between prison officers and between external organisations and institutions, including magistrates and Boards of Superintendence, visiting committees and local asylums, as was the impact of particular individuals, such as Chaplain James Nugent at Liverpool who continued to push moral agendas designed to reduce the prison's population and

[39] RGPBI, 1901–02 (1902) [Cd. 1241], p. 14.
[40] Forsythe, *The Reform of Prisoners 1830–1900*, p. 202.

reform its inmates in the final decades of the nineteenth century.[41] While a number of prison medical officers, notably Dr David Nicolson, forged their identities as specialists in the practice of prison psychiatry in the pages of medical journals, others, such as Dr Robert McDonnell, through their day-to-day work and presentation of evidence via reports and parliamentary inquiries, emphasised the importance of their roles in individual prisons and that they were creating a new form of psychiatry in criminal justice settings.

It was suggested in Chapter 1 that the prison has loomed small in terms of the scholarship on the history of psychiatry, and our book is intended to go some way in developing this area of scholarship, while acknowledging the scope for further comparative inquiries through exploration of different periods and geographical contexts. Our study has demonstrated the ways in which psychiatry expanded its professional influence beyond lunatic asylums into prisons during the nineteenth century, largely in the hands of the prison medical officers who insisted that they were creating new forms of psychiatric knowledge and expertise distinct from psychiatric practice outside the criminal justice system. By the close of the century prison medical officers and asylum superintendents were, however, increasingly working together to tackle the broader issue of the placing of mentally disordered offenders, in a situation hampered by overcrowding and limited resources in both sets of institutions. In many ways the prison and asylum had run along parallel tracks, in terms of sharing a reformist agenda in the mid-nineteenth century, involving control of the prisoner or patient under conditions of enforced confinement and isolation in specially designed environments.[42] While the purpose of the asylum was to cure its patients, the prison's mission was to punish and rehabilitate. However, both sought the production of improved and more able individuals, no longer a burden to the state. Both sets of institutions emphasised the critical role of self-management, whether this was under the direction of the chaplains with their efforts at redeeming prisoners in their cells through their admonishments or shaped by the philosophy and practice of moral therapy in asylums, which aimed at self-control and conformity to particular forms of behaviour. It could even be argued that for a brief period

---

[41] See also Catherine Cox and Hilary Marland, '"Unfit for Reform or Punishment": Mental Disorder and Discipline in Liverpool Borough Prison in the Late Nineteenth Century', *Social History*, 44:2 (2019), 173–201.

[42] For the role of chaplains, see Sean Grass, *The Self in Cell: Narrating the Victorian Prisoner* (New York: Routledge, 2003), ch. 1. See, for seclusion in asylum practice, Leslie Topp, 'Single Rooms, Seclusion and the Non-Restraint Movement in British Asylums, 1838–1844', *Social History of Medicine*, 31:4 (2018), 754–73.

in the mid-nineteenth century the prison chaplains were more ambitious than their asylum doctor counterparts, aiming at inner reflection resulting in deep-seated and genuine redemption, whereas moral treatment less actively pursued the identification of the root causes of mental disturbance.[43] So too the shift to a more penal approach in the 1860s and 1870s, accompanied by interest in establishing the links between mental decline and criminal behaviour was mirrored by the increased influence of theories of degeneration and heredity in late nineteenth-century asylums, as they too faced the problems of overcrowded conditions and huge pressure on resources and staff.[44] In both contexts, claims to authority rested increasingly on psychiatry's alliance with degeneration theory, though equally it can be questioned how influential this theory was in practice, as asylums and prisons continued to focus on individual cases of mental deterioration and to acknowledge the impact of environmental factors.[45]

'We Are Recreating Bedlam': The Crisis in Prison Mental Health Services

While the Gladstone Report prompted changes in responses to mentally ill prisoners, shaking off the preoccupation with positivist approaches, and opening the door once again to reform, this emphasis was diluted in the years that followed and, as Bailey has so aptly put it, post Gladstone, 'the pace of progress in humanizing prisons was glacial'.[46] Today the situation regarding mentally ill people in prison is far from resolved. Indeed as the number of cases of diagnosed mental illness among

---

[43] See Foucault's searing critique of moral therapy: Michel Foucault, *Madness and Civilization: A History of Insanity in the Age of Reason* (London: Tavistock, 1967), ch. 9, 'The Birth of the Asylum' and Andrew Scull, 'Moral Treatment Reconsidered: Some Sociological Comments on an Episode in the History of British Psychiatry', in Andrew Scull (ed.), *Madhouses, Mad-Doctors, and Madmen: The Social History of Psychiatry in the Victorian Era* (London: Athlone, 1981), pp. 105–20.

[44] Laurence Ray, 'Models of Madness in Victorian Asylum Practice', *European Journal of Sociology*, 22:2 (1981), 229–64; Janet Saunders, 'Quarantining the Weak-Minded: Psychiatric Definitions of Degeneracy and the Late-Victorian Asylum', in W.F. Bynum, Roy Porter and Michael Shepherd (eds), *Anatomy of Madness: Essays in the History of Psychiatry*, vol. 3 (London: Routledge, 1988), pp. 273–96; Andrew Scull, *The Most Solitary of Afflictions: Madness and Society in Britain 1700–1900* (New Haven, CT and London: Yale University Press, 2005), ch. 6; Andrew Scull, *Madness in Civilisation* (London: Thames & Hudson, 2015), ch. 8.

[45] See Tony Ward, 'An Honourable Regime of Truth? Foucault, Psychiatry and English Criminal Justice', in Helen Johnston (ed.), *Punishment and Control in Historical Perspective* (Houndmills: Palgrave Macmillan, 2008), pp. 56–75, at p. 63.

[46] Bailey, 'English Prisons, Penal Culture, and the Abatement of Imprisonment, 1895–1922', p. 322.

inmates has soared in recent decades, and, with few alternatives to prison, in some regards their opportunities for effective treatment have deteriorated. Media reports continue to highlight the plight of mentally ill prisoners and the strain they place on overburdened prisons, prompting *The Guardian* to claim in 2014 that 'We are recreating Bedlam'.[47]

The Gladstone Committee was meant to have swept aside 'the old-fashioned idea that separate confinement was desirable on the grounds that it enables the prisoner to meditate on his misdeeds', and, although there were further modifications and the length of separation was reduced for many prisoners in English and Irish prisons, it endured. In 1909 the author and playwright John Galsworthy, reviving earlier campaigns, felt compelled to lobby the Prison Commission and government for its abolition.[48] In a letter to the Home Secretary, Herbert Gladstone, later reproduced in *The Nation*, Galsworthy urged 'the complete abandonment of this closed cellular confinement'.[49] He described how in the year ending March 1907 1,035 persons, of whom 691 had never been sentenced to penal servitude before, were to endure 4,000-odd hours of 'agony and demoralisation', in a 'smothering process to which the mind must adapt itself or perish'.[50] Echoing Dickens in 1842, Galsworthy argued that far from causing reflection and sober self-examination, separate confinement led to mental vacuity and put at risk 'that terribly intricate and hidden thing, the mind'.[51] Interviewing sixty prisoners at Lewes Prison, which had adapted separation so that convicts worked in roofless cells and could see the warders and prison officers though they could not speak to each other, Galsworthy reported how some were 'driven crazy' and complained of sleeplessness. Several men were in tears throughout the interview. The prisoners described how, 'I didn't hardly know how to keep myself together. I thought I should go mad', 'It made me very nervous, the least thing upsets me', and 'It destroys a man'.[52]

[47] Anon., '"We Are Recreating Bedlam": The Crisis in Prison Mental Health Services', *The Guardian*, 24 May 2014.
[48] Webb, *English Prisons*, p. 223.
[49] TNA, HO 45/13658, Prisons and Prisoners: Separate or Cellular Confinement, 1909–30, Solitary Confinement: An Open Letter to the Home Secretary, p. 1 (emphasis in original).
[50] Ibid., pp. 16, 13–14; *The Nation*, 8 May 1909; R.H.G., 'Mr John Galsworthy on Prison Reform', *Journal of the American Institute of Criminal Law and Criminology*, 2:5 (1912), 756–8. See also Jamie Bennett, 'The Man, the Machine and the Myths: Reconsidering Winston Churchill's Prison Reforms', in Johnston (ed.), *Punishment and Control in Historical Perspective*, pp. 95–114.
[51] TNA, HO 45/13658, Prisons and Prisoners: A Letter to Sir Evelyn Ruggles Brise, Prison Commission, 23 July 1909, p. 25.
[52] Ibid.: A Minute on Separate Confinement forwarded to the Home Secretary and Prison Commissioners, Compiled from visits paid to 60 convicts undergoing confinement, 22

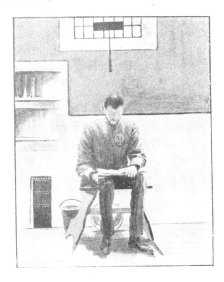

Figure 6.1 Sunday in cell, Wormwood Scrubs, c. 1891
Credit: Archives Howard League for Penal Reform, Modern Records Centre,
University of Warwick

Again in 1922, Stephen Hobhouse and Archibald Fenner Brockway's masterly account *English Prisons Today*, drawing on their own prison experiences and the recollections of prison staff and inmates, illuminated the endurance of the system of separate confinement, which they defined as one of the greatest flaws in an overall bankrupt prison system, 'driving the man more and more into himself'.[53] Political prisoners held in Ireland also highlighted the persistence of separate confinement and harsh prison conditions. While Ernest Blythe noted that the prison regime was not as severe as that endured by the Fenians in the 1860s

Sept. 1909, pp. 35–7, 39–40. See also Forsythe, *Penal Discipline*, pp. 64–7 for Galsworthy's campaigns for prison reform.
[53] Stephen Hobhouse and A. Fenner Brockway, *English Prisons Today: Being the Report of the Prison System Enquiry Committee* (London: Longmans, Green and Co., 1922), p. 571.

and 1880s, Herbert Moore Pim, who was held in Belfast Prison with Blythe in 1915, published a polemical prison memoir under the pseudonym A. Newman in which he slated the 'English jail system'.[54] An author, Quaker and separatist nationalist, he described prison life as 'a series of humiliations' as prisoners were 'forced night after night to recall with horrible vividness the evils of the past'.[55] He noted how 'Men go mad in prison at the end of three months' and that prison was 'one mass of preventions against suicide'.[56] He also commented on the architecture of the prison cell: 'The oppression of being shut in, and the abominably constructed door, whose every nail seemed to be a symbol declaring the idea of jaildom.'[57]

Toby Seddon has summarised changes in the early twentieth-century prison, and efforts to clear out various categories of mentally ill prisoners, including the weak-minded, in order to focus on 'responsible prisoners', capable of reform. He has also highlighted the further shift towards psychological and psychoanalytic approaches in the 1920s and 1930s, with many doctors arguing that all crime had 'mental origins'. In the post-war period there was a further shift towards penal-welfarism and correctional crime control, though most of this work, as in the nineteenth century, remained diagnostic.[58] Though, as Chapter 3 illuminated, the weak-minded became the focus of increased concern in the late nineteenth century, efforts to move those thus identified from prison were hampered by the lack of institutional facilities, an early illustration of what was also to become a persistent problem during the twentieth century for the mentally ill. In Liverpool 'feeble-minded' prisoners ended up in lunatic asylums and workhouses owing to the absence of services, and, while both prisoners classified as insane or mentally defective were transferred, as in 1917 when eight prisoners were removed to asylums and six to 'Mental Deficiency Institutions', demand for places was far from being fully met.[59] In Ireland there were no separate state-run

[54] Murphy, *Political Imprisonment and the Irish*, p. 45.
[55] A. Newman, *What It Feels Like* (Dublin: Whelan & Son, 1915), p. 4.   [56] Ibid., p. 5.
[57] Ibid., p. 19.
[58] Toby Seddon, *Punishment and Madness: Governing Prisoners with Mental Health Problems* (Abingdon: Routledge-Cavendish, 2007), pp. 6–7. See Janet Weston, *Medicine, the Penal System and Sexual Crimes in England, 1919–1960s: Diagnosing Deviance* (London: Bloomsbury Academic, 2017), ch. 2 for the change from punishment to rehabilitation in scrutinising the mental state of sexual offenders in the 1920s and 1930s. See also Clive Emsley, *Crime and Society in Twentieth-Century England* (Harlow: Longman, 2011), for shifting attitudes to crime and imprisonment more broadly.
[59] Liverpool Record Office, 347 MAG 1/3/5, Proceedings at the Meetings of the Visiting Committee of Liverpool Prison, Nov. 1904–Sept. 1912, Annual Meeting of the Visiting Committee, 5 Jan. 1911, p. 352; 347 MAG 1/3/6, Proceedings at the Meetings of the Visiting Committee of Liverpool Prison, Oct. 1912–Dec. 1919, Annual Meeting of the

institutional facilities for 'feeble-minded' prisoners established in this period, and these offenders continued to accumulate in prisons, work-houses and lunatic asylums in the early twentieth century.

After World War II, 'deinstitutionalisation' saw significant numbers of mentally ill people confined in prison as mental hospitals began to close or reduce provision.[60] In England, the closure of the large Victorian asylums in the 1960s and 1970s led to a drastic decline in the number of psychiatric hospital beds, and in 1978, J.H. Orr, Director of Prison Medical Services in England, described how

Mentally disordered offenders are entering prisons not because the net is insufficiently wide or discriminating but because hospital places are not forthcoming ... we imprison more mentally disordered offenders than under the old Lunacy and Mental Deficiency Acts. In 1931 (when the average prison population was about 12,500) 105 sentenced prisoners were recognized as suffering from mental *illness* and transferred to hospital. In 1976 the number of sentenced prisoners recognized as suffering from mental illness was more than double this figure, but the number transferred ... less than half.[61]

Psychiatric hospitals, meanwhile, were unwilling to take prisoners and lacked suitable facilities and secure units for managing 'difficult patients'.[62] At Pentonville in 1959, out of the 4,000 received into the prison, around twenty-four men were referred to the psychiatric unit at Wormwood Scrubs for medical treatment for mental disorders or to psychiatric treatment agencies on release. A similar proportion each year were certified insane. Certification was unpopular with one member of the medical staff at Pentonville who 'firmly believed that medical super-intendents of mental hospitals were very reluctant to receive offenders', tending to decertify them and send them back to prison as soon as possible.[63]

In Ireland, deinstitutionalisation and the closure of the Victorian asylums occurred at a slower pace, but the provision of psychiatric beds was still under pressure. Consequently, psychiatric hospitals were severely overcrowded. At the same time, the prison estate and prison

Visiting Committee, 14 Jan. 1918, Report to the Secretary of State for the Year 1917, p. 193.

[60] Andrew Scull, *Decarceration: Community Treatment and the Deviant – A Radical View*, 2nd edn (Oxford: Polity Press and New Brunswick, NJ: Rutgers University Press, 1984).

[61] J.H. Orr, 'The Imprisonment of Mentally Disordered Offenders', *British Journal of Psychiatry*, 133:3 (1978), 194–9, at p. 195.

[62] Richard Smith, 'The Mental Health of Prisoners: II The Fate of the Mentally Abnormal in Prison', *British Medical Journal* (*BMJ*), 288:386 (4 Feb. 1984), 386–8, at p. 386.

[63] Terence Morris and Pauline Morris, *Pentonville: A Sociological Study of an English Prison* (London and New York: Routledge, 1963), pp. 202–3.

population remained small until the 1960s, while there were very limited prison psychiatric services. The 1966 *Report of the Commission of Inquiry on Mental Illness* noted that the transfer of prisoners certified to be 'insane' to local psychiatric hospitals was not always suitable and recommended the use of Dundrum for this purpose.[64] They also proposed that the prison service make appropriate arrangements with relevant local health authorities to provide psychiatric services for prisoners.[65] Yet, in 1972 most major prisons did not employ psychiatric staff, though Mountjoy Prison's medical officer was a trained psychiatrist.[66] Prisons remained heavily dependent for psychiatric services on local hospitals as well as the Central Mental Hospital, Dundrum, which was also operating at full capacity. It took until the 1980s for the recommendation of the 1966 Commission of Inquiry to be implemented, and by then prisoners were only accepted at Dundrum as psychiatric facilities outside prison shrank further. Meanwhile prisons continued to be criticised for failing to provide psychological and psychiatric services.[67]

In 1991 the Home Office published a study by Professor John Gunn on mental health problems in English and Welsh prisons, based on interviews with just over 2,000 prisoners or 5 per cent of the sentenced prison population. Some 37 per cent of men and 56 per cent of women serving sentences of over six months were reported to have a medically identifiable mental health problem. It was estimated that over 9,000 prisoners were suffering from a significant mental disturbance, many of whom were in urgent need of transfer to hospital. At the same time, patients who did not need to be in psychiatric hospitals could not be moved to community facilities because of the shortfall in provision. As a result of this and with mental hospital services in England so lacking, 'mentally disordered people continue to accumulate in the prison system'.[68] In England and Wales the number of people in prison continued to rise dramatically, by 25,000 between 1995 and 2005, making many prisons very overcrowded, and prompting one *Guardian* report to

---

[64] *Report of the Commission of Inquiry on Mental Illness* (Dublin: Stationery Office, 1966), p. 93.
[65] Ibid., p.94.
[66] Oisín Wall, '"Embarrassing the State": The "Ordinary" Prisoner Rights Movement in Ireland, 1972–6', *Journal of Contemporary History*, 55:2 (2020), 388–410.
[67] Art O'Connor and Helen O'Neill, 'Male Prison Transfers to the Central Mental Hospital, a Special Hospital (1983–1988)', *Irish Journal of Psychological Medicine*, 7:2 (1990), 118–20,
[68] Wellcome Library, MIND Archive, SAMIN/B/91 Prisons, p. 4. See also J. Gunn, T. Maden and M. Swinton, 'Treatment Needs of Prisoners with Psychiatric Disorders', *BMJ*, 303:6798 (10 Aug. 1991), 338–41; J. Gunn, T. Maden and M. Swinton, *Mentally Disordered Prisoners* (London: Home Office, 1991).

assert that the UK was determined to emulate the US with its conditions of 'terrifying harshness'.[69] In 2005 *Troubled Inside*, a series of reports commissioned by the Prison Reform Trust, concluded that 72 per cent of male and 70 per cent of female sentenced prisoners suffered from two or more mental disorders.[70]

One of the striking features of late twentieth-century Irish prisons has been the build-up of mentally disordered offenders; in 1993 it was estimated that 5 per cent of prisoners in the Republic were mentally ill and there was a waiting list for admission to Dundrum.[71] Initiatives to improve poor psychiatric provision within prisons included the introduction of in-reach psychiatric teams to prisons in England and Ireland, and a diversion scheme was developed at Cloverhill remand prison in Ireland.[72] Yet, the problem persisted; in 2018 Michael Donnellan, Director General of the Irish Prison Service, informed a parliamentary committee that 8 per cent of prisoners had a diagnosed psychiatric condition and that managing 'people with severe and enduring mental illness posed a major challenge' to the Irish Prison Services. A departmental 'taskforce' was appointed to consider the mental health and addiction challenges of persons interacting with the criminal justice system in April 2021.[73]

Meanwhile, prison medical officers and prison medical services have in recent decades become more open and engaged, joining in critiques of the prison medical services and highlighting obstacles to the care of their prisoner patients. In parliamentary inquiries undertaken in the 1980s in the UK, prison medical officers reflected more openness on the issue of dual loyalty and expressed an eagerness to work with the rest of the medical profession.[74] Duvall has argued that this shift to collaboration began to replace assertions that prison medical officers have some form of particular knowledge and special experience in treating mentally ill prisoners.[75] Nonetheless, many reports remained critical of their role.

---

[69] Cited in Dora Rickford and Kimmett Edgar, *Troubled Inside: Responding to the Mental Health Needs of Men in Prison* (London: Prison Reform Trust, 2005), p. viii.

[70] Ibid., p. ix.

[71] Trish Hegarty, 'Study Finds 5% of Prison Inmates are Mentally Ill', *The Irish Times*, 24 Mar. 1993.

[72] Brendan Kelly, *'Hearing Voices': The History of Psychiatry in Ireland* (Dublin: Irish Academic Press, 2016), pp. 266–7.

[73] Mark Hilliard, 'Prisons Unable to Meet Rising Population's Need for Mental Healthcare', *The Irish Times*, 6 June 2020, http://justice.ie/en/JELR/Pages/PR21000071 [accessed 16 Apr. 2021].

[74] Nicholas Duvall, '"From Defensive Paranoia to … Openness to Outside Scrutiny": Prison Medical Officers in England and Wales in the 1970s and 1980s', *Medical History*, 62:1 (2018), 112–31.

[75] Ibid.

Richard Smith described in a series of articles in the *British Medical Journal* in 1983 the isolation of prison doctors, and, facing pressures of overcrowding, the loss of interest in reform and the role of psychiatric techniques in this process, even though it was acknowledged by mid-century that 'the greater part of the work lies in the psychiatric field'.[76] Still referring in 2005 to the crisis in the prison medical service, Gunn, for example, found many doctors excessively preoccupied with the problem of malingering, as well as a huge level of unmet psychiatric need and overuse of psychotropic drugs, while there were fewer opportunities for doctors to keep up with developments in medicine and many struggled to resolve the tension between managerial and physician roles; 'it is difficult for doctors to separate their responsibility to patients as a doctor from the need to adapt medical care to meet the requirements of the current prison system'.[77] In England responsibility for commissioning all health care services for prisoners was transferred to the National Health Service in 2013, but still as prison populations continue to grow, so too do the number of people in prison who are reported as having mental health diagnoses, and efforts to achieve an equivalent health service flounder in a situation of general shortfalls in psychiatric services. In Ireland too integration of prison medical services with general health systems remains the goal, and in 2016 Judge Michael Reilly, Inspector of Prisons, produced a report on prison health care that strongly advocated for the incorporation of prison health care into the Irish Health Service Executive.[78]

The residue of the nineteenth-century prison system remains with us today, not only in the physical structures of prison estates in England and Ireland, but also in prison disciplines that still emphasise order and uniformity, and in the imposition of solitary confinement, no longer a philosophy and method of reform, but a form of protection, or means of dealing with disruptive behaviour among prisoners, the poor physical state of prisons, overcrowding and the shortage of prison staff and resources. Many prisoners continue to be confined in restricted regimes spending most of their day in cellular isolation. Some request removal to these restricted regimes, 'prisons within prisons', for protection from other violent inmates or to get away from drugs, though they may not

---

[76] Richard Smith, 'History of the Prison Medical Services', *BMJ*, 287:6407 (10 Dec. 1983), 1786–8, at p. 1787.

[77] Adam Sampson, 'Crisis in the Prison Medical Service', in Rickford and Edgar, *Troubled Inside*, n.p.

[78] Michael Reilly, *Healthcare in Irish Prisons* (Nenagh: Inspector of Prisons, 2016).

be fully aware of the extent of their isolation, and 'segs' can become 'a breeding ground for mental health problems'.[79]

A recent report on Wormwood Scrubs Prison in London revealed that many prisoners had less than two hours a day 'unlocked' and all had only forty minutes of outdoor exercise a day, less than the time prescribed at Pentonville in 1842.[80] Despite the Irish Prison Service's commitment to reduce solitary confinement and restricted regimes, in April 2017, 430 prisoners were on restricted regimes, defined as a minimum of nineteen hours locked in cells.[81] In 2001, the study *Out of Sight, Out of Mind* found that 78 per cent of prisoners in solitary confinement in Irish prisons were mentally ill.[82] The Irish Penal Reform Trust's 2018 report on solitary confinement in Irish prisons highlighted the 'exceptional and devastating harm to prisoners' mental health that can be caused by extended periods of isolation', and sought the abolition of 'the practice of holding any category of prisoner on 22- or 23-hour lock-up' and that such restrictive regimes should be an implemented as an 'exceptional measure'.[83] They noted that the Irish Prison Service anticipated 11 per cent of the prison population would be subject to restricted regimes in the coming years and that designated parts of Mountjoy Male Prison and the Midlands Prison would be classed as 'protection prisons'. This included a unit at the Midlands Prison for a small number of 'violent and disruptive' prisoners, managed jointly by the Prison Psychological Service and the prison's operational staff.[84] In the late nineteenth century, as detailed in Chapter 4, violent behaviour on the part of mentally ill prisoners that disrupted prison discipline was likely to trigger removals to lunatic asylums. Nowadays that opportunity rarely exists and forensic hospitals, including Dundrum Central Mental Hospital, operate at full capacity. Prisoners with severe psychiatric conditions, some of whom are violent, suicidal or liable to self-harm, are inappropriately retained in prisons in Safety Observation Cells, a practice criticised by the European

---

[79] Erwin James, 'Prison Segregation Units are a Breeding Ground for Mental Health Problems', *The Guardian*, 17 Dec. 2015.

[80] HM Prisons Inspectorate, *Report of Announced Inspection of HMP Wormwood Scrubs 30 November–4 December 2015* (London: HM Inspectorate of Prisons, 2016): www.justiceinspectorates.gov.uk/hmiprisons/wp-content/uploads/sites/4/2016/04/Wormwood-Scrubs-web2015.pdf [accessed 28 Nov. 2017].

[81] Irish Penal Reform Trust, *Submission to the Second Periodic Review of Ireland under the United Nations Convention against Torture and Other Cruel, Inhuman or Degrading Treatment or Punishment* (Dublin: Irish Penal Reform Trust, 2017), p. 17.

[82] Cited in Nuala Haughey, '78% of Solitary Prisoners Mentally Ill', *The Irish Times*, 20 Feb. 2001.

[83] Agnieszka Martynowicz and Linda Moore, *Behind the Door: Solitary Confinement in the Irish Penal System* (Dublin: Irish Penal Reform Trust, 2018), p. 3.

[84] Ibid., pp. 6–7.

Committee for the Prevention of Torture during an inspection of Irish prisons in 2015.[85]

While there is no question that in many regards conditions have improved, and that prison psychiatry and the intention to treat and care for mentally ill prisoners effectively has moved on considerably, some prisons remain desperately overcrowded, resources are scarce and psychiatric support limited both within and outside prisons. People in prison had and still have higher rates of mental illness than the general population, those with mental health problem are more likely to be admitted to prison, and prisons exacerbate mental health problems. The Irish Penal Reform Trust report extensively referenced *Deep Custody*, produced by the English Prison Reform Trust in 2015, which also highlighted the toxic effects of segregation, 'social isolation, reduced sensory input/ enforced idleness and increased control of prisoners'.[86] The findings of the report and particularly the responses of prisoners subjected to isolation, echo and reproduce the observations of prison authors in the late nineteenth century, and those collected by John Galsworthy at Lewes Prison in 1909, with the prisoners he spoke to describing how the 'Walls seem to close in.... I get blankness in the brain – have to stop reading', 'Its hell upon earth', and 'Almost unbearable depression'.[87] In a similar way the prisoners interviewed for the report *Deep Custody* explained 'The longer you're here, the more you develop disorders. Being in such a small space has such an effect on your social skills.... Its isolation to an extreme', 'All my mental health problems start kicking in – been really depressed listening to all the voices a lot more, just stuck in my thoughts' and 'Your head does go ... only so many times you can speak to four walls'.[88]

---

[85] *Report to the Government of Ireland on the Visit to Ireland Carried Out by the European Committee for the Prevention of Torture and Inhuman or Degrading Treatment or Punishment (CPT)* (Strasbourg: Council of Europe, 2015), www.coe.int/en/web/cpt/ireland [accessed 14 Feb. 2020].

[86] Sharon Shalev and Kimmett Edgar, *Deep Custody: Segregation Units and Close Supervision Centres in England and Wales* (London: Prison Reform Trust, 2015), p. 91.

[87] TNA, HO45/13658, Prisons and Prisoners, A Minute on Separate Confinement, forwarded to the Home Secretary and Prison Commissioners, pp. 39–40.

[88] Shalev and Edgar, *Deep Custody*, pp. 54–5, 94.

Bibliography

Primary Sources

National Archives of Ireland (NAI)

Government Prison Office (GPO):
GPO/Letter Books (LB), 'A' Series, Vols 1–10, May 1846–July 1874.
GPO/LB, 'B' Series, Vols 12–25, July 1849–July 1874.
GPO/LB, Vol. 33, Convict Removal Book, 1857–60.
GPO/Incoming Correspondence Registers and Indexes, Vols 2–46, 1851–79.
GPO/Incoming Correspondence (CORR), 1851–79:
GPO/CORR/1851/Mountjoy.
GPO/CORR/1853/Antrim.
GPO/CORR/1853/Mountjoy.
GPO/CORR/1853/Spike Island.
GPO/CORR/1853/Philipstown.
GPO/CORR/1854/Antrim.
GPO/CORR/1854/Mountjoy.
GPO/CORR/1854/Spike Island.
GPO/CORR/1854/Philipstown.
GPO/CORR/1855/Mountjoy.
GPO/CORR/1855/Philipstown.
GPO/CORR/1855/Spike Island.
GPO/CORR/1856/Antrim.
GPO/CORR/1856/Mountjoy.
GPO/CORR/1856/Philipstown.
GPO/CORR/1856/Spike Island.
GPO/CORR/1857/Antrim.
GPO/CORR/1857/Mountjoy.
GPO/CORR/1857/Philipstown.
GPO/CORR/1857/Spike Island.
GPO/CORR/1858/Antrim.
GPO/CORR/1858/Mountjoy (Male).
GPO/CORR/1858/Philipstown.
GPO/CORR/1858/Spike Island.
GPO/CORR/1859/Antrim.
GPO/CORR/1859/Mountjoy (Male) Prison.

GPO/CORR/1859/Mountjoy (Female) Prison.
GPO/CORR/1859/Philipstown.
GPO/CORR/1859/Spike Island.
GPO/CORR/1860/Antrim.
GPO/CORR/1860/Mountjoy (Male) Prison.
GPO/CORR/1860/Mountjoy (Female) Prison.
GPO/CORR/1860/Philipstown.
GPO/CORR/1861/Antrim.
GPO/CORR/1861/Mountjoy (Male) Prison.
GPO/CORR/1861/Mountjoy (Female) Prison.
GPO/CORR/1861/Philipstown.
GPO/CORR/1862/Antrim.
GPO/CORR/1862/Mountjoy (Male) Prison.
GPO/CORR/1862/Mountjoy (Female) Prison.
GPO/CORR/1862/Philipstown.
GPO/CORR/1863/Antrim.
GPO/CORR/1863/Mountjoy (Male) Prison.
GPO/CORR/1863/Mountjoy (Female) Prison.
GPO/CORR/1864/Mountjoy (Male) Prison.
GPO/CORR/1864/Mountjoy (Female) Prison.
GPO/CORR/1865/Mountjoy (Male) Prison.
GPO/CORR/1865/Mountjoy (Female) Prison.
GPO/CORR/1866/Mountjoy (Male) Prison.
GPO/CORR/1866/Mountjoy (Female) Prison.
GPO/CORR/1867/Mountjoy (Male) Prison.
GPO/CORR/1867/Mountjoy (Female) Prison.
GPO/CORR/1868/Mountjoy (Male) Prison.
GPO/CORR/1868/Mountjoy (Female) Prison.
GPO/CORR/1869/Mountjoy (Male) Prison.
GPO/CORR/1869/Mountjoy (Female) Prison.
GPO/CORR/1872/Government.
GPO/CORR/1872/Mountjoy (Male) Prison.
GPO/CORR/1872/Spike Island Prison.
GPO/CORR/1873/Mountjoy (Male) Prison.
GPO/CORR/1873/Mountjoy (Female) Prison.
GPO/CORR/1873/Spike Island Prison.
GPO/CORR/1874/nos. 1–588.
GPO/CORR/1875/nos. 589–1259.
GPO/Philipstown Prison (PN):
GPO/PN/2, Headmaster's Journal, June 1857–July 1866.
GPO/PN/4, Philipstown Character Book, 1847–62.
GPO/PN/5, Philipstown Character Book, 1851–59.
GPO/Miscellaneous (XB)/3, Convict Prisons Minute Book, 1846–48.
Inspectors General of Prisons (IGP):
IGP/Correspondence/Boxes 1–11, Administrative, 1843–56.
IGP/Letter Books (LB), Vols 1–2, Jan. 1857–Dec. 1865.
General Prisons Board (GPB):
GPB/Minute Books (MB)/Vols 1–12, Nov. 1877–Feb. 1920.

GPB/Incoming Correspondence Registers and Indexes, Vols 1–133, 1878–1919.
GPB/Incoming Correspondence (CORR), 1878–1925:
GPB/CORR/1883/12222–12949 [Box].
GPB/CORR/1883/12950–13189 [Box].
GPB/CORR/1884/5381.
GPB/CORR/1884/4270–4871 [Box].
GPB/CORR/1884/7152–7742 [Box].
GPB/CORR/1884/11045.
GPB/CORR/1884/15050.
GPB/CORR/1884/15924.
GPB/CORR/1885/571.
GPB/CORR/1885/881.
GPB/CORR/1885/7084.
GPB/CORR/1885/7123.
GPB/CORR/1886/6836.
GPB/CORR/1886/6837.
GPB/CORR/1886/6969.
GPB/CORR/1886/6971.
GPB/CORR/1886/7036.
GPB/CORR/1886/7076.
GPB/CORR/1887/9419.
GPB/CORR/1887/9575.
GPB/CORR/1887/9688.
GPB/CORR/1887/13203–13883 [Box].
GPB/CORR/1888/927.
GPB/CORR/1888/942.
GPB/CORR/1888/1072.
GPB/CORR/1888/1195.
GPB/CORR/1888/1365.
GPB/CORR/1888/3881.
GPB/CORR/1888/4798.
GPB/CORR/1888/4924.
GPB/CORR/1888/4927.
GPB/CORR/1888/4929.
GPB/CORR/1888/4991.
GPB/CORR/1888/5280.
GPB/CORR/1888/5468.
GPB/CORR/1888/6679.
GPB/CORR/1888/8013–8487 [Box].
GPB/CORR/1888/12875–13307 [Box].
GPB/CORR/1888/13247.
GPB/CORR/1889/5730–6147 [Box].
GPB/CORR/1889/11098–11365 [Box].
GPB/CORR/1889/9135–9621 [Box].
GPB/CORR/1890/851–1100 [Box].
GPB/CORR/1890/3621–4171 [Box].
GPB/CORR/1890/6943–7457 [Box].

GPB/CORR/1890/8069–9156 [Box].
GPB/CORR/1890/9157–9720 [Box].
GPB/CORR/1890/12165–12730 [Box].
GPB/CORR/1891/571–1084 [Box].
GPB/CORR/1891/7937–8444 [Box].
GPB/CORR/1891/10701–11023 [Box].
GPB/CORR/1891/11024–11672 [Box].
GPB/CORR/1891/1683–2129 [Box].
GPB/CORR/1892/6030–6328 [Box].
GPB/CORR/1892/10799–11400 [Box].
GPB/CORR/1893/1650–1949 [Box].
GPB/CORR/1893/14806–15229 [Box].
GPB/CORR/1893/14183–14805 [Box].
GPB/CORR/1894/1–636 [Box].
GPB/CORR/1894/2039–2500 [Box].
GPB/CORR/1894/2235.
GPB/CORR/1894/3415–3912 [Box].
GPB/CORR/1894/5030–5543 [Box].
GPB/CORR/1895/1650–2136 [Box].
GPB/CORR/1898/10490–11000 [Box].
GPB/CORR/1908/3855–4557 [Box].
GPB/CORR/1908/1358–2200 [Box].
GPB/CORR/1908/11337–11735 [Box].
GPB/CORR/1909/13636–13975 [Box].
GPB/CORR/1918/498–1007 [Box].
GPB/CORR/1918/5538–5863 [Box].
GPB/CORR/1918/8307–8330 [Box].
GPB/Incoming Correspondence (CORR)/Supplementary (SUPP):
GPB/CORR/SUPP/1879–1880 [Year].
GPB/CORR/SUPP/1879/18466.
GPB/CORR/SUPP/1881–82.
GPB/Rules and Instructions (RL):
GPB/RL/1, General Prisons Board Circulars, 1877–84.
GPB/RL/2, General Prisons Board Circulars, 1886–1909.
GPB/RL/3, General Prisons Board Circulars, 1893–1902.
GPB/RL/4, General Prisons Board Circulars, 1902–06.
GPB/RL/5, General Prisons Board Circulars, 1907–11.
GPB/RL/6, General Prisons Board Circulars, 1917–21.
GPB/RL/11, Instructions to Inspectors, 1878–1911.
GPB/RL/13, General Orders and Instructions, 1879–1917.
GPB/RL/14, Office Handbook, 1908.
GPB/Penal Files (PEN):
GPB/PEN/3/8 (Catherine Murray).
GPB/PEN/3/12 (Bridget Magrath).
GPB/PEN/3/13 (Patrick Gordon).
GPB/PEN/3/14 (William Hurley).
GPB/PEN/3/15 (Lawrence Murphy).
GPB/PEN/3/17 (Samuel Hogan).

GPB/PEN/3/19 (Mary Mulroy).
GPB/PEN/3/20 (John McNally).
GPB/PEN/3/21 (Michael Kennedy).
GPB/PEN/3/23 (Edward Fox).
GPB/PEN/3/25 (Thomas Dignam).
GPB/PEN/3/26 (John Lalor).
GPB/PEN/3/27 (Edward Sullivan).
GPB/PEN/3/28 (John Walsh).
GPB/PEN/3/29 (Timothy Horgan).
GPB/PEN/3/30 (Thomas Kearney).
GPB/PEN/3/31 (Thomas Harrison).
GPB/PEN/3/32 (William Reilly).
GPB/PEN/3/33 (Lawrence McLeavy).
GPB/PEN/3/34 (Patrick Sheridan).
GPB/PEN/3/39 (Andrew Martin).
GPB/PEN/3/40 (Thomas McCune).
GPB/PEN/3/41 (William Williamson, otherwise John O'Hare).
GPB/PEN/3/42 (John Gibbons).
GPB/PEN/3/43 (Bryan Cormican).
GPB/PEN/3/44 (Patrick Bowens).
GPB/PEN/3/45 (John McCaffrey).
GPB/PEN/3/46 (Malachy Bowens).
GPB/PEN/3/47 (Anne Cooney).
GPB/PEN/3/48 (Bridget Hayes, otherwise Bridget O'Neill).
GPB/PEN/3/49 (Mary Dwyer).
GPB/PEN/3/50 (John Kelly).
GPB/PEN/3/51 (James McLaughlin).
GPB/PEN/3/52 (Edward Mathews).
GPB/PEN/3/53 (John Herbert).
GPB/PEN/3/54 (James Byrne).
GPB/PEN/3/55 (John Byrne).
GPB/PEN/3/56 (Anne Hall, otherwise Mary McCabe).
GPB/PEN/3/57 (James Markey).
GPB/PEN/3/58 (Denis Flanagan).
GPB/PEN/3/60 (William Doherty).
GPB/PEN/3/61 (James Slattery).
Chief Secretary's Office Registered Papers (CSORP):
CSORP/1874/4814, Weakminded Prisoners.
CSORP/1905/12904, *Report on the Committee of Inquiry into Certain Doubtful Cases of Insanity Amongst Convicts and Person Detained,* 1905.

The National Archives (TNA)

Home Office and Prison Commission (PCOM): Prisons Records:
PCOM 2/84–89, Pentonville Prison, Middlesex: Minute Books, 1842–50.
PCOM 2/90, Pentonville Prison, Middlesex: Commissioner's Visiting Book, 1843–54.

PCOM 2/93, Pentonville Prison, Middlesex: Visitors' Book, 1862–63.
PCOM 2/94, Pentonville Prison, Middlesex: Visitors' Book, 1842–49.
PCOM 2/96, Pentonville Prison, Middlesex: Visitors' Order Book, 1849–50.
PCOM 2/353, Pentonville Prison, Middlesex: Chaplain's Journal, May 1846–Mar. 1851.
Ministry of Health (MH) Papers:
MH 51/754, Insane or Imbecile Prisoners: Duties of Magistrates, 1861.
Home Office (HO) Papers:
HO 45/1451, Lunacy: Poor Law and Paupers; Prisons and Prisoners, Sept. 1846–Jan. 1849.
HO 45/9525, Lunacy: Report on Accommodation at Broadmoor Asylum and Question of Removing Lunatic Convicts from Woking Prison to Broadmoor, 1874–87.
HO 45/9632/A26128, Lunacy: Salaries of Drs. Gover and Orange. Arrangements and Fees for Examinations of Prisoners on Capital Charge, as to Insanity, 1883–86.
HO 45/9640/A34434, Prisons and Prisoners (4) Other: Medical Examination of Prisoners Unfit for Prison Discipline with a View to Decreasing Number of Deaths in Prisons, 1884–89.
HO 45/9695/A9757, Prisons and Prisoners (3) Prisoners – Visiting Committees and Boards of Visitors: Liverpool Prison. Annual Reports of Visiting Committee, 1892–95.
HO 45/9955/V10698, Lunacy: Prison Department Reports on Criminal Lunatics Not under Definite Sentence Whose Maintenance Is Chargeable to Prison Vote, 1888–96.
HO 45/13658, Prisons and Prisoners: Separate or Cellular Confinement, 1909–30.
HO 114/513/X66658, Lunacy: Edward Cox. Injuries to Insane Prisoner Inquiry, 1897–98.
HO 144/469/X6313, Lunacy: Removal to Asylum of Prisoners Certified Insane, 1885.
HO 144/477/X22478, Lunacy: Prisoner Admitted to Lunatic Asylum on the Day Following His Discharge from Prison, 1889 (1897).
HO 144/658/V/12914, Prisons and Prisoners (4) Other: Committal to Prison of Prisoners Medically or Mentally Unfit for Prison Discipline, 1889–1902.
Treasury Board Papers:
T 1.13216, Lunacy Commission: Dundrum Criminal Lunatic Asylum Dublin, Report upon Dundrum Lunatic Asylum (printed), n.d. (stamped by Treasury, 20 Feb. 1882).
Admiralty Papers (ADM):
ADM 101/69/6, Medical Journal of the *Stratheden*, Convict Ship, from 22 July 1845 to 7 Jan. 1846 by Henry Baker, Surgeon and Superintendent.
ADM 101/49/10, Medical Journal of the *Marion*, Convict Ship, for 1 Sept. 1847 to 5 Feb. 1848 by John Anderson, Surgeon and Superintendent.

National Library of Ireland

Bye-laws for the City of Dublin Prisons by the Board of Superintendence (Dublin, 1862).
Bye-laws, Rules and Regulations of the County of Londonderry Gaol (Londonderry, 1862).
Bye-laws, Rules and Regulations of the County of Kildare Gaol (Naas, 1861).
Rules to be Observed in Mountjoy Male Prison (Dublin, 1867).
Mayo Papers, MS 43,817/1, Letter from Walter Crofton to Lord Naas, 8 Oct. 1866.

Berkshire Record Office (BRO)

BRO, Q/SO/22–25, County of Berkshire Sessions Order Books, 1849–58.

Dublin City Archives

Dublin City Council, Board of Superintendence of the City of Dublin Prisons, Minute Books:
BSP/mins/02, Minute Book, 2 Oct. 1851–14 Dec. 1853.
BSP/mins/03, Minute Book, 14 Dec. 1853–23 Dec. 1856.
BSP/mins/04, Minute Book, 7 Jan. 1857–12 July 1859.
Dublin City Council (DCC), Visiting Committee to Dublin City Prisons, Minute Books:
DCC/Prisons/Mins/01, Minute Book, 16 July 1878–25 Mar. 1887.
DCC/Prisons/Mins/02, Minute Book, 21 Jan. 1888–11 July 1900.
DCC/Prisons/Mins/03, Minute Book, 8 Aug. 1900–10 Feb. 1916.
DCC/Prisons/Mins/04, Minute Book, 31 Jan. 1916–15 Apr. 1920: Mountjoy Prison.
Trustees of Newgate Prison (NP):
DCC/NP/Abst/01, Abstract of Minutes, 4 Feb. 1865–21 Feb. 1872.
Richmond Female Penitentiary/Grangegorman Prison:
BSP/Rich/Abst/01, Abstracts of Minutes of Commissioners, 1864–69.
BSP/Rich/Abst/02, Abstracts of Minutes of Commissioners, 1874–75.
Printed Reports:
DCC/Prisons/Reports/01, Printed Reports, 1845–59.
DCC/Prisons/Reports/03, Printed Reports, 1866–70.
DCC/Prisons/Reports/04, Printed Reports, 1870–74.
Report of the Visiting Committee of Justices on the City Prisons (Report No. 130, submitted 29 June 1881).
Report of the Visiting Committee of Justices on the City Prisons (Report No. 15, submitted 10 Dec. 1882).
Report of the Visiting Committee of City Prisons, 1887–1918.

Minutes of the Municipal Council of the City of Dublin, Jan.–Dec. 1881.

Minutes of the Municipal Council of the City of Dublin, Jan.–Dec. 1882.

Lancashire Archives

Lancashire Archives, QAM 4/2, Register of Class 1 Lunatics, Covering Admissions 4 Feb. 1869–15 Feb. 1893.

Liverpool Record Office (LRO)

H365.3 ANN, *Kirkdale Gaol Chaplain's Annual Report* (Preston, 1848). Liverpool Borough Gaol:

347 JUS/4/2/1, *Rules and Regulations for the Government of the Liverpool Borough Gaol and House of Correction at Walton-on-the-Hill, Near Liverpool* (1855).

347 JUS/4/2/2, *By-laws of the Liverpool Borough Prison for the Regulation of All Such Matters as Lie within the Discretion of the Visiting Justices* (1865–74).

347 JUS 4/1/1, Minutes of Justices Sessions Gaol and House of Correction, Oct. 1837–Jan. 1851.

347 JUS 4/1/2, Minutes of Justices Sessions Gaol and House of Correction, Oct. 1864–Jan. 1870.

365.32 BOR (loose reports):

Reports of the Governor, Chaplain, Prison Minister and Surgeon, of the Liverpool Borough Prison, Presented to the Court of Gaol Sessions, Holden on the 28th Day of October, 1869.

Report of Visiting Justices of the Borough Gaol, n.d., 1868–69.

H352 COU, Borough of Liverpool. Proceedings of the Council, 1863–64.

H352 COU, Borough of Liverpool. Proceedings of the Council, 1876–77.

347 MAG/1/2/1, Minutes of the Quarterly and Annual Meetings of the Visiting Justices of the Borough Gaol and House of Correction, also Special Gaol Sessions, 1852–64.

347 MAG 1/2/2, Proceedings of the Meetings of the Liverpool Justices of the Peace, Minutes, 1870–78.

347 MAG 1/3/1A, Proceedings of the Meetings of the Liverpool Justices of the Peace, Minute Book, Feb. 1856–Sept. 1866.

347 MAG 1/3/3, Proceedings of the Meetings of the Visiting Committee, Liverpool Borough Gaol, Apr. 1878–June 1897.

347 MAG 1/3/4, Proceedings at the Meetings of the Visiting Committee, Visiting Committee Minutes, July 1897–Oct. 1904.

347 MAG 1/3/5, Proceedings at the Meetings of the Visiting Committee of Liverpool Prison, Nov. 1904–Sept. 1912.

347 MAG 1/3/6, Proceedings at the Meetings of the Visiting Committee of Liverpool Prison, Oct. 1912–Dec. 1919.

Rainhill Asylum:
M614 RAI/40/2/1, *Annual Reports of the Lancashire Asylums, 1866–70.*
M614 RAI/40/2/2, *Annual Reports of the Lancashire Asylums, 1871–74.*
M614 RAI/40/2/3, *Annual Reports of the Lancashire Asylums, 1875–78.*
M614 RAI/40/2/4, *Reports of the County Lunatic Asylums at Rainhill, Lancaster, Prestwich and Whittingham, 1879–82.*
M614 RAI/40/2/5, *Reports of the County Lunatic Asylums at Lancaster, Rainhill, Prestwich, and Whittingham, 1883–86.*
M614 RAI/40/2/6, *Reports of the County Lunatic Asylums at Lancaster, Rainhill, Prestwich, and Whittingham, 1887–90.*
M614 RAI/8/5, Rainhill Asylum Female Casebook, Feb. 1865–Jan. 1870.
M614 RAI/8/6, Rainhill Asylum Female Casebook, Jan. 1870–Oct. 1873.
M614 RAI/8/7, Rainhill Asylum Female Casebook, Oct. 1873–July 1878.
M614 RAI/8/8, Rainhill Asylum Female Casebook, July 1878–July 1882.
M614 RAI/8/9, Rainhill Asylum Female Casebook, July 1882–Sept. 1885.
M614 RAI/8/16, Rainhill Asylum Female Casebook, July 1892–Mar. 1894.
M614 RAI/8/18, Rainhill Asylum Female Casebook, Oct. 1895–July 1897.
M614 RAI 8/25, Rainhill Asylum Female Casebook, Feb. 1905–May 1906.
M614 RAI/11/2, Rainhill Asylum Male Casebook, Feb. 1857–May 1861.
M614 RAI/11/4, Rainhill Asylum Male Casebook, June 1865–May 1870.
M614 RAI/11/5, Rainhill Asylum Male Casebook, May 1870–Dec. 1873.
M614 RAI 11/6, Rainhill Asylum Male Casebook, Dec. 1873–July 1877.
M614 RAI/11/7, Rainhill Asylum Male Casebook, July 1877–June 1881.
M614 RAI/11/16, Rainhill Asylum Male Casebook, Dec. 1894–June 1896.
M614 RAI/11/17, Rainhill Asylum Male Casebook, June 1896–Nov. 1897.
M614 RAI/11/20, Rainhill Asylum Male Casebook, June 1899–July 1900.
M614 RAI/11/21, Rainhill Asylum Male Casebook, July 1900–Nov. 1901.

London Metropolitan Archives (LMA)

New Prison or House of Detention, Clerkenwell (later Clerkenwell Prison):
MA/G/CLE/114–679, Box containing correspondence in seven bundles.
MA/G/CLE/114–177/Item no. 147, Return of the number of prisoners charged with attempting to commit suicide from 1847 to 1859.
MA/G/CLE/114–177/Item no. 156, *Annual Report of the Governor, and of the Surgeon and Chaplain,* 1859.
MA/G/CLE/190/Item no. 184, *Report of the Visiting Justices of the House of Correction,* 1859.
MA/G/CLE/205–319 [Jan.–Dec. 1860]/Item no. 210, Police court charge, Marylebone Police Court, 28 Jan. 1860.
MA/G/CLE/205–319 [Jan.–Dec. 1860]/Item no. 212, Letter from John Skaife, Clerk, Visiting Justices to Middlesex House of Detention, Clerkenwell, 16 Feb. 1860.
MA/G/CLE/205–319 [Jan.–Dec. 1860]/Item no. 215, Letter from Home Secretary to Visiting Justices, approval of Elizabeth Livermore removal, 17 Feb. 1860.

MA/G/CLE/205–319 [Jan.–Dec. 1860]/Item no. 218, Letter from John Skaife, Clerk, Visiting Justices to Middlesex House of Detention, Clerkenwell, 28 Feb. 1860.

ACC/3588, Burt J. (Warder at H.M. Prison, Wormwood Scrubs), Reminiscences of Twenty-Nine and Half Years as an Officer in H. M. Prison Wormwood Scrubs.

Modern Records Centre, University of Warwick

Howard League Papers:
MSS.16A/7/1/William Tallack: Manuscript Notebook Recording Visit to Ireland and Inspections of *Irish Prisons*, June 1895.

MSS.16X/1/7, Annual Reports of the Howard Association, 1897–1901, with Pamphlets of the Howard Association, c. 1865–1901.

Royal College of Physicians of Ireland, Heritage Centre

Conolly Norman Lectures, 1905–07:
CN/1, First Series, March–May 1905, Lecture, 'The Maniacal State', 3 Mar. 1905.

TPCK/5, Kirkpatrick Medical Biographies.

Wakefield County Record Office

QS 10/54–60, Quarter Sessions Order Books, 1841–66.

Wellcome Library

Reports of the Superintendent and Chaplain of Broadmoor Criminal Lunatic Asylum, for the Years 1864–70 (1865–71).

Reports of the Superintendent and Chaplain of Broadmoor Criminal Lunatic Asylum, for the Year 1873 (1874).

Reports upon Broadmoor Criminal Lunatic Asylum, with Statistical Tables, for the Year 1885 (1887).

County Lunatic Asylums Reports Lancashire (Lancaster, Prestwich, Rainhill) (1851–58).

MIND Archive, SAMIN/B/91 Prisons.

Wolfson Centre for Archival Research, Birmingham Central Library

LS11/2/5/13, *Regulations for the Government of the Prison, Provided and Established at Birmingham, in and for the Borough of Birmingham, 1849*.

LS11/2/5/12, *Rules and Regulations for the Government of the Common Gaol and House of Correction of the Borough of Birmingham, 1860*.

Birmingham Vol. 16 [pamphlets], 64872 System of Discipline in Borough Gaol:

J. Allday, *True Account of the Proceedings Leading to, and a Full & Authentic Report of, The Searching Inquiry, by Her Majesty's Commissioners, into the Horrible System of Discipline Practised at the Borough Gaol of Birmingham* [1853].

Official Papers

Statutes

27 Geo.III, c.39, Prisoners (Ireland) Act (1787).

57 Geo.III, c.106, Asylums for the Lunatic Poor (Ireland) Act (1817).

1&2 Geo. IV, c.33, Lunacy (Ireland) Act (1821).

7 Geo. IV, c.74, Prisons (Ireland) Act (1826).

1&2 Vict., c.27, Criminal Lunatics (Ireland) Act (1838).

2&3 Vict., c.56, Prisons Act (1839).

3&4 Vict., c.44, Prisons (Ireland) Act (1840).

3&4 Vict., c.54, Insane Prisoners Act (1840).

5&6 Vict., c.29, Pentonville Prison Act (1842).

17&18 Vict., c.76, Convict Prisons Act (1854).

19&20 Vict., c.68, Prisons (Ireland) Act (1856).

28&29 Vict., c.126, Prison Act (1865).

36&37 Vict., c.49, General Prisons (Ireland) Act (1877).

38&39 Vict., c.67, Lunatic Asylums Act (1875).

40&41 Vict., c.21, Prison Act (1877).

47&48 Vict., c.64, Criminal Lunatics Act (1884).

Hansard Parliamentary Debates (HL and HC).

Annual Reports

Report of Inspectors of Prisons of Great Britain, Part 1 (1837–38) [141].

Reports of the Inspectors of Prisons of Great Britain, Northern and Eastern District, 1836–57.

Reports of the Inspectors of Prisons of Great Britain, Northern District, Annual Reports, 1858–78.

Annual Reports of the Commissioners for the Government of the Pentonville Prison (RCGPP), 1843–50.

Annual Reports of the Commissioners in Lunacy, 1846–98.

Annual Reports of the Directors of Convict Prisons (RDCP), 1850–95.

Annual Reports of the Commissioners of Prisons, 1878–95.

Annual Reports of the Commissioners of Prisons and the Directors of Convict Prisons, 1895–1900.

Annual Reports of the Inspector of Government Prisons in Ireland, 1850–52.

Annual Reports of the Directors of Convict Prisons in Ireland (RDCPI), 1854–77.

Annual Reports of the Inspectors General of Prisons in Ireland (RIGPI), 1818–76.
Annual Reports of the General Prisons Board (RGPBI), 1879–1911.
Annual Reports of the District, Local and Private Lunatic Asylums in Ireland, 1843–49.
Annual Reports of the District, Criminal and Private Lunatic Asylums in Ireland, 1851–99.
Annual Report of Commissioners of Public Works (Ireland), 1847–48 (1848) [983].

Rules
Rules for Local Prisons, Ireland (1878–79) [261].
Copies of Two Orders in Council Approving of Rules and Special Rules Made by the General Prisons Board for Ireland, 1885 (1884–85) [132].

Commissions, Reports and Inquiries
Report from the Select Committee on the Penitentiary at Millbank (1824) [408].
Report of the Commissioners Directed by the Lord Lieutenant of Ireland to Inquire into the State of the Richmond Penitentiary in Dublin (1826–27) [335].
Report of William Crawford, Esq., on the Penitentiaries of the United States (1834) [593].
Report from the Select Committee of the House of Lords Appointed to Consider the State of the Lunatic Poor in Ireland (1843) [625].
Joshua Jebb, Second Report of the Surveyor-General of Prisons (1847) [867].
Report from the Select Committee on Prison Discipline Together with the Proceedings of the Committee, Minutes of Evidence, Appendix and Index [Grey Committee] (1850) [632].
Royal Commission of Inquiry into the Condition and Treatment of the Prisoners Confined in Birmingham Borough Prison (1854) [1809].
Convict Prisons (Ireland). Copies of Correspondence Relative to the Management and Discipline of Convict Prisons, and the Extension of Prison Accommodation, with Reports of Commissioners (1854) [344].
Prisons (Separate Confinement) (1856) [163].
Report from the Select Committee of the House of Lords on the Present State of Discipline in Gaols and Houses of Correction [Carnarvon Committee] (1863) [499].
Royal Commission to Inquire into Operation of Acts Relating to Transportation and Penal Servitude. Report, Appendix, Minutes of Evidence [Royal Commission on Transportation and Penal Servitude] (1863) [3190] [3190–I].
Correspondence between the Secretary of State for the Home Department and the Directors of Convict Prisons, on the

Recommendations of the Royal Commission on the Penal Servitude Acts (1864) [61].

Report of Commissioners in Lunacy on the Present Condition of Broadmoor Criminal Lunatic Asylum and Its Inmates (1864) [216].

Report on the District, Criminal and Private Lunatics Asylums in Ireland, 1866 (1866) [3721].

Correspondence Relative to Change in Medical Management of Mountjoy Convict Prison 1868 (1867–68) [502].

Report of the Committee on Dietaries in County and Borough Gaols, Ireland (1867–68) [3981].

Copy of a Report Made by the Commissioners of Lunacy, on the 14th October 1868 upon Broadmoor Criminal Lunatic Asylum (1868–69) [244].

Report of the Committee Appointed to Inquire into the Dietaries of the Prisons in England and Wales Subject to the Prison Acts 1865 and 1877 (1878) [C.95].

Report from a Committee Appointed to Inquire into Certain Matters Relating to the Broadmoor Criminal Lunatic Asylum (1877) [C.1674].

Royal Commission into Penal Servitude Acts, Minutes of Evidence [Kimberley Commission] (1878–79) [C.2368] [C.2368–I] [C.2368–II].

Report of the Commission to Inquire into the Subject of Criminal Lunacy (1882) [C.3418].

Royal Commission on Prisons in Ireland, Second Report (1884) [C.4145].

Royal Commission on Prisons in Ireland, Vol. 1. Reports, Digest of Evidence, Appendices; Minutes of Evidence, 1884 (1884–85) [C.4233] [C.4233–I].

Report from the Departmental Committee on Prisons [Gladstone Committee] (1895) [C.7702] [C.7702–1].

Medical Journals

Asylum Journal
British Medical Journal
Dublin Journal of Medical Science
Dublin Medical Press
Journal of Mental Science
Lancet
Medical Press and Circular

Periodicals

Chambers's Journal
Fortnightly Review

Illustrated London News
Journal of the Statistical and Social Inquiry Society of Ireland
Journal of the Statistical Society of London
The Nation
Quarterly Review

Newspapers

Belfast Newsletter
Daily Chronicle
Freeman's Journal
Liverpool Mercury
Manchester Evening News
Manchester Guardian
The Irish Times
The Times

Primary Printed

Anon., 'Lunatic Asylums in Ireland', *Dublin Medical Press*, 25:633 (Feb. 1851), 124.
'Influence of Prison Discipline on Health', *Lancet*, 72:1820 (17 July 1858), 70–1.
'Criminal Responsibility of the Insane', *British Medical Journal*, 2:104 (25 Dec. 1858), 1068; 1:105 (1 Jan. 1859), 17–18.
'Criminal Responsibility of the Insane', *Dublin Medical Press*, 41:1044 (Jan. 1859), 13.
'The Psychology of Punishments', *British Medical Journal*, 1:330 (27 Apr. 1867), 484–5.
'Death of a Convict at Spike Island', *Medical Press and Circular* (9 Mar. 1870), 193–7.
'Criminal Lunatics: Broadmoor and Dundrum', *British Medical Journal*, 1:699 (23 May 1874), 686–7.
'Criminal Lunatics and Lunatic Convicts', *British Medical Journal*, 2:705 (4 July 1874), 14–16.
'The Medical Department of the Convict Service', *Lancet*, 110:2810 (7 July 1877), 18.
'The British Medical Association: Psychological Section', *Medical Press and Circular* (15 Aug. 1877), 138.
'Insane or Lunatic', *Lancet*, 110:2820 (15 Sept. 1877), 401–2.
'Criminal Lunacy in 1877. Broadmoor Criminal Lunatic Asylum. Annual Report for the Year 1877. 32nd Report of Commissioners in Lunacy', *Journal of Mental Science*, 24:108 (Jan. 1879), 643–9.
'Irish Prison Surgeons', *Medical Press and Circular* (22 Nov. 1882), 451.
'Prison Surgeons', *Medical Press and Circular* (14 Mar. 1883), 233–4.
'Irish Prison Surgeons and Their Grievances', *Medical Press and Circular* (12 Sept. 1883), 223–4.

'Royal Commission on Prisons in Ireland', *Medical Press and Circular* (31 Oct. 1883), 381.

'The Dublin Trials', *Lancet*, 124:3182 (23 Aug. 1884), 347.

'Retrospect of 1884 – The Irish Prison Service', *Medical Press and Circular* (31 Dec. 1884), 578.

'The Medical Department of the Irish Prisons Board', *Medical Press and Circular* (4 Mar. 1885), 200.

'The Prison Reports', *Lancet*, 132:3395 (22 Sept. 1888), 589.

'Report of the Commissioners of Prisons', *Lancet*, 134:3455 (16 Nov. 1889), 1012.

'Plea of Insanity in Criminal Cases', *Journal of Mental Science*, 37:157 (Apr. 1891), 260–3.

'General Prisons Board Report', *Lancet*, 140:3617 (24 Dec. 1892), 1472.

'Crime and Insanity', *Journal of Mental Science*, 42:78 (July 1896), 602–4.

'Insanity in Prison', *Journal of Mental Science*, 43:80 (Jan. 1897), 115–16.

'Malingery', *Lancet*, 165:4545 (7 Jan. 1905), 45–7.

'Recent Works on Malingering', *Dublin Journal of Medical Science*, 144:2 (Aug. 1917), 119–21.

B.2.15 [R.A. Castle], *Among the Broad-Arrow Men: A Plain Account of English Prison Life* (London: A. and C. Black, 1924).

Baker, John, 'Cases of Incendiarism with Commentary', *Journal of Mental Science*, 35:149 (Apr. 1889), 45–54.

'Some Points Connected with Criminals', *Journal of Mental Science*, 38:162 (July 1892), 364–9.

'Insanity in English Local Prisons, 1894–95', *Journal of Mental Science*, 42:177 (Apr. 1896), 294–302.

Balfour, Jabez Spencer, *My Prison Life* (London: Chapman and Hall, 1907).

Balfour-Browne, J.H., 'Feigned Insanity', *Medical Press and Circular* (19 Oct. and 2 Nov. 1870), 301–5, 345–7.

Bentham, Jeremy, *The Rationale of Punishment* (London: Robert Heward, 1830).

Bidwell, Austin, *From Wall Street to Newgate via the Primrose Way* (Hartford, CT: Bidwell Publishing Co., 1895).

Blandford, G. Fielding, *Insanity and Its Treatment: Lectures on the Treatment, Medical and Legal of Insane Patients* (Edinburgh: Oliver and Boyd; London: Simpkin, Marshall, Hamilton, Kent, and Co., 1892).

Bucknill, John Charles, *An Inquiry into the Proper Classification and Treatment of Criminal Lunatics* (London: John Churchill, 1852).

Unsoundness of Mind in Relation to Criminal Acts (London: Samuel Highley, 1854).

Bucknill, John Charles and Daniel Hack Tuke, *A Manual of Psychological Medicine Containing the History, Nosology, Description, Statistics, Diagnosis, Pathology, and Treatment of Insanity, with an Appendix of Cases*, 2nd edn (London: John Churchill, 1862).

Burman, J. Wilkie, 'Some Further Cases of General Paralytics Committed to Prison for Larceny', *Journal of Mental Science*, 20:90 (July 1874), 246–54.

'On the Separate Care and Special Medical Treatment of the Acute and Curable Cases in Asylums', *Journal of Mental Science*, 25:111 (Oct. 1879), 315–25; 25:112 (Jan. 1880), 468–80.

Burt, John T., *Results of the System of Separate Confinement as Administered at the Pentonville Prison, London* (London: Longman, Brown, Green and Longmans, 1852).

Irish Facts and Wakefield Figures in Relation to Convict Discipline in Ireland (London: Longman and Co., 1863).

Cameron, Charles Alexander, *History of the Royal College of Surgeons in Ireland* (Dublin: Fanin and Company, 1916).

Campbell, John, *Thirty Years' Experience of a Medical Officer in the English Convict Service* (London, Edinburgh and New York: T. Nelson and Sons, 1884).

Carpenter, Mary, *Our Convicts*, vol. 2 (London: Longman, Green, Longman, Roberts & Green, 1864).

Chesterton, George Laval, *Revelations of Prison Life*, 2 vols (London: Hurst and Blackett, 1856).

Clay, Reverend W.L., *The Prison Chaplain: A Memoir of the Reverend John Clay* (Cambridge: Macmillan, 1861).

Our Convict Systems (Cambridge: Macmillan and Co., 1862).

Collie, Sir John, *Malingering and Feigned Sickness* (London: Edward Arnold, 1913).

Davitt, Michael, *Leaves from a Prison Diary; Or, Lectures to a 'Solitary' Audience* (London: Chapman and Hall, 1885), reprinted with introduction by T.W. Moody (Shannon: Irish University Press, 1972), vol. 1.

Dickens, Charles, *American Notes for General Circulation*, Vol. 1 (London: Chapman and Hall, 1842; with an Introduction and Notes by Patricia Ingham, London: Penguin Classics, 2002).

Douglas, Archibald Robertson, 'Penal Servitude and Insanity', *Journal of Mental Science*, 44:185 (Apr. 1898), 271–7.

Editorial, 'Lunatics in Prisons', *British Medical Journal*, 2:1035 (30 Oct. 1880), 710–11.

Falkiner, Frederick Richard, 'Our Habitual Criminals', *Journal of the Statistical and Social Inquiry Society of Ireland*, 8:60 (Aug. 1882), 317–30.

Field, John, *The Advantages of the Separate System of Imprisonment* (London: Longman, 1846).

Fitzpatrick, Jeremiah, *An Essay on Gaol Abuses* (Dublin: Byrne and Brown, 1784).

Thoughts on Penitentiaries (Dublin: H. Fitzpatrick, 1790).

Fletcher, Susan Willis, *Twelve Months in an English Prison* (Boston, MA: Lee and Shephard; New York: Charles T. Dillingham, 1884).

Fry, Elizabeth, *Memoirs of the Life of Elizabeth Fry*, vol. 2 (London: John Hatchard, 1847).

Gibson, Charles Bernard, *Life Among Convicts* (London: Hurst and Blackett, 1863).

Gibson, Edward, 'Penal Servitude and Tickets of Leave', *Journal of the Statistical and Social Inquiry Society of Ireland*, 3:23 (Apr. 1863), 332–43.

Gordon, Mary, *Penal Discipline* (London: Routledge, 1922).

Gray, Francis, *Prison Discipline in America* (London: John Murray, 1848).

Griffiths, Arthur, *Memorials of Millbank, and Chapters in Prison History* (London: Henry S. King & Co., 1875).

Gunn, John, Anthony Madden and Mark Swinton, 'Treatment Needs of Prisoners with Psychiatric Disorders', *British Medical Journal*, 303:6798 (10 Aug. 1991), 338–41.

Mentally Disordered Prisoners (London: Home Office, 1991).

Guy, William A., 'On Insanity and Crime; and on the Plea of Insanity in Criminal Cases', *Journal of the Statistical Society of London*, 32:2 (June 1869), 159–91.

Guy, William A. and David Ferrier, *Principles of Forensic Medicine*, 7th edn, rev. William R. Smith (London: Henry Renshaw, 1895).

Hanway, Jonas, *Solitude in Prison* (London: J. Bew, 1776).

Hobhouse, Stephen and Archibald Fenner Brockway, *English Prisons Today: Being the Report of the Prison System Enquiry Committee* (London: Longmans, Green and Co., 1922).

Holtzendorff, Baron Von, *Reflections and Observations on the Present Condition of the Irish Convict System translated by Mrs Lentaigne* (Dublin: J.M. O'Toole and Son, 1863).

Hood, W. Charles, *Suggestions for the Future Provision of Criminal Lunatics* (London: John Churchill, 1854).

Criminal Lunatics: A Letter to the Chairman of the Commissioners in Lunacy (London: John Churchill, 1860).

'Criminal Lunatics. A Letter to the Chairman of the Commissioners in Lunacy', *Journal of Mental Science*, 6:34 (July 1860), 513–19.

Hopkins, Tighe, *The Silent Gate: A Voyage into Prison* (London: Hurst & Blackett, 1900).

Howard, John, *The State of the Prisons in England and Wales* (Warrington: William Eyres, 1780).

[Jebb, Joshua], *Reports and Observations on the Discipline and Management of Convict Prisons, by the Late Major-General Sir Joshua Jebb, K.C.B., Surveyor General of Prisons, &c., &c.* (London: Hatchard and Co., 1863).

Kingsmill, Reverend Joseph, *Chapters on Prisons and Prisoners*, 3rd edn (London: Longman, Brown, Green, and Longmans, 1854).

Kirkdale Gaol: Twelve Months Imprisonment of a Manchester Merchant (Manchester: Heywood & Son, 1880).

Lalor, Joseph, 'On the Use of Education and Training in the Treatment of the Insane in Public Lunatic Asylums', *Journal of the Statistical and Social Inquiry Society of Ireland*, 7:54 (Aug. 1878), 361–73.

Laurie, Peter, *"Killing no Murder;" or the Effects of Separate Confinement on the Bodily and Mental Condition of Prisoners in the Government Prisons and Other Gaols in Great Britain and America* (London: John Murray, 1846).

[Lee, John], *The Man They Could Not Hang: The Life Story of John Lee*, Told by Himself (London: Mellifont Press, 1936).

MacDonnell, Hercules, 'A Review of Some of the Subjects in the Report of the Royal Commission on Prisons in Ireland', *Journal of the Statistical and Social Inquiry Society of Ireland*, 8:63 (July 1885), 617–23.

'Notes on Some Continental Prisons', *Journal of the Statistical and Social Inquiry Society of Ireland*, 9:64 (July 1886), 81–95.

'Prisons and Prisoners. Suggestions as to Treatment and Classification of Criminals', *Journal of the Statistical and Social Inquiry Society of Ireland*, 10:79 (Apr. 1899), 441–52.

Maudsley, Henry, 'Stealing as a Symptom of General Paralysis', *Lancet*, 106:2724 (13 Nov. 1875), 693–5.

Maybrick, Florence Elizabeth, *Mrs. Maybrick's Own Story: My Fifteen Lost Years* (New York and London: Funk & Wagnalls, 1905).

Mayhew, Henry and John Binny, *The Criminal Prisons of London* (London: Griffin, Bohn & Co., 1862).

McDonnell, Robert, 'Observations on the Case of Burton, and So-called Moral Insanity in Criminal Cases', *Journal of the Statistical and Social Inquiry Society of Ireland*, 3:25 (Dec. 1863), 447–56.

Morris, Terence and Pauline Morris, *Pentonville: A Sociological Study of an English Prison* (London and New York: Routledge, 1963).

Morrison, William Douglas, 'Are Our Prisons a Failure?', *The Fortnightly Review*, 55:328 (Apr. 1894), 459–69.

Murray, James, 'The Life History of a Malingering Criminal', *Journal of Mental Science*, 36:154 (July 1890), 347–54.

Neild, James, *State of the Prisons in England, Scotland and Wales* (London: John Nichols, 1812).

Newman, A., *What It Feels Like* (Dublin: Whelan & Son, 1915).

Nicolson, David, 'Feigned Attempts at Suicide', *Journal of Mental Science*, 17:80 (Jan. 1872), 484–99.

'Parliamentary Blue Books: Reports of Directors of Convict Prisons, in England, Ireland and Scotland, for the year 1870', *Journal of Mental Science*, 18:82 (July 1872), 256–62.

'The Morbid Psychology of Criminals', *Journal of Mental Science*, 19:87 (Oct. 1873), 398–409; 20:89 (Apr. 1874), 20–37; 21:94 (July 1875), 225–50.

'A Chapter in the History of Criminal Lunacy in England', *Journal of Mental Science*, 23:102 (July 1877), 165–85.

'Presidential Address at Fifty-Fourth Annual Meeting of the Medico-Psychological Association', *Journal of Mental Science*, 41:175 (Oct. 1895), 567–91.

'Can the Reproachful Differences of Medical Opinion in Lunacy Cases be Obviated?', *British Medical Journal*, 2:2020 (16 Sept. 1899), 699–702.

Norman, Conolly, 'Feigned Insanity', in Daniel Hack Tuke (ed.), *A Dictionary of Psychological Medicine: Giving the Definition, Etymology and Synonyms of the Terms Used in Medical Psychology with the Symptoms, Treatment, and Pathology of Insanity and the Law of Lunacy in Great Britain and Ireland* (London: J.&A. Churchill, 1892), pp. 502–5.

O'Connor, Art and Helen O'Neill, 'Male Prison Transfers to the Central Mental Hospital, a Special Hospital (1983–1988)', *Irish Journal of Psychological Medicine*, 7:2 (1990), 118–20.

One Who Has Endured It, *Five Years of Penal Servitude* (London: Richard Bentley & Son, 1878).

One Who Has Tried It, 'What Prison Life Is Really Like', *The Windsor Magazine* (2 July 1895), 197–201.

One Who Has Tried Them, *Her Majesty's Prisons: Their Effects and Defects*, vols 1 and 2 (London: Sampson Low, Marsten, Searle & Rivington, 1881).

Orange, William, 'Presidential Address, Delivered at the Annual Meeting of the Medico-Psychological Association, held at the Royal College of Physicians,

London, July 27th, 1883', *Journal of Mental Science*, 29:127 (Oct. 1883), 329–54.

Ormsby, Lambert Hepenstal, *Medical History of the Meath Hospital and County Dublin Infirmary* (Dublin: Fannin and Co., 1888).

Orr, J.H., 'The Imprisonment of Mentally Disordered Offenders', *British Journal of Psychiatry*, 133:3 (1978), 194–9.

Patmore, Tennyson, 'Some Points Bearing on "Malingering"', *British Medical Journal*, 1:1727 (3 Feb. 1894), 238–9.

Quinton, Richard Frith, *Crime and Criminals 1876–1910* (London: Longmans, Green and Co., 1910).

Pitcairn, John James, 'The Detection of Insanity in Prison', *Journal of Mental Science*, 43: 180 (Jan. 1897), 58–63.

Reilly, Michael, *Healthcare in Irish Prisons* (Nenagh: Inspector of Prisons, 2016).

Report of the Commission of Inquiry on Mental Illness (Dublin: Stationery Office, 1966).

Report to the Government of Ireland on the Visit to Ireland Carried Out by the European Committee for the Prevention of Torture and Inhuman or Degrading Treatment or Punishment (CPT) (Strasbourg: Council of Europe, 2015).

R.H.G., 'Mr John Galsworthy on Prison Reform', *Journal of the American Institute of Criminal Law and Criminology*, 2:5 (1912), 756–8.

Rickford, Dora and Kimmett Edgar, *Troubled Inside: Responding to the Mental Health Needs of Men in Prison* (London: Prison Reform Trust, 2005).

Robertson, Alex, 'Case of Feigned Insanity', *Journal of Mental Science*, 29:125 (Apr. 1883), 81–5.

[Robinson, Frederick], *Female Life in Prison*, vol. I (London: Hurst & Blackett, 1863).

Rossa, Jeremiah O'Donovan, *Six Years in Six English Prisons* (New York: P.J. Kennedy, 1874).

Shalev, Sharon and Kimmett Edgar, *Deep Custody: Segregation Units and Close Supervision Centres in England and Wales* (London: Prison Reform Trust, 2015).

Shipley, Reverend Orby, *The Purgatory of Prisoners: or, An Intermediate Stage between the Prison and the Public, Being Some Account of the New System of Penal Reformation Introduced by the Board of Directors of Convict Prisons in Ireland* (London: John Henry and James Parker, 1857).

Smith, Richard, 'The Mental Health of Prisoners: II The Fate of the Mentally Abnormal in Prison', *British Medical Journal*, 288:386 (4 Feb. 1984), 386–8.

Sullivan, William Charles and Stewart Scholar, 'Alcoholism and Suicidal Impulses', *Journal of Mental Science*, 44:185 (Apr. 1898), 259–71.

Taylor, Alfred Swaine (the late), *The Principles and Practice of Medical Jurisprudence*, 6th edn (London: J.&A. Churchill, 1910), vol. 2.

Thomson, James Bruce, 'The Hereditary Nature of Crime', *Journal of Mental Science*, 15:72 (Jan. 1870), 487–98.

Turner, J. Horsfall, *The Annals of Wakefield House of Correction* (Bingley: privately printed, 1904).

W.B.N., *Penal Servitude* (London: William Heinemann, 1903).

Webb, Sidney and Beatrice, *English Prisons under Local Government* (London: Longmans, Green and Co., 1922).

Wheatley, Edward Balme, *Observations on the Treatment of Convicts in Ireland with Some Remarks on the Same in England by Four Visiting Justices of the West Riding Prison at Wakefield* (London: Simpkin, Marshall and Co., 1862).

Wilde, Oscar, *Children in Prison and Other Cruelties of Prison Life* (London: Murdoch and Co., 1898).

[Wilde, Oscar], *Oscar Wilde: The Soul of Man and Prison Writings*, edited with an Introduction by Isobel Murray (Oxford: Oxford University Press, 1990).

Winslow, Forbes, 'Medical Society of London: Prison Discipline', *Lancet*, 57:1439 (29 Mar. 1851), 357–60.

Winslow, L. Forbes, *Mad Humanity: Its Forms Apparent and Obscure* (London: C. A. Pearson, 1898).

Winslow, Lyttelton S., *Manual of Lunacy: A Handbook Relating to the Legal Care and Treatment of the Insane*, with a preface by Forbes Winslow (London: Smith, Elder & Co., 1874).

Secondary Sources

Books

Andrews, Jonathan, Asa Briggs, Roy Porter, Penny Tucker and Keir Waddington, *The History of Bethlem* (London and New York: Routledge, 1997).

Bailey, Victor, *Delinquency and Citizenship: Reclaiming the Young Offender 1914–18* (New York: Oxford University Press, 1987).

Policing and Punishment in Nineteenth-Century Britain (Abingdon: Routledge, 2016).

Bailey, Victor (ed.), *Nineteenth-Century Crime and Punishment*, 4 vols (Abingdon: Routledge, 2021).

Bartlett, Peter, *The Poor Law of Lunacy: The Administration of Pauper Lunatics in Mid-Nineteenth-Century England* (London and New York: Leicester University Press, 1999).

Becker, Peter and Richard F. Wetzell (eds), *Criminals and Their Scientists: The History of Criminology in International Perspective* (Cambridge: Cambridge University Press, 2006).

Berrios, German and Roy Porter (eds), *A History of Clinical Psychiatry: The Origin and History of Psychiatric Disorders* (London and New Brunswick, NJ: Athlone, 1995).

Bourke, Joanna, *Dismembering the Male: Men's Bodies, Britain, and the Great War* (Chicago: Chicago University Press, 1996).

Brennan, Damien, *Irish Insanity* (London and New York: Routledge, 2014).

Brown, Alyson, *English Society and the Prison: Time, Culture and Politics in the Development of the Modern Prison, 1850–1920* (Woodbridge: Boydell, 2003).

Inter-war Penal Policy and Crime in England: The Dartmoor Convict Prison Riot, 1932 (Basingstoke: Palgrave Macmillan, 2013).

Butler, Richard, *Building the Irish Courthouse and Prison: A Political History, 1750–1850* (Cork: Cork University Press, 2020).

Carey, Tim, *Mountjoy: The Story of a Prison* (Dublin: Collins Press, 2000).

Carroll-Burke, Patrick, *Colonial Discipline: The Making of the Irish Convict System* (Dublin: Four Courts Press, 2000).

Coakley, Davis, *Irish Masters of Medicine* (Dublin: Town House, 1992).

Collins, Philip, *Dickens and Crime* (New York: St Martin's Press, 1994).

Cox, Catherine, *Negotiating Insanity in the Southeast of Ireland, 1820–1900* (Manchester: Manchester University Press, 2012).

Creese, Richard, W.F. Bynum and J. Bearn (eds), *The Health of Prisoners* (Amsterdam and Atlanta, GA: Rodopi, 1995).

Crone, Rosalind with Lesley Hoskins and Rebecca Preston, *Guide to the Criminal Prisons of Nineteenth-Century England*, vol. 1 (London: London Publishing Partnership, 2018).

Crowther, M. Anne and Marguerite W. Dupree, *Medical Lives in the Age of Surgical Revolution* (Cambridge: Cambridge University Press, 2007).

Davie, Neil, *Tracing the Criminal: The Rise of Scientific Criminology in Britain, 1860–1918* (Oxford: Bardwell Press, 2006).

Davis, Gayle, *'The Cruel Madness of Love': Sex, Syphilis and Psychiatry in Scotland, 1880–1930* (Amsterdam and New York: Rodopi, 2008).

DeLacy, Margaret, *Prison Reform in Lancashire, 1700–1850: A Study in Local Administration* (Stanford, CA: Stanford University Press, 1986).

Digby, Anne, *Madness, Morality, and Medicine: A Study of the York Retreat, 1796–1914* (Cambridge: Cambridge University Press, 1985).

Eigen, Joel Peter, *Mad-Doctors in the Dock: Defending the Diagnosis, 1760–1913* (Baltimore, MD: Johns Hopkins University Press, 2016).

Witnessing Insanity: Madness and Mad-Doctors in the English Court (New Haven, CT: Yale University Press, 1995).

Emsley, Clive, *Crime and Society in Twentieth-Century England* (Harlow: Longman, 2011).

Evans, Robin, *The Fabrication of Virtue: English Prison Architecture, 1750–1840* (Cambridge: Cambridge University Press, 1982).

Farrell, Elaine, *Women, Crime and Punishment in Ireland: Life in the Nineteenth-Century Convict Prison* (Cambridge: Cambridge University Press, 2020).

Finnane, Mark, *Insanity and the Insane in Post-Famine Ireland* (London: Croom Helm, 1981).

Forsythe, William James, *The Reform of Prisoners 1830–1900* (London and Sydney: Croom Helm, 1987).

Penal Discipline, Reformatory Projects and the English Prison Commission 1895–1939 (Exeter: University of Exeter Press, 1991).

Foucault, Michel, *Madness and Civilization: A History of Insanity in the Age of Reason* (London: Tavistock, 1967).

Discipline and Punish: The Birth of the Prison, translated from the French by Alan Sheridan (London: Allen Lane, 1977).

Foxhall, Katherine, *Health, Medicine and the Sea: Australian Voyages c. 1815–1860* (Manchester and New York: Manchester University Press, 2012).

Garland, David, *Punishment and Modern Society: A Study in Social Theory* (Oxford: Clarendon, 1990).

Godfrey, Barry, Pamela Cox, Heather Shore and Zoe Alker, *Young Criminal Lives: Life Courses and Life Chances from 1850* (Oxford: Oxford University Press, 2017).

Goldman, Lawrence, *Science, Reform and Politics in Victorian Britain: The Social Science Association, 1857–1886* (Cambridge: Cambridge University Press, 2002).

Grass, Sean, *The Self in Cell: Narrating the Victorian Prisoner* (New York: Routledge, 2003).

Guenther, Lisa, *Solitary Confinement: Social Death and Its Afterlives* (Minneapolis, MN and London: University of Minnesota Press, 2013).

Higgins, Peter McRorie, *Punish or Treat?: Medical Care in English Prisons 1770–1850* (Victoria, BC and Oxford: Trafford, 2007).

Hoppen, K. Theodore, *Governing Hibernia: British Politicians and Ireland 1800–1921* (Oxford: Oxford University Press, 2016).

Hunter, Richard and Ida Macalpine, *Three Hundred Years of Psychiatry* (London: Oxford University Press, 1963).

Ignatieff, Michael, *A Just Measure of Pain: The Penitentiary in the Industrial Revolution 1750–1850* (New York: Pantheon Books, 1978).

Jackson, Mark, *The Borderland of Imbecility: Medicine, Society and the Fabrication of the Feeble Mind in Late Victorian and Edwardian England* (Manchester: Manchester University Press, 2000).

Jacob, Jean Daniel, Amélie Perron and Dave Holmes (eds), *Power and the Psychiatric Apparatus: Repression, Transformation and Assistance* (London and New York: Routledge, 2014).

Johnston, Helen (ed.), *Punishment and Control in Historical Perspective* (Houndmills: Palgrave Macmillan, 2008).

Crime in England 1815–1880: Experiencing the Criminal Justice System (London and New York: Routledge, 2015).

Jones, Kathleen, *Lunacy, Law, and Conscience 1744–1845* (London: Routledge & Kegan Paul, 1955).

Kavanagh, Joan and Dianne Snowden, *Van Diemen's Women: A History of Transportation to Tasmania* (Dublin: The History Press, 2015).

Kelly, Brendan, *Custody, Care & Criminality: Forensic Psychiatry and Law in 19th Century Ireland* (Dublin: History Press, 2014).

'Hearing Voices': The History of Psychiatry in Ireland (Dublin: Irish Academic Press, 2016).

Kilcommins, Shane, Ian O'Donnell, Eoin O'Sullivan and Barry Vaughan, *Crime, Punishment and the Search for Order in Ireland* (Dublin: Institute of Public Administration, 2004).

Lande, Gregory, *Madness, Malingering, and Malfeasance: The Transformation of Psychiatry and the Law in the Civil War* (Washington, DC: Brassey's, 2003).

Luddy, Maria, *Women and Philanthropy in Nineteenth-Century Ireland* (Cambridge: Cambridge University Press, 1995).

MacDonagh, Oliver, *The Inspector General: Sir Jeremiah Fitzpatrick and the Politics of Social Reform, 1783–1802* (London: Croom Helm, 1981).

Marland, Hilary, *Medicine and Society in Wakefield and Huddersfield 1780–1870* (Cambridge: Cambridge University Press, 1987).

Dangerous Motherhood: Insanity and Childbirth in Victorian Britain (Houndmills: Palgrave Macmillan, 2004).

Martynowicz, Agnieszka and Linda Moore, *Behind the Door: Solitary Confinement in the Irish Penal System* (Dublin: Irish Penal Reform Trust, 2018).

Mauger, Alice, *The Cost of Insanity in Nineteenth-Century Ireland: Public, Voluntary and Private Asylum Care* (Cham: Palgrave Macmillan, 2018).

McCarthy, Cal and Barra O'Donnabhain, *Too Beautiful for Thieves and Pickpockets: A History of the Victorian Convict Prison on Spike Island* (Cork: Cork County Library, 2016).

McConville, Seán, *A History of English Prison Administration, Vol. 1, 1750–1877* (London, Boston and Henley: Routledge & Kegan Paul, 1981).

   English Local Prisons 1860–1900: Next Only to Death (London and New York: Routledge, 1995).

   Irish Political Prisoners, 1920–1962: Pilgrimage of Desolation (New York: Routledge, 2014).

Melling, Joseph and Bill Forsythe (eds), *Insanity, Institutions and Society, 1800–1914* (London and New York: Routledge, 1999).

Miller, Ian, *Reforming Food in Post-Famine Ireland: Medicine, Science and Improvement, 1845–1922* (Manchester: Manchester University Press, 2014).

   A History of Force Feeding: Hunger Strikes, Prisons and Medical Ethics, 1909–1974 (Houndmills: Palgrave Macmillan, 2016).

Morris, Norval and David J. Rothman (eds), *The Oxford History of the Prison: The Practice of Punishment in Western Society* (New York and Oxford: Oxford University Press, 1998).

Murphy, William, *Political Imprisonment and the Irish, 1912–1921* (Oxford: Oxford University Press, 2014).

O'Donnell, Ian, *Prisoners, Solitude, and Time* (New York and Oxford: Oxford University Press, 2014).

O'Sullivan, Eoin and Ian O'Donnell, *Coercive Confinement in Ireland: Patients, Prisoners and Penitents* (Manchester: Manchester University Press, 2012).

Pick, Daniel, *Faces of Degeneration: A European Disorder, c.1848–1918* (Cambridge: Cambridge University Press, 1989).

Porter, Roy, *Mind-Forg'd Manacles: A History of Madness in England from the Restoration to the Regency* (London: Athlone, 1987; Penguin edn, 1990).

Priestley, Philip, *Victorian Prison Lives: English Prison Biography, 1830–1914* (London: Pimlico, 1985).

Prior, Pauline M., *Madness and Murder: Gender, Crime and Mental Disorder in Nineteenth-Century Ireland* (Dublin: Irish Academic Press, 2008).

Radzinowicz, Leon and Roger Hood, *History of English Criminal Law and Its Administration, Volume 5: The Emergence of Penal Policy* (London: Stevens, 1986).

Rafter, Nicole Hahn, *Creating Born Criminals* (Champaign, IL: University of Illinois Press, 1997).

Sargent, Paul, *Wild Arabs and Savages: A History of Juvenile Justice in Ireland* (Manchester: Manchester University Press, 2014).

Scull, Andrew, *Museums of Madness: The Social Organization of Insanity in 19th Century England* (London: Allen Lane, 1979).

   Decarceration: Community Treatment and the Deviant – A Radical View, 2nd edn (Oxford: Polity Press and New Brunswick, NJ: Rutgers University Press, 1984).

   The Most Solitary of Afflictions: Madness and Society in Britain 1700–1900 (New Haven, CT and London: Yale University Press, 1993).

   Madness in Civilisation (London: Thames & Hudson, 2015).

Scull, Andrew, Charlotte MacKenzie and Nicholas Hervey, *Masters of Bedlam: The Transformation of the Mad-Doctoring Trade* (Princeton, NJ: Princeton University Press, 1996).

Seddon, Tony, *Punishment and Madness: Governing Prisoners with Mental Health Problems* (Abingdon: Routledge-Cavendish, 2007).

Sim, Joe, *Medical Power in Prisons: The Prison Medical Service in England 1774–1989* (Milton Keynes and Philadelphia, PA: Open University Press, 1990).

Smith, Leonard, '*Cure, Comfort and Safe Custody*': *Public Lunatic Asylums in Early Nineteenth-Century England* (London and New York: Leicester University Press, 1999).

Private Madhouses in England, 1640–1815: Commercialised Care for the Insane (Cham: Palgrave Macmillan, 2020).

Smith, Richard, *Prison Health Care* (London: British Medical Association, 1984).

Smith, Roger, *Trial by Medicine: Insanity and Responsibility in Victorian Trials* (Edinburgh: Edinburgh University Press, 1981).

Stevens, Mark, *Broadmoor Revealed: Victorian Crime and the Lunatic Asylum* (Barnsley: Pen & Sword, 2013).

Thomas, James Edward, *The English Prison Officer since 1850* (London and Boston: Routledge & Kegan Paul, 1972).

Torrey, E. Fuller and Judy Miller, *The Invisible Plague: The Rise of Mental Illness from 1750 to the Present* (New Brunswick, NJ and London: Rutgers University Press, 2002).

Walker, Nigel, *Crime and Insanity in England, Volume One: The Historical Perspective* (Edinburgh: Edinburgh University Press, 1968).

Walker, Nigel and Sarah McCabe, *Crime and Insanity in England, Volume Two: New Solutions and New Problems* (Edinburgh: Edinburgh University Press, 1973).

Wallis, Jennifer, *Investigating the Body in the Victorian Asylum: Doctors, Patients, and Practices* (Cham: Palgrave Macmillan, 2017).

Watson, Katherine, *Medicine and Justice: Medico-Legal Practice in England and Wales, 1700–1914* (Abingdon: Routledge, 2019).

Weston, Janet, *Medicine, the Penal System and Sexual Crimes in England, 1919–1960s: Diagnosing Deviance* (London: Bloomsbury Academic, 2017).

Wiener, Martin J., *Reconstructing the Criminal: Culture, Law, and Policy in England, 1830–1914* (Cambridge: Cambridge University Press, 1990).

Williams, Lucy, *Wayward Women: Female Offending in Victorian England* (Barnsley: Pen & Sword, 2016).

Wright, David, *Mental Disability in Victorian England: The Earlswood Asylum, 1847–1901* (Oxford: Oxford University Press, 2001).

Wright, Jonathan Jeffrey, *Crime and Punishment in Nineteenth-Century Belfast: The Story of John Linn* (Dublin: Four Courts Press, 2020).

Zedner, Lucia, *Women, Crime and Custody in Victorian England* (Oxford: Clarendon, 1991).

Articles and Chapters in Books

Allderidge, Patricia, 'Bethlem to Broadmoor', *Proceedings of the Royal Society of Medicine*, 67:9 (Sept. 1974), 897–9.

Anderson, Clare and Hamish Maxwell-Stewart, 'Convict Labour and the Western Empires, 1415–1954', in Robert Aldrich and Kirsten McKenzie (eds), *Routledge History of Western Empires* (London and New York: Routledge, 2014), pp. 102–17.

Anderson, Sarah and John Pratt, 'Prisoner Memoirs and Their Role in Prison History', in Helen Johnston (ed.), *Punishment and Control in Historical Perspective* (Houndmills: Palgrave Macmillan, 2008), pp. 179–98.

Bailey, Victor, 'English Prisons, Penal Culture, and the Abatement of Imprisonment, 1895–1922', *Journal of British Studies*, 36:3 (1997), 285–324.

Bennett, Jamie, 'The Man, the Machine and the Myths: Reconsidering Winston Churchill's Prison Reforms', in Helen Johnston (ed.), *Punishment and Control in Historical Perspective* (Houndmills: Palgrave Macmillan, 2008), pp. 95–114.

Bennett, Rachel, '"Bad for the Health of the Body, Worse for the Health of the Mind": Female Responses to Imprisonment in England, 1853–1869', *Social History of Medicine*, 34:2 (2021), 532–52.

Bogacz, Ted, 'War Neurosis and Cultural Change in England, 1914–22: The Work of the War Office Committee of Enquiry into "Shell Shock"', *Journal of Contemporary History*, 24:2 (1989), 227–56.

Breathnach, Ciara, 'Medical Officers, Bodies, Gender and Weight Fluctuation in Irish Convict Prisons, 1877–95', *Medical History*, 58:1 (2014), 67–86.

Butler, Richard, 'Rethinking the Origins of the British Prisons Act of 1835: Ireland and the Development of Central-Government Prison Inspection, 1820–35', *The Historical Journal*, 59:3 (2016), 721–46.

Byrne, Fiachra, '"In Humanity's Machine": Prison Health and History', *ECAN Bulletin: Howard League for Penal Reform*, 33 (July 2017), 14–20.

Chaney, Sarah, 'Useful Members of Society or Motiveless Malingerers? Occupation and Malingering in British Psychiatry, 1870–1940', in Waltraud Ernst (ed.), *Work Therapy, Psychiatry and Society, c. 1750–2010* (Manchester: Manchester University Press, 2016), pp. 277–97.

Charleroy, Margaret and Hilary Marland, 'Prisoners of Solitude: Bringing History to Bear on Prison Health Policy', *Endeavour*, 40:3 (2016), 141–7.

Coleborne, Catharine, '"His Brain Was Wrong, His Mind Astray": Families and the Language of Insanity in New South Wales, Queensland and New Zealand 1800–1920', *Journal of Family History*, 31:1 (2006), 45–65.

Cooter, Roger, 'Malingering in Modernity: Psychological Scripts and Adversarial Encounters during the First World War', in Roger Cooter, Mark Harrison and Steve Sturdy (eds), *War, Medicine and Modernity* (Stroud: Sutton, 1999), pp. 125–48.

Cox, Catherine and Hilary Marland, '"A Burden on the County": Madness, Institutions of Confinement and the Irish Patient in Victorian Lancashire', *Social History of Medicine*, 28:2 (2015), 263–87.

'"He Must Die or Go Mad in This Place": Prisoners, Insanity and the Pentonville Model Prison Experiment, 1842–1852', *Bulletin of the History of Medicine*, 92:1 (2018), 78–109.

'"Unfit for Reform or Punishment": Mental Disorder and Discipline in Liverpool Borough Prison in the Late Nineteenth Century', *Social History*, 44:2 (2019), 173–201.

Cox, Catherine, Hilary Marland and Sarah York, 'Emaciated, Exhausted and Excited: The Bodies and Minds of the Irish in Nineteenth-Century Lancashire Asylums', *Journal of Social History*, 46:2 (2012), 500–24.

Crone, Rosalind, 'The Great "Reading" Experiment: An Examination of the Role of Education in the Nineteenth-century Gaol', *Crime, History & Societies*, 16:1 (2012), 47–74.

Crossman, Virginia, 'Workhouse Medicine in Ireland: A Preliminary Analysis, 1850–1914', in Jonathan Reinarz and Leonard Schwarz (eds), *Medicine and the Workhouse* (Rochester, NY: University of Rochester Press, 2013), pp. 123–39.

Davie, Neil, 'The Role of Medico-legal Expertise in the Emergence of Criminology in Britain (1870–1918)', *Criminocorpus, revue hypermédia* [Online], *Archives d'anthropologie criminelle* and related subjects, 3 [11 Oct. 2010], criminocorpus.revues.org/316

'"Business as Usual?" Britain's First Women's Convict Prison, Brixton 1853–1869', *Crimes and Misdemeanours*, 4:1 (2010), 37–52.

Duvall, Nicholas, '"From Defensive Paranoia to ... Openness to Outside Scrutiny": Prison Medical Officers in England and Wales in the 1970s and 1980s', *Medical History*, 62:1 (2018), 112–31.

Eigen, Joel Peter, '"I Answer As a Physician": Opinion as Fact in Pre-McNaughtan Insanity Trials', in Michael Clark and Catherine Crawford (eds), *Legal Medicine in History* (Cambridge: Cambridge University Press, 1994), pp. 167–99.

Ellis, Robert, 'The Asylum, the Poor Law, and a Reassessment of the Four-Shilling Grant: Admission to the County Asylums of Yorkshire in the Nineteenth Century', *Social History of Medicine*, 19:1 (2006), 55–71.

Farrell, Elaine, '"Having an Immoral Conversation" and Other Prison Offenses: The Punishment of Convict Women', in Christina S. Brophy and Cara Delay (eds), *Women, Reform and Resistance in Ireland, 1850–1950* (Houndmills: Palgrave Macmillan, 2015), pp. 101–18.

Finnane, Mark, 'Asylums, Family and the State', *History Workshop Journal*, 20:1 (1985), 134–48.

Forsythe, Bill, 'Centralisation and Local Autonomy: The Experience of English Prisons 1820–1877', *Journal of Historical Sociology*, 4:3 (1991), 317–45.

Gibbons, Pat, Niamh Mulryan and Art O'Connor, 'Guilty but Insane: The Insanity Defence in Ireland, 1850–1995', *British Journal of Psychiatry*, 170:5 (1997), 467–72.

Gibson, Mary, 'Global Perspectives on the Birth of the Prison', *American Historical Review*, 116:4 (2011), 1040–63.

Harding, Christopher, '"The Inevitable End of a Discredited System"? The Origins of the Gladstone Committee Report on Prisons, 1895', *The Historical Journal*, 31:3 (1988), 591–608.

Hardy, Anne, 'Development of the Prison Medical Service, 1774–1895', in Richard Creese, W.F. Bynum and J. Bearn (eds), *The Health of Prisoners* (Amsterdam and Atlanta, GA: Rodopi, 1995), pp. 59–82.

Heaney, Henry, 'Ireland's Penitentiary 1820–1831: An Experiment that Failed', *Studia Hibernica*, 14 (1974), 28–39.

Henriques, Ursula R.Q., 'The Rise and Decline of the Separate System of Prison Discipline', *Past & Present*, 54:1 (1972), 61–93.

Johnston, Helen, '"Reclaiming the Criminal": The Role and Training of Prison Officers in England, 1877 to 1914', *The Howard Journal of Criminal Justice*, 47:3 (2008), 297–312.

'Moral Guardians? Prison Medical Officers, Prison Practice and Ambiguity in the Nineteenth Century', in Helen Johnston (ed.), *Punishment and Control in Historical Perspective* (Houndmills: Palgrave Macmillan, 2008), pp. 77–94.

Kane, Jacqueline L., 'Prison Palace or "Hell upon Earth": Leicester County Gaol under the Separate System, 1846–1865', *Transactions of the Leicestershire Archaeological and Historical Society*, 70 (1996), 128–46.

Kelly, Brendan, 'Poverty, Crime and Mental Illness: Female Forensic Psychiatric Committal in Ireland, 1910–1948', *Social History of Medicine*, 21:2 (2008), 311–28.

Marland, Hilary, '"Close Confinement Tells Very Much Upon a Man": Prisoner Memoirs, Insanity and the Late Nineteenth- and Early Twentieth-Century Prison', *Journal of the History of Medicine and Allied Sciences*, 74:3 (2019), 267–91.

Maxwell-Stewart, Hamish, 'Transportation from Britain and Ireland, 1615–1875', in Clare Anderson (ed.), *A Global History of Convicts and Penal Colonies* (London: Bloomsbury, 2018), pp. 183–210.

McConville, Seán, 'The Victorian Prison', in Norval Morris and David J. Rothman (eds), *The Oxford History of the Prison: The Practice of Punishment in Western Society* (New York and Oxford: Oxford University Press, 1998), pp. 131–67.

McGowen, Randall, 'The Well-Ordered Prison: England, 1780–1865', in Norval Morris and David J. Rothman (eds), *The Oxford History of the Prison: The Practice of Punishment in Western Society* (New York and Oxford: Oxford University Press, 1998), pp. 71–99.

Moran, James, 'The Signal and the Noise: The Historical Epidemiology of Insanity in Antebellum New Jersey', *History of Psychiatry*, 14:3 (2003), 281–301.

Murphy, William, 'Dying, Death and Hunger Strike: Cork and Brixton, 1920', in James Kelly and Mary Ann Lyons (eds), *Death and Dying in Ireland, Britain, and Europe: Historical Perspectives* (Dublin: Irish Academic Press, 2013), pp. 297–316.

Nichol, N., '"Malingering" and Convict Protest', *Labour History*, 47 (1984), 18–27.

O'Brien, Sean T., 'The Prison Writing of Michael Davitt', *New Hibernia Review*, 14:3 (2010), 16–32.

Ogborn, Miles, 'Discipline, Government and Law: Separate Confinement in the Prisons of England and Wales, 1830–1877', *Transactions of the Institute of British Geographers*, 20:3 (1995), 295–311.

Pickstone, John V., 'Ways of Knowing: Towards a Historical Sociology of Science, Technology and Medicine', *British Journal for the History of Science*, 36:4 (1993), 433–58.

Porter, Roy, 'Howard's Beginning: Prisons, Disease, Hygiene', in Richard Creese, W.F. Bynum and J. Bearn (eds), *The Health of Prisoners* (Amsterdam and Atlanta, GA: Rodopi, 1995), pp. 5–26.

'Madness and Its Institutions', in Andrew Wear (ed.), *Medicine in Society* (Cambridge: Cambridge University Press, 1992), pp. 277–301.

Prior, Pauline M., 'Mad, Not Bad: Crime, Mental Disorder and Gender in Nineteenth-Century Ireland', *History of Psychiatry*, 8:32 (1997), 501–16.

'Prisoner or Patient? The Official Debate on the Criminal Lunatic in Nineteenth-Century Ireland', *History of Psychiatry*, 15:2 (2004), 177–92.

Ramsey, Matthew, 'Conscription, Malingering, and Popular Medicine in Napoleonic France', in Robert Holtman (ed.), *The Consortium on Revolutionary Europe, 1750–1850: Proceedings, 1978* (The Consortium on Revolutionary Europe: Athens, GA, 1978), pp. 188–99.

Ray, Laurence, 'Models of Madness in Victorian Asylum Practice', *European Journal of Sociology*, 22:2 (1981), 229–64.

Reinarz, Jonathan and Alistair Ritch, 'Exploring Medical Care in the Nineteenth-Century Provincial Workhouse: A View from Birmingham', in Jonathan Reinarz and Leonard Schwarz (eds), *Medicine and the Workhouse* (Rochester, NY: University of Rochester Press, 2013), pp. 140–63.

Rothman, David J., 'Perfecting the Prison: United States, 1789–1865', in Norval Morris and David J. Rothman (eds), *The Oxford History of the Prison: The Practice of Punishment in Western Society* (New York and Oxford: Oxford University Press, 1998), pp. 100–16.

Rubin, Ashley T., 'A Neo-Institutional Account of Prison Diffusion', *Law and Society Review*, 49:2 (2015), 365–99.

Saunders, Janet, 'Magistrates and Madmen: Segregating the Criminally Insane in Late-Nineteenth-Century Warwickshire', in Victor Bailey (ed.), *Policing and Punishment in Nineteenth Century Britain* (London: Croom Helm, 1981), pp. 217–41.

'Quarantining the Weak-Minded: Psychiatric Definitions of Degeneracy and the Late-Victorian Asylum', in W.F. Bynum, Roy Porter and Michael Shepherd (eds), *Anatomy of Madness: Essays in the History of Psychiatry*, vol. 3 (London: Routledge, 1988), pp. 273–96.

Scull, Andrew, 'Moral Treatment Reconsidered: Some Sociological Comments on an Episode in the History of British Psychiatry', in Andrew Scull (ed.), *Madhouses, Mad-Doctors, and Madmen: The Social History of Psychiatry in the Victorian Era* (London: Athlone, 1981), pp. 105–20.

Seddon, Toby, *Punishment and Madness: Governing Prisoners with Mental Health Problems* (Abingdon: Routledge, 2007).

Shepherd, Jade, '"I Am Very Glad and Cheered When I Hear the Flute": The Treatment of Criminal Lunatics in Late Victorian Broadmoor', *Medical History*, 60:4 (2016), 473–91.

'Feigning Insanity in Late-Victorian Britain', *Prison Service Journal*, 232 (2017), 17–23.

Sim, Joe, 'The Future of Prison Health Care: A Critical Analysis', *Critical Social Policy*, 22:2 (2002), 300–23.

Smith, Beverly A., 'The Irish General Prisons Board, 1877–1885: Efficient Deterrence or Bureaucratic Ineptitude?', *Irish Jurist*, 15:1 (1980), 122–36.

'Irish Prison Doctors – Men in the Middle, 1865–90', *Medical History*, 26:4 (1982), 371–94.

'The Female Prisoner in Ireland, 1855–1878', *Federal Probation*, 54:4 (1990), 69–81.

Smith, Richard, 'History of the Prison Medical Services', *British Medical Journal*, 287:6407 (10 Dec. 1983), 1786–8.

Smith, Roger, 'The Boundary Between Insanity and Criminal Responsibility in Nineteenth-Century England', in Andrew Scull (ed.), *Madhouses, Mad-Doctors, and Madmen: A Social History of Psychiatry in the Victorian Era* (London: Athlone, 1981), pp. 363–84.

Stack, John A., 'Deterrence and Reformation in Early Victorian Social Policy: The Case of Parkhurst Prison, 1838–1864', *Historical Reflections/Réflexions Historiques*, 6:2 (1979), 387–404.

Summers, Anne, 'Elizabeth Fry and Mid-Nineteenth Century Reform', in Richard Creese, W.F. Bynum and J. Bearn (eds), *The Health of Prisoners* (Amsterdam and Atlanta, GA: Rodopi, 1995), pp. 83–101.

Teagarden, Ernest, 'A Victorian Prison Experiment', *Journal of Social History*, 2:4 (1969), 357–65.

Tomlinson, Heather, 'Design and Reform: The "Separate System" in the Nineteenth Century English Prison', in Anthony D. King (ed.), *Buildings and Society: Essays on the Social Development of the Built Environment* (London: Routledge, 1984), pp. 94–119.

Topp, Leslie, 'Single Rooms, Seclusion and the Non-Restraint Movement in British Asylums, 1838–1844', *Social History of Medicine*, 31:4 (2018), 754–73.

Wall, Oisín, '"Embarrassing the State": The "Ordinary" Prisoner Rights Movement in Ireland, 1972–6', *Journal of Contemporary History*, 55:2 (2020), 388–410.

Walsh, Oonagh, '"The Designs of Providence": Race, Religion and Irish Insanity', in Joseph Melling and Bill Forsythe (eds), *Insanity, Institutions and Society, 1800–1914* (London and New York: Routledge, 1999), pp. 223–42.

'Lunatic and Criminal Alliances in Nineteenth-Century Ireland', in Peter Bartlett and David Wright (eds), *Outside the Walls of the Asylum: The History of Care in the Community 1750–2000* (London and New Brunswick, NJ: Athlone, 1999), pp. 132–52.

'"A Person of the Second Order": The Plight of the Intellectually Disabled in Nineteenth-Century Ireland', in Laurence Geary and Oonagh Walsh (eds), *Philanthropy in Nineteenth-Century Ireland* (Dublin: Four Courts Press, 2015), pp. 161–80.

Walton, John K., 'Lunacy in the Industrial Revolution: A Study of Asylum Admissions in Lancashire 1848–50', *Journal of Social History*, 13:1 (1979), 1–122.

'Casting Out and Bringing Back in Victorian England: Pauper Lunatics, 1840–70', in W.F. Bynum, Roy Porter and Michael Shepherd (eds), *The Anatomy of Madness: Essays in the History of Psychiatry*, vol. II (London and New York: Tavistock, 1985), 132–46.

Walton, John Kimmons, Martin Blinkhorn, Colin Pooley, David Tidswell and Michael J. Winstanley, 'Crime, Migration and Social Change in North-West

England and the Basque Country, c. 1870–1930', *British Journal of Criminology*, 39:1 (1999), 90–112.

Ward, Tony, 'Law, Common Sense and the Authority of Science: Expert Witnesses and Criminal Insanity in England, ca. 1840–1940', *Social and Legal Studies*, 6:3 (1997), 343–62.

'Legislating for Human Nature: Legal Responses to Infanticide, 1860–1938', in Mark Jackson (ed.), *Infanticide: Historical Perspectives on Child Murder and Concealment, 1550–2000* (Aldershot: Ashgate, 2002), pp. 249–69.

'An Honourable Regime of Truth? Foucault, Psychiatry and English Criminal Justice', in Helen Johnston (ed.), *Punishment and Control in Historical Perspective* (Houndmills: Palgrave Macmillan, 2008), pp. 56–75.

Watson, Stephen, 'Malingerers, the "Weakminded" Criminal and the "Moral Imbecile": How the English Prison Officer Became an Expert in Mental Deficiency, 1880–1930', in Michael Clark and Catherine Crawford (eds), *Legal Medicine in History* (Cambridge: Cambridge University Press, 1994), pp. 223–41.

Wessely, Simon, 'Malingering: Historical Perspectives', in P.W. Halligan, Christopher Bass and David A. Oakley (eds), *Malingering and Illness Deception* (Oxford: Oxford University Press, 2003), pp. 31–41.

Wiener, Martin J., 'The Health of Prisoners and the Two Faces of Benthanism', in Richard Creese, W.F. Bynum and J. Bearn (eds), *The Health of Prisoners* (Amsterdam and Atlanta, GA: Rodopi, 1995), pp. 44–58.

'Murderers and "Reasonable Men": The "Criminology" of the Victorian Judiciary', in Peter Becker and Richard F. Wetzell (eds), *Criminals and Their Scientists: The History of Criminology in International Perspective* (Cambridge: Cambridge University Press, 2006), pp. 43–60.

Wilson, David, 'Millbank, the Panopticon and Their Victorian Audiences', *The Howard Journal of Criminal Justice*, 41:4 (2002), 364–81.

'Testing a Civilisation: Charles Dickens on the American Penitentiary System', *The Howard Journal of Criminal Justice*, 48:3 (2009), 280–96.

Wright, David, 'Getting out of the Asylum: Understanding the Confinement of the Insane in the Nineteenth Century', *Social History of Medicine*, 10:1 (1997), 137–55.

Unpublished theses and dissertations

Andrews, Emily, 'Senility before Alzheimer: Old Age in British Psychiatry, c. 1835–1912' (unpublished University of Warwick PhD thesis, 2014).

Reid, Peter, 'Children, Mental Deficiency and Institutions in Dublin, 1900 to 1911' (unpublished University College Dublin MLitt thesis, 2018).

Saunders, Janet, 'Institutionalised Offenders: A Study of the Victorian Institution and Its Inmates, with Special Reference to Late Nineteenth Century Warwickshire' (unpublished University of Warwick PhD thesis, 1983).

Sellers, Laura, 'Managing Convicts, Understanding Criminals: Medicine and the Development of English Convict Prisons, c. 1837–1886' (unpublished University of Leeds PhD thesis, 2017).

Online Sources

McGuire, James and Quinn, James (eds), *Dictionary of Irish Biography* (Cambridge: Cambridge University Press, 2009) (*DIB*).

Matthew, Colin (ed.), *Dictionary of National Biography* (Oxford: Oxford University Press, 2004) (*DNB*).

Old Bailey Proceedings Online (www.oldbaileyonline.org, version 8.0, 1 Aug. 2019).

Royal College of Physicians Munk's Roll: http://munksroll.rcplondon.ac.uk/Biography/Details/1843

Voices from Broadmoor: Crime, Madness and the Asylum: https://voicesfrombroadmoor.wordpress.com/2015/06/22/broadmoors-victorian-superintendents/

Index

acquittal on grounds of insanity, 154, 156, 161, 167, 173

Act for Consolidating and Amending the Law Relating to Prisons in Ireland (1826). *See* Prisons (Ireland) Act (1826)

Act for the Better Care and Maintenance of Lunatics, Being Paupers or Criminals in England. *See* County Asylum (Wynn's) Act (1808)

Act for the Formation, Regulation and Government of Convict Prisons (1854). *See* Convict Prisons (Ireland) Act (1854)

alienists. *See* psychiatry

archival and official sources, 3–7, 27–28, 108–9, 207, 231–32, 235, 256

assessing lunacy, 205, 237
  expert witnesses, 4, 151, 167–74, 198
  judges, 167
  prison medical officers, 52–54, 168–74, 212, 241, 251
  psychiatrists, 167, 228–32
  removal to 'specialist' facilities, 139–41, 174

Association for the Improvement of Prisons and Prison Discipline in Ireland, 5, 25, 34

Association of Gaol Surgeons (Ireland), 105, 114

asylums
  asylum design. *See* prison and asylum design
  Broadmoor Asylum. *See* Broadmoor Asylum
  county and district asylums, 11, 156–59, 180–82, 222–24; *see also* County Asylum (Wynn's) Act (1808); Irish Lunatic Asylums for the Poor Act (1817); Lunacy (Ireland) Act (1821)
  Dundrum Criminal Lunatic Asylum. *See* Dundrum Criminal Lunatic Asylum

  perceived benefits
    early release, 224
    milder discipline, 204, 222
    relative ease of escape, 222–24
  private asylums, 11–12, 159
  public asylums, 3, 11, 81, 162, 179–82, 205, 222–24
  voluntary asylums, 11–12

Auburn Penitentiary (USA), 32

authority and decision-making, 4, 28–29, 60–62, 152, 251–52
  asylum doctors, 192
  boards of superintendence, 251
  local magistrates, 175–77, 182
  prison chaplains, 42–43, 51–52, 54–55, 61, 76, 214
  prison medical officers, 52–54, 62–64, 80–81, 192, 251

Baker, Henry
  transportation and mental health, 46

Baker, Dr John, 240
  Lombrosian theories, rejection of, 145

Belfast House of Correction, 17, 39
  separate confinement, 28

Bentham, Jeremy
  criminal mind, 26
  panopticon, 14, 32, 35

Bethlem Hospital, 12, 46–47, 121
  conditions, 159
  removals to, 161, 213, 224
  specialist facilities, 154–56, 160–62

Better Government of Convict Prisons Act (1850), 61

Birmingham Borough Gaol
  excessive punishment, 114
  implementation of separate confinement, 49, 51, 61

Blaker, Dr E.S.
  real or feigned insanity, 233–34

CPSIA information can be obtained
at www.ICGtesting.com
Printed in the USA
LVHW080916020322
712332LV00004B/369